T0192213

Despite numerous international declarations and conventions prohibiting human rights violations, torture remains a major problem in many countries of the world. Progress on the humanitarian front has not been adequately paralleled by efforts in the scientific world to achieve a better understanding of the various forms of political repression and their effects on individuals, communities and societies.

This book reveals in some detail the medical, psychiatric and psychological problems confronting survivors of torture, and reviews the various treatment approaches available to those involved in their care. Comparisons are made, where appropriate, with other violent acts or situations, by reference to the experience of treating prisoners of war, Holocaust survivors, and other survivors of violence in the military or civilian arenas. Contributions are drawn both from host countries treating refugees who have experienced torture and also from a number of countries where treatment and rehabilitation of torture survivors has taken place in a setting of continuing political repression.

The importance of this work lies in its emphasis on a scientific approach to the problem of torture while also giving due consideration to its social and political dimensions. As a source of theoretical and practical information it is unrivalled, addressing the needs of all health workers helping survivors of torture, and reviewing issues in the sociology and psychobiology of organized violence that will command the attention of a much wider readership.

*Torture and its consequences:
current treatment approaches*

Torture
and
its consequences:

CURRENT TREATMENT APPROACHES

EDITED BY METİN BAŞOĞLU
Institute of Psychiatry, University of London, UK

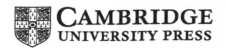

CAMBRIDGE
UNIVERSITY PRESS

CAMBRIDGE UNIVERSITY PRESS
Cambridge, New York, Melbourne, Madrid, Cape Town, Singapore, São Paulo

Cambridge University Press
The Edinburgh Building, Cambridge CB2 8RU, UK

Published in the United States of America by Cambridge University Press, New York

www.cambridge.org
Information on this title: www.cambridge.org/9780521392990

© Cambridge University Press 1992

This publication is in copyright. Subject to statutory exception
and to the provisions of relevant collective licensing agreements,
no reproduction of any part may take place without the written
permission of Cambridge University Press.

First published 1992
First paperback edition 1998
Re-issued in this digitally printed version 2007

A catalogue record for this publication is available from the British Library

Library of Congress Cataloguing in Publication data

Torture and its consequences : current treatment approaches /
edited by Metin Başoğlu.
p. cm.
Includes bibliographical references.
ISBN 0–521–39299–3 (hc)
1. Torture victims – Mental health.
2. Torture victims – Rehabilitation.
3. Torture – Psychological aspects.
4. Post-traumatic stress disorder – Treatment.
I. Başoğlu, Metin.
[DNLM: 1. Psychotherapy – methods.
2. Stress Disorders, Post-Traumatic – therapy.
4. Torture – psychology.   WM 170 T712]
RC451.4.T67T68   1992
616.85′21–dc20
DNLM/DLC
for Library of Congress   92–13560   CIP

ISBN 978-0-521-39299-0 hardback
ISBN 978-0-521-65954-3 paperback

Dedicated to all sufferers of torture

'I didn't mind the pain so much.
It was the cries next door I couldn't bear.'

A SURVIVOR

CONTENTS

Part I: Torture and its consequences

Part II: Theory

Part III: Assessment, diagnosis, and classification

Part IV: Rehabilitation programmes for torture survivors

Part V: Psychotherapy

Part VII: Modern ethics and international law

CONTRIBUTORS

Anne Marie Albano, PhD, Clinical Psychologist, National Center for PTSD, Boston VA Medical Center, Tufts University School of Medicine, USA

Ron Baker, (Professor), International Consultant in Training and Senior Research Associate in the Refugee Studies Programme, Oxford University, UK

Metin Başoğlu, MD, Lecturer in Psychiatry, Institute of Psychiatry, University of London, UK

Dudley David Blake, PhD, Clinical Psychologist, National Center for PTSD, Boston VA Medical Center, Tufts University School of Medicine, USA

Søren Bøjholm, MD, The Rehabilitation and Research Centre for Torture Victims (RCT), Copenhagen, Denmark

Enrique Bustos, BA, BSc, MSc, Certified Psychologist and Psychotherapist, Swedish Red Cross, Stockholm

Ma. Victoria Cabildo, RN, Former Program Coordinator, Philippine Action Concerning Torture, Medical Action Group, Inc., Manila, Philippines

Yael Caspi-Yavin, MA, MPH, PhD Candidate, Department of Behavioral Science, Harvard School of Public Health, USA

Terence Dowdall, Senior Lecturer in Clinical Psychology, Child Guidance Clinic, University of Cape Town, South Africa

Lucila Edelman, MD, The Psychological Assistance Team of the Mothers of the Plaza de Mayo, Argentina

Sylvia Estrado-Claudio, MD, Health Action Information Network, Quezon City, Philippines

Inge Kemp Genefke, MD, DMSchc, Medical Director, The Rehabilitation and Research Centre for Torture Victims (RCT), Copenhagen, Denmark

Mirta Groshaus, MD, The Psychological Assistance Team of the Mothers of the Plaza de Mayo, Argentina

Marianne Kastrup, MD, PhD, Psychiatrist, The Rehabilitation and Research Centre for Torture Victims (RCT), Copenhagen, Denmark

Terence M. Keane, PhD, Professor of Psychiatry (Psychology), National Center for PTSD, Boston VA Medical Center, Tufts University, School of Medicine, USA

Daniel Kersner, MD, The Psychological Assistance Team of the Mothers of the Plaza de Mayo, Argentina

Diana Kordon, MD, The Psychological Assistance Team of the Mothers of the Plaza de Mayo, Argentina

Dario Lagos, MD, The Psychological Assistance Team of the Mothers of the Plaza de Mayo, Argentina

Inge Lunde, MD, Chief Psychiatrist, ETICA Treatment Centre, Copenhagen, Denmark

Richard McNally, PhD, Associate Professor, Department of Psychology, Harvard University, Department of Psychology, Cambridge, Massachusetts, USA

Mahboob Mehdi, MBBS, Medical Director, Voice Against Torture and Rehabilitation and Health Centre for Torture Victims, Islamabad, Pakistan

Thomas W. Miller, PhD, ABPP, Chief, Psychology Service, Professor, Department of Psychiatry, Veterans Administration and University of Kentucky Medical Centers, Lexington, Kentucky, USA

Susan Mineka, PhD, Professor of Psychology, Department of Psychology, Northwestern University, Evanston, IL, USA

Richard F. Mollica, MD, MAR, Director, Harvard Program in Refugee Trauma, Harvard School of Public Health, Clinical Director, Indochinese Psychiatry Clinic, St Elizabeth's Hospital, USA

Elena Nicoletti, Psychologist, The Psychological Assistance Team of the Mothers of the Plaza de Mayo, Argentina

Jørgen Ortmann, MD, Chief Psychiatrist, ETICA Treatment Centre, Copenhagen, Denmark

June Pagaduan-Lopez, MD, Program Consultant, Philippine Action Concerning Torture, Medical Action Group, Inc. Manila, Philippines.

Murat Paker, MD, MSc Student in Psychology, Department of Psychology, Boğaziçi University, Istanbul, Turkey

Özgün Paker, MD, MSc Student in Psychology, Department of Psychology, Boğaziçi University, Istanbul, Turkey

Aurora A. Parong, MD, Executive Director, Medical Action Group, Inc., Manila, Philippines

Elizabeth Protacio-Marcelino, PhD, Executive Director, Children's Rehabilitation Center, Quezon City, Philippines

José A. Saporta, Jr., MD, Clinical Associate in Psychiatry, Massachusetts General Hospital, Instructor in Psychiatry, Harvard Medical School, USA

Grethe Skylv, MD, MA, The Rehabilitation and Research Centre for Torture Victims (RCT), Copenhagen, Denmark

Norman Solkoff, PhD Distinguished Professor, Department of Psychology and Psychiatry, New York State University at Buffalo, USA

Finn Somnier, MD, Neurologist, The Rehabilitation and Research Centre for Torture Victims (RCT), Copenhagen, Denmark

Bent Sørensen, MD (Professor), Member of United Nations Committee Against Torture and Member of the European Committee for the Prevention of Torture, The Rehabilitation and Research Centre for Torture Victims (RCT), Copenhagen, Denmark

Bessel A. van der Kolk, MD, Director, Trauma Clinic, General Hospital Massachusetts, Instructor in Psychiatry, Harvard Medical School, USA

Loes H. M. van Willigen, MD, Director, Refugee Health Care Centre, Rijswijk, The Netherlands

Peter Vesti, MD, Psychiatrist, The Rehabilitation and Research Centre for Torture Victims (RCT), Copenhagen, Denmark

Şahika Yüksel, MD, Professor of Psychiatry, Department of Psychiatry, University of Istanbul, Turkey

PREFACE

In recent years, there has been a proliferation of publications on traumatic stress responses in many traumatized groups including survivors of war violence, rape, accidents, and natural disasters. There are, however, relatively few scientific publications on the trauma of torture and other forms of organised violence, despite the health implications of torture being practised systematically in more than 100 countries. The purpose of this book is to fill a gap in the scientific literature on torture and its treatment.

The selection of the topics for this book has been guided by several considerations. The proliferation of knowledge over the last decade concerning other types of trauma could be of benefit to the study of torture. Thus, in an attempt to bridge the gap between these related fields, some space is devoted to psychobiological theories of traumatic stress and the recent advances in assessment, classification, and treatment of traumatic stress responses, in general.

Since torture is only one of the many forms of organized violence suffered by survivors, an exclusively torture-oriented approach would overlook the importance of other associated traumas before and after torture. The focus of this book, as the title suggests, is on torture but due attention has been paid to the multi-faceted problems of torture survivors.

Current views among health workers concerning torture and its treatment are varied and at times conflicting. Much debate centres around issues of assessment, diagnostics, organization of health care services, treatment, outcome evaluation, and research. In selecting the topics for this volume, care has been taken to represent as closely as possible the diverse views surrounding these issues.

One section is devoted to chapters by workers who help non-refugee survivors of torture living in their home country. The experience of these workers is particularly valuable for mental health professionals in countries where systematic torture is widespread. The authors in this section also provide an analysis of the socio-political context of human rights violations in their countries to help achieve a better understanding of the complex phenomenon of torture.

Although this book is primarily intended for mental health professionals, its wide scope covering both medical and socio-political aspects of torture should make it of interest to all those involved in human rights issues.

I would like to extend my gratitude to all those who have contributed directly or indirectly to the preparation of this volume. Aslí Göksel, Ayşe Bircan and my colleagues and friends at the Institute of Psychiatry in London, Isaac Marks, Homa Noshirvani, and Seda Şengün gave me generous support and encouragement throughout the project and provided valuable comments on parts of the book. Norman Solkoff (New York State University at Buffalo), Richard Mollica (Director of Harvard Program in Refugee Trauma, Harvard School of Public Health and Clinical Director of Indochinese Psychiatry Clinic, St Elizabeth Hospital), Richard McNally (Department of Psychology, Harvard University), Lenia Palazidou from the Maudsley Hospital in London, and Cengiz and Emine Kılıç from Ankara reviewed some of the chapters and provided comments that were of great help in the difficult process of editing.

Thanks are also due to Anne Burley and James Welsch from Amnesty International in London for providing me with AI publications and keeping me updated on Human Rights issues over the years. I should also like to thank James Welsch for his valuable comments, Loes van Willigen (Refugee Health Care Centre, Rijswijk, The Netherlands) for her kind help and guidance in organizing some of the contributors for this volume, and Ron Baker (Senior Research Associate in the Refugee Studies Programme, Oxford University) for the support and encouragement he has given me in the planning of this book from the very beginning. I am grateful to all of the authors in the book for their contribution and particularly for their patience with my endless editorial nagging. Special thanks are due to Susan Mineka (Department of Psychology, Northwestern University, Evanston) for sharing her extensive knowledge and expertise in learning theory with me and for co-authoring with me the difficult chapter on the parallels between the experimental models of anxiety/depression and human experience under torture. I am particularly indebted to Richard Barling of Cambridge University Press for his constant support and encouragement throughout the preparation of this book. Kate Fleet went beyond her duty as a proof-reader and generously spent endless hours to ensure a uniform standard of English in the book. Finally, I am deeply grateful to all the survivors of torture, some of them close friends, whom I have interviewed over the years for sharing their painful memories with me. I have learned a great deal from them.

INTRODUCTION

Considering the wide range of situations which involve human induced physical and psychological suffering, a clear-cut definition of torture is problematic. In his history of torture, Peters (1985) noted that, since the Romans in the second and third century, the various legal definitions of torture have emphasized one common element: 'torment inflicted by a public authority for ostensibly public purposes'. Peters also wrote (p. 2):

> Yet it is likely that people using the term in the second half of the twentieth century may find these definitions too narrow. Is not the key to torture simply the physical or mental suffering deliberately inflicted upon a human being by any other human being? In many respects the meaning of the term in the common usage of most western languages might well support such a question. From the seventeenth century on, the purely legal definition of torture was slowly displaced by a moral definition; from the nineteenth century, the moral definition of torture has been supplanted largely by a sentimental definition, until 'torture' may finally mean whatever one wishes it to mean, a moral–sentimental term designating the infliction of suffering, however defined, upon anyone for any purpose – or for no purpose.

Any scientific treatment of this subject must therefore be based on a clearly stated definition of the term torture. For the purposes of this book the definition adopted is that of the World Medical Association in its Tokyo declaration (1975):

> deliberate, systematic or wanton infliction of physical or mental suffering by one or more persons acting alone or on the orders of any authority, to force another person to yield information, to make a confession, or for any other reason.

PREVALENCE OF THE PROBLEM

Despite numerous international declarations and conventions prohibiting human rights violations, torture remains a major problem. The 1991 Report of Amnesty International (AI) listed 144 countries known for some form of human rights violation in the previous year. During 1990, AI initiated 823 Urgent Action appeals on behalf of 3626 people in 90 countries, following reports of torture, prisoners in a critical state of health, arbitrary arrest, prolonged incommunicado detention, detention without charge or trial or unfair trial, extrajudicial killings or 'disappearances', death sentences, death threats, amputation, hunger-strike, and political executions (Amnesty International, 1991 Report). Reliable estimates of the prevalence of torture are difficult to obtain due to the politically sensitive nature of such information which is all too often either suppressed or denied by the governments concerned. AI figures are thus likely to reflect a fraction of the true magnitude of human rights violations and torture throughout the world.

It is important to note that not all torture is carried out for political purposes. The human rights problem that arises from the ill-treatment or torture of non-political detainees and prisoners may easily be overlooked due to the relatively less media attention given to such cases. Many of the countries listed in the 1991 AI Report, including some Western European and North American countries, are also known for allegations of torture and ill-treatment in police custody or in prisons. Some of the statistics provided in the AI Report are indeed sobering. In Austria, for example, 'The Interior Minister stated in January that between 1984 and 1989 he had received 2622 allegations of ill-treatment by the police, of which 1142 had resulted in criminal complaints against officers leading to 33 convictions. He said that disciplinary investigations were carried out concerning 120 officers and disciplinary measures were taken against 26 of them' (p. 36). The ill-treatment at times allegedly took the form of undressing, pushing sharp objects under the fingernails, burning with a cigarette, and beating of the genitals with a ruler (p. 37).

TORTURE: A NEGLECTED PROBLEM

In the last decade there has been a worldwide surge of interest in, and awareness of, human rights issues. Numerous rehabilitation centres have been set up in both Western and developing countries to provide multidisciplinary help for torture survivors. In 1981, the United Nations Voluntary Fund for Victims of Torture was founded to support projects providing medical, psychological, social, legal, and economic aid to torture survivors. These developments, however, have not been adequately paralleled by efforts in the scientific world to achieve a better understanding of the various forms of political repression and their effects on individuals, communities and societies.

The reasons for the relative lack of scientific attention to the problem of torture are varied and complex. Although no political system or ideology can claim immunity from human rights violations and torture, the systematic practice of torture is more prevalent in developing countries and other parts of the world troubled by regional conflicts, civil strife or other religious or political unrest. Political repression and lack of facilities and financial resources in such countries make any kind of work with survivors of torture a risky and difficult task.

Western academics studying human responses to traumatic stress have focused mainly on traumas such as war violence, natural disasters, accidents and rape. The problem of torture has been largely neglected. Nevertheless its serious health implications are evident as 5% to 35% of the world's 14 million refugee population (700 000 to 4.9 million refugees) are estimated to have had at least one experience of torture (Baker, this volume). These figures do not take into account non-tortured refugees who may have been severely traumatized for other reasons. Interest among the academic community in the needs of traumatized refugees may be partly discouraged in Western countries by unfavourable governmental refugee policies and by political preferences in defining national mental health priorities (see Baker, this volume, for a discussion of refugee policies in Western Europe).

WHY STUDY TORTURE?

Study of torture and care of tortured individuals is not merely a humanitarian concern; it is also an effective political statement against the most abhorrent form of human rights violation. Such political statements are essential in preserving hard-earned human rights in democratic societies. Torture is thus not a problem confined to a remote dictatorship or a totalitarian regime but one that concerns the very moral fabric of the democratic societies in which we live.

Effective measures against torture require a scientific analysis of the factors which generate and sustain the problem. Social, political, and behavioural sciences can contribute much to our understanding of the factors that are associated with a high prevalence of torture in various parts of the world. Torture seems to be most commonly associated with struggle for social change and reform against militaristic, totalitarian regimes in areas marked by socio-cultural, economic, and political deprivation. Effective preventive work also requires due attention to the role of international economic and political dynamics which contribute to the maintenance of the repressive regimes and the conditions that breed deprivation, human misery, injustice, violence, and wars.

The emergence of a new science in this field could make significant contributions to the political struggle against torture. The knowledge generated by this science could be used as a powerful instrument in increasing public awareness of the problem and in directing this awareness to bring pressure upon governments and international organizations such as the United Nations to take more effective measures against the practice of torture. In a rapidly changing world and particularly after the historic changes which brought an end to the the Cold War in the world, scientists have an important role to play in ensuring that respect of human rights is an indispensable component of the 'New World Order'. Mental health professionals are in a unique position to promote this case since the health effects of torture and other similar forms of organized violence on the individual fall mainly into the realm of psychiatry and psychology. Considering the important role played by some doctors, psychiatrists, and psychologists in the state machinery which perpetrates and sustains the problem of torture, mental health professionals are also under an additional moral obligation to concern themselves with this human rights issue. Despite their unique position, however, they have so far been left out of important decision-making processes in the international struggle against torture.

As is amply documented in this volume, torture may lead to serious medical, psychiatric and psychological problems that need professional attention. Before we can begin to understand how best to treat these problems, there are important scientific issues that need to be explored. We still, for example, know little about the personality variables, coping strategies under torture and other situational factors which determine short- and long-term psychological responses to torture, the relationship between various types of torture and subsequent psychological problems, and the efficacy and the therapeutic ingredients of current treatments for survivors of torture. Furthermore, as international pressure on torturers grows, more and more sophisticated methods of torture, mainly of a psychological nature, are being developed to avoid leaving physical scars on the tortured individuals. We need a better understanding of these methods and their psychological effects.

As noted earlier, no society is free from human rights violations and in any country there will be, to a greater or lesser extent, individuals who suffer from some form of ill-treatment or torture. Furthermore, as long as there is violence in the world, there will be sufferers of violent acts or situations sharing common elements with torture in terms of their psychological impact on the individual. Child abuse, sexual or otherwise, domestic/marital violence, rape, kidnapping, ill-treatment of non-political detainees or prisoners, hostage-taking, terrorist acts, and captivity during war are but a few examples. Despite the apparent differences between these situations, the ensuing 'core' psychological symptoms are remarkably similar, suggesting commonalities in the way the traumatic effects of these events are mediated in the central nervous system. A better understanding of torture and its effects would thus benefit not only survivors of torture but also those who have suffered other related traumas.

CURRENT ISSUES IN WORK WITH SURVIVORS OF TORTURE

An important issue of debate among workers helping survivors of torture concerns political as opposed to medical focus on the problem of torture. Torture is viewed by some as primarily, or even solely, a political issue and medical, psychiatric or psychological approaches to the problem are regarded as reductionist 'medicalizing.' There are also concerns that the study of torture would amount to a new discipline, 'torturology', the very existence of which might imply a passive acceptance of the practice of torture. These views have generated considerable resistance in the field to scientific approaches to the problem.

Considering the 'neutrality' or indifference of traditional health care systems to the social and political dimensions of medical and psychiatric problems, these anxieties are not unfounded. Mollica points out in the opening chapter of this volume that 'Barriers to access, inequities in treatment and quality of care, cultural insensitivity and increased social ostracization are well-documented aspects of Western medicine's care of poor, minority and seriously disabled patients.' It is indeed difficult not to acknowledge the '. . . problems inherent in medicine and psychiatry's traditional relationship to emarginated social groups'. Furthermore, examples of blatant abuse of scientific research for political purposes are not too far in human memory. These considerations, however, do not justify a categorical rejection of all scientific approaches to the problem. A critical distinction has to be

made, on the one hand, between scientific work that would be of value
in the combat against torture and the treatment of its effects and, on
the other, work devoid of a useful purpose.

Another issue concerns whether torture survivors with psychological problems can be regarded as 'psychiatric patients'. Some maintain
that torture survivors have been previously 'healthy' individuals and
that their psychological problems are nothing more than a 'normal
response to an abnormal situation'; they cannot thus be classified and
treated as 'psychiatric patients'. This view does not take into account
the duration of psychological problems after torture. Most tortured
individuals experience some degree of psychological distress after the
trauma. Many, however, recover from these effects after a period of
time and thus cannot be regarded as 'psychiatric patients'. Their
response is indeed a 'normal' one to extreme stress. This may not,
however, apply to those survivors who continue to have severely
disabling problems many years after the trauma. Similar situations
arise for other traumatic events. For instance, loss of a loved one is a
trauma often followed by a grief reaction. This is a normal reaction
which often resolves after some time and therefore does not require
treatment. But this normal reaction turns into a 'morbid grief' situation
when the grief reaction persists for many years after the loss and leads
to psychological and social disability. Clearly, duration of the problem
and the degree of incapacitation are important criteria in deciding if,
and when, there is a problem which requires attention.

The assertion that torture survivors were previously 'healthy' individuals before the trauma seems to imply that other individuals with
psychiatric problems were previously 'unhealthy'. This is not necessarily true. For instance, certain specific phobias are known to be
associated with a traumatic event. Some people bitten by a dog may
develop a dog phobia. Others who get trapped in an enclosed space
may develop claustrophobia. They are not disqualified as 'psychiatric
patients' just because they were 'healthy' before the incident. Perhaps
one might argue that psychiatric patients have a genetic, constitutional
and developmental predisposition to psychiatric illness while this is
not the case for survivors of torture. Such 'vulnerability' factors,
however, could also explain why some individuals among torture
survivors are less able to cope with stress and thus are more likely to
develop psychological problems after torture than others. While it is
true that a massive trauma such as torture could overwhelm the
coping resources of even the most resilient person, it may also be true
that, given the same intensity of traumatic stress, some individuals are
more prone to psychological problems than others. Clearly ambiguous

descriptions of psychological functioning such as 'healthy' or 'unhealthy' do not contribute much to our understanding of the issue.

Another much debated issue concerns the nosological classification of psychological consequences of torture. There are three main arguments concerning classification: 1) Torture is a political phenomenon and thus cannot be classified in psychiatric terms, 2) The term post-traumatic stress disorder (PTSD) does not apply to torture because torture is only part of a series of ongoing traumatic situations for the survivor, 3) Psychiatric labels are stigmatizing and therefore should be avoided.

The first argument essentially concerns the question of validity in psychiatric classification. Problems of validity apply to the classification of all psychiatric disorders and not only of torture-related psychological problems. All traumatic events, whether political or non-political, have a psychological impact which may evolve into chronic, disabling symptoms. In this respect, there seems to be no sufficient grounds for singling out torture among other extreme life events. A more plausible stance would be to strive towards improving the validity of the existing diagnostic categories by, for instance, including definitional criteria which acknowledge the political and cultural dimensions of the problem, rather than a categorical rejection of all classification attempts.

Torture as a traumatic event is often only one in a series of stressful life events experienced by survivors. Most authors in this volume agree on the shortcomings of the term PTSD as applied to torture survivors. The term *post-* indeed seems to fail to capture the real nature of traumatization in torture survivors. As is amply documented in this volume, adverse events resulting from political repression span a relatively long period of time, leading to repeated traumatization of individuals. So perhaps '*ongoing*-traumatic stress' is indeed a more appropriate term for survivors of organised violence.

Should psychiatric diagnoses of torture-related problems be avoided because they are stigmatizing and lead to discrimination? The question of labelling is indeed a difficult one which applies not only to psychiatric problems but also to other medical conditions such as AIDS, venereal or infectious diseases, genetic illnesses, cancer, physical disabilities and so on. Diagnostic terms are nevertheless unavoidable since they enable research and communication among health professionals. In the case of torture survivors psychiatric terminology should only be used to define the chronic, severely disabling psychological problems following torture and not the immediate transient psychological reactions.

An important advantage of inclusion of torture-related signs and
symptoms in major international classification systems is the recognition of the fact that torture as a form of political repression is an
important mental health problem. Mollica and Caspi-Yavin in this
volume point out that 'PTSD is a unique diagnosis since it is one of the
few diseases in DSM-IIIR which relate symptoms directly to a psychosocial event'. The recognition of torture as a psychosocial event that
may lead to psychiatric illness may help direct the attention of
academics, mental health professionals, politicians and the world
media to this problem. The message would then be clear: the mental
health implications of torture may be prevented by eradicating torture.
The dissemination of this awareness would certainly be an important
step in the political struggle against torture.

In conclusion, the alternative to a purely political approach to
torture is an integrated model which gives due weight to all relevant
aspects of the problem. It should be clear from the preview of contents
below that the selection of the topics for this volume is based on the
understanding that torture is a complex phenomenon with interacting
social, cultural, political, medical, psychological, and biological dimensions. It is hoped that the broad perspective of the book and its
integrated approach to the problem will achieve some synthesis
between the widely divergent views in the field.

PREVIEW OF CONTENTS

The contents are organized into seven sections. There may be some overlap among the chapters and the sections with respect to the various issues covered. This is not entirely undesirable since one of the main purposes is to bring together the experience of health professionals working with survivors of torture in different social, political and cultural settings.

PART I: TORTURE AND ITS CONSEQUENCES

In the opening chapter Mollica (Chapter 1) emphasizes the need for the development of a new science in order to address two major issues concerning torture: its prevention and the rehabilitation of survivors. In his review of political versus medical focus in work with survivors of torture, he concludes that 'The potential benefits of a research agenda can occur in spite of the acknowledged dangers of medical science if the basic commitment of patients and practitioners remains directed at protecting human rights and eliminating torture.' He also puts forward those '. . . principles and concepts that must underlie a program of research capable of respecting the integrity of the survivor as well as contributing socially useful findings and outcomes'. He reviews certain important epistemological issues in scientific research concerning the development of theory, formulation of hypotheses, the validation of causal mechanisms, and the interpretation of results. A concluding statement sums up the integrated approach to the problem of torture discussed earlier; 'Scientific investigations are in fact crucial elements of an integrated triad of *advocacy, clinical care* and *applied research* necessary to eliminate torture and successfully treat its victims.'

Two chapters by contributors from the Rehabilitation Centre for Torture Victims (RCT) in Denmark review the physical and psychosocial consequences of torture.

Skylv from RCT (Chapter 2) provides valuable information about the physical sequelae of torture, a step towards relating particular physical signs to particular forms of torture. Are there physical signs that can be an evidence of particular forms of torture? The author acknowledges the difficulties, 'even with the most careful history taking and physical examination', in defining 'the symptoms and signs that have been caused by a particular form of torture in an individual victim'. The difficulty arises from the fact that individuals are often subjected to more than one form of torture, thereby suffering overlapping injuries. An understanding of the correlation between the physical injuries and various methods of torture, the author points out, is also important in planning treatment.

Somnier, Vesti, Kastrup, and Genefke (Chapter 3) provide an extensive and up-to-date review of the social and psychological consequences of torture. The review covers 46 reports on torture published in English. This is a timely review given the recent increase in publications on this topic and the need for setting new directions for future research. The authors briefly discuss the shortcomings of the DSM-III diagnosis of post-traumatic stress disorder as it relates to torture-related psychological symptoms and the methodological problems that plague studies of torture survivors. The authors conclude that '. . . despite the methodological shortcomings of the studies reviewed . . . there is sufficient evidence to suggest a relationship between torture and subsequent psychological sequelae.'

Chapter 4 by Paker, Paker, and Yüksel presents findings from a recent systematic study of 246 non-political prisoners in a prison in Turkey. This study has attempted to overcome some of the methodological shortcomings of other similar studies reviewed in the previous chapter. It is based on a fairly large sample of subjects, the entire prison population, who were serving their term in prison at the time of the study. The sample is therefore relatively homogenous with respect to the life circumstances during and following the trauma and the nature of ill-treatment received from the prison authorities. Information on the psychological state of the prisoners has been gathered using a semi-structured interview scale and other standardized rating instruments. Furthermore, the data have been analysed using multivariate statistical techniques (e.g. multiple regression analysis), thereby controlling for intervening variables in examining the effects of torture per se. The investigators have found that a history of torture was predictive of greater psychopathology among the prisoners.

The psychosocial problems arising from asylum-seeking and refugee status are discussed by Baker (in Chapter 5) who also provides a critical account of current refugee policies in European countries. The author states 'In a range of generally informative material on refugees and situations that create them such as war, political instability and genocidal threat, the special needs and experiences of the tortured refugee are rarely discussed. This represents serious neglect of a substantial proportion of the world's refugees.' An important question raised is whether it requires 'too much stretch of the imagination to suggest that current ways in which asylum and refugee status seekers are handled border on what is inhuman and degrading, and constitutes a breach of Article 5' of the UN Declaration of Human Rights ('No one shall be subjected to torture or to cruel inhuman or degrading treatment or punishment'). Finally, the author formulates three survival patterns for traumatized refugees: negative, adaptive, and constructive.

The two other chapters in this Part concern prisoners-of-war and Holocaust survivors. These chapters highlight the long-term consequences of torture and provide a review of the experience gained with ex-POWs and concentration camp survivors over the last 45 years. Many of the issues reviewed in these two chapters are highly relevant to work with survivors of political torture today.

Miller (Chapter 6), in his review of the literature on captivity as a stressful life event, concludes that 'Subsequent to severe trauma such as a prisoner of war experience, residual difficulties are likely to occur as long as 40 years after the event.' The author presents a detailed review of the literature on POW experience during World War II and the Korean war, with particular focus on psychological consequences of captivity, mediating variables in the development of PTSD, impact of torture during captivity, captor–captive relationship, methodological issues in research, and treatment prospects.

Much has been written about the Holocaust but relatively little attention is paid to its implications for the problem of torture today. There are important reasons in reviewing the experience of Holocaust survivors in a book on the current problem of torture. These are stated by Solkoff (Chapter 7) in his introduction: 'With the steady rise in neo-fascist, religious fundamentalistic, antisemitic, and jingoistic nationalist movements, it behoves us to look again at the genocidal actions of the Nazi system . . . It is hoped that this review of past experiences with Holocaust survivors will help inform our understanding of how to deal with current problems of torture.' After a brief review of the concentration camp experience, the author focuses on the coping strategies used by the survivors both during and after the traumatic experience. Also presented is a review of the methodological flaws that characterize the research on the 'survivor syndrome'. The

author concludes 'Although the ideal study, from a scientific standpoint cannot be conducted on such a complex topic, fraught with
emotion, the methodological ideal must at least be approached if we
are to understand the diversity of effects of exposure to any intense
trauma.'

PART II: THEORY

This section consists of two chapters dealing with the theoretical
aspects of human response to trauma and issues in the classification of
trauma responses.

Saporta and van der Kolk (Chapter 8) provide a detailed review of
the literature on the psychobiology of traumatic stress response syndromes and discuss the treatment implications of recent findings in
this area. The authors aim to '... introduce the reader to the complex
interaction between biological, psychological, and social factors that
converge and perpetuate the long term consequences of trauma'. After
a brief discussion of four primary features of trauma – incomprehensi-
bility, disrupted attachment, traumatic bonding, and inescapability –
the authors review three animal models for PTSD: inescapable stress,
forced isolation, and disruption of attachments in nonhuman primates. Also reviewed are the role of endogenous opiods in trauma
responses and the psychobiology of reliving and reenactment. The
chapter ends with a discussion of treatment implications.

Başoğlu and Mineka (Chapter 9) review the animal and human
literature on the role of uncontrollable and unpredictable stress in
post-traumatic stress responses and examine the parallels between
experimental models of anxiety/depression and human experience
under torture and their implications for treatment. The authors
propose that '. . . the human experience with closest parallels to
experimental models in animals is the experience of humans undergoing torture. Although these parallels cannot provide a comprehensive
account of human behaviour, they could nevertheless contribute to
our understanding of the mechanisms involved in the development of
posttrauma stress symptoms and help us in identifying the principles
of effective treatment in torture survivors.'

PART III: ASSESSMENT, DIAGNOSIS, AND CLASSIFICATION

The two chapters in this Part deal with issues in assessment, diagnosis
and classification of trauma responses with a focus on two related

questions concerning a) the validity of post-traumatic stress disorder as a diagnostic category and b) its validity in relation to post-torture psychological problems. They thus complement each other.

McNally (Chapter 10) deals with the first question. The author reviews the evidence on PTSD as a coherent syndrome, its prevalence, longitudinal course, and the risk factors for developing PTSD. Also discussed are data from family studies, patterns of comorbidity, delimitation from other disorders, the implications of psychophysiological research for the validity of the syndrome. The chapter ends with a discussion of several questions of central importance in the preparation for the publication of DSM-IV in 1993: 'Should the stressor criterion be altered?' 'Should there be a duration requirement for diagnosing PTSD?' 'Where should PTSD be classified in DSM-IV?'

Mollica and Caspi-Yavin (Chapter 11) focus on the assessment and diagnosis of torture survivors. They review the definitional problems concerning torture and the variability of what is regarded as torture from culture to culture. 'Clinicians who care for torture survivors must learn the types of horrific human abuses that are perpetrated by different regimes in various geopolitical regions.' The authors, in their discussion of the usefulness of the DSM-IIIR diagnosis of PTSD in torture survivors, state that '... the high prevalence of torture in many non-western cultures and the entry of ethnically diverse survivors into torture treatment centers world-wide raise additional problems as to the cultural validity of the PTSD criteria . . . Cross-cultural research suggests that assessment of psychiatric illness should begin with local phenomenological descriptions of folk diagnoses which then can be compared to Western psychological criteria.' The authors conclude that 'The accurate assessment of torture events and symptoms and the proper classification of this information into a diagnostic system is fundamental to the effective treatment of torture survivors.'

PART IV: REHABILITATION PROGRAMMES FOR TORTURE SURVIVORS

This Part consists of chapters on the treatment of torture survivors. Over the last decade or so numerous rehabilitation centres for torture survivors have been established throughout the world. Some of these centres are based in host countries serving refugees in exile while others are situated in the home country of traumatized individuals in need of care. Due to different socio-political circumstances in which these centres operate, they have adopted different models in organising their work with survivors. Although there seems to be a general

consensus on the need for some kind of organized services for
survivors, there is less agreement on the desirable models of organization.

van Willigen (Chapter 12) presents factual details about the organization of some of the rehabilitation centres throughout the world and
reviews the differences and the similarities in the fundamental principles underlying their approach. One of the important issues raised in
this chapter is the distinction between 'torture' and 'organized violence'. The author argues for greater emphasis on the latter concept.
Since uprooting and exile are closely associated with organized violence, '. . . it must be relevant to consider all refugees victims of
organized violence'. Too much emphasis on torture 'may, by relegating other forms of organized violence and their psychological
impact on the individual to a position of secondary importance,
inadvertently result in the neglect of people who, though not tortured,
are nevertheless highly traumatized'. The chapter ends with the
author's recommendations on a multi-disciplinary approach designed
to deal with the consequences of organized violence.

Two examples of a multi-disciplinary or integrative approach in the
care of torture survivors are provided in this Part. Bøjholm and Vesti
(Chapter 13) give an account of the multi-disciplinary rehabilitation of
torture survivors as practised in the Rehabilitation Centre for Torture
Victims (RCT) in Copenhagen. The RCT accepts only tortured refugees
on grounds that they constitute a different population from non-
tortured refugees. Is there a need for specialised centres for torture
survivors? Some believe not. Bøjholm and Vesti argue that 'Torture
survivors suffer from many of the same severe psychological problems
as do other refugees, but have also other distinguishing characteristics
which make it possible for experienced medical personnel to identify
them among refugees . . . Previous experience with survivors, particularly concentration camp survivors, indicated a need for a
treatment centre with specialised treatment programmes undertaken
by specially trained personnel. Similarly, work with torture survivors
requires a wide knowledge of torture methods and their effects.'

The last chapter in this Part is on sexual torture, an aspect of the
problem that has so far received relatively little attention. Lunde and
Ortmann (ETICA) (Chapter 14) define sexual torture as violence
against the sexual organs, physical sexual assault, 'mental sexual
assault', or a combination of the three. The authors review the
literature on the physical and psychological effects of sexual torture
and present a treatment model within a multi-disciplinary approach
involving medical treatment, psychotherapy, physiotherapy, social

counselling, and family therapy. The chapter ends with a discussion of various issues in treatment outcome evaluation and research. The authors conclude that 'Accumulation of knowledge could be enhanced and achieved more speedily if multi-centre research were to be conducted in accordance with a common protocol. This should involve professionals from different countries with different cultural back-grounds and experiences in the examination and treatment of torture survivors.'

PART V: PSYCHOTHERAPY

Bustos (Chapter 15) presents a psychodynamic formulation of psychological responses to torture, a description of the psychodynamic therapy model, and a discussion of various issues in treatment including regression, human relatedness, transference, countertransference, and verbal and non-verbal communication. Also discussed are three additional forms of countertransference specific to work with refugee torture survivors: culturally determined, colonial and ethnoidentificative countertransference. The author concludes that 'New theoretical and clinical findings concerning torture trauma necessitate a revision of the traditional psychodynamic therapy strategies in the treatment of torture survivors.'

Vesti and Kastrup (Chapter 16) describe 'insight therapy' as it is practised in the RCT in Denmark. The treatment consists of five phases and is '. . . based on the assumption that being able to confront the traumatic experience has a therapeutic effect'. Also discussed are various issues in psychotherapy such as resistance to treatment, transference, countertransference, contraindications for 'insight therapy' and alternative psychotherapies, and the use of interpreters in therapy. The authors conclude that little is known about the relative efficacy of different psychotherapies and point to the need for research on the short- and long-term outcome of psychotherapy.

Keane, Albano and Blake (Chapter 17) present a detailed review of the current trends in the treatment of PTSD. These include direct therapeutic exposure, desensitization, implosive therapy and flooding, cognitive behavioural therapy, cognitive therapy, pharmacotherapy, skills training, family therapy, group therapy, and stress inoculation training. The authors provide the rationale for their chapter appearing in a book on torture: 'The study of trauma secondary to torture can clearly benefit from an integration with the combat literature. With little extant information on torture, it is relevant to consider the conditions of combatants and prisoners of war in trying to develop a

comprehensive understanding of the clinical technology that might be
of some assistance to the treatment of torture victims. While some of
the sociopolitical issues surrounding torture may differ from those
related to combat trauma, the issues of helplessness, terror, bodily
injury, and guilt (or responsibility) over the experience seem especially
common to both forms of trauma.'

In the last chapter of this Part (Chapter 18), Başoğlu gives a
description of the behavioural and cognitive treatment of torture
survivors and discusses various theoretical and practical issues in
therapy. This chapter thus complements the chapter by Keane, Albano
and Blake by providing an account of behavioural and cognitive
approach in the treatment of survivors of torture. The author reviews
some of the moral and political issues that are often raised in therapy
and discusses how they can be dealt with using a cognitive restructuring approach. The chapter also includes a brief review of the common
elements between cognitive-behavioural treatment and other psychotherapies frequently used with torture survivors. 'The psychotherapy
methods used in treating torture survivors ... have an important
element in common: getting the survivor to talk about his/her traumatic experiences and encourage free emotional expression in a
therapeutic context ... It is thus conceivable that a therapeutic ingredient common to all these therapies may be extinction of anxiety
through exposure to painful memories, followed (or accompanied) by
cognitive change which ultimately enables integration of the traumatic
experience.'

PART VI: TORTURE IN PARTICULAR COUNTRIES: EXPERIENCE WITH SURVIVORS OF TORTURE IN THEIR HOME COUNTRY

This Part consists of four chapters by authors who help survivors of
organized violence living in their home country (Argentina, South
Africa, Pakistan, the Philippines). These countries are not selected
from among others for any special reason. Nor are they meant to be a
representative sample for the problem of torture in the world. They are
merely some examples of countries where there are systematic efforts
to help torture survivors.

The authors in this Part provide an account of their work and
experience with survivors of organized violence. Their experience is of
special importance for several reasons. The majority of torture survivors in the world live in developing countries and work with survivors
in those areas is quite different from that in Western countries. Much

of the care services are undertaken by health professionals who are often themselves active in the ongoing political struggle, at least by virtue of helping tortured political activists, and therefore have to conduct their work under considerable political oppression. Further, the client population served by these workers is probably different in some ways, being perhaps, for example, more physically and psychologically disabled, from those who manage to find their way to specialized centres in Western countries. In addition, much of the rehabilitation work may need to be carried out while the clients are still at serious risk of further victimization. Such experience is therefore valuable and complements specialized rehabilitation work with tortured refugees in Western countries. Furthermore, these chapters provide an account of the socio-economic and political context of torture and other human rights violations – an account without which it would be difficult to understand the individual, social and political dimensions of the phenomenon.

Kordon, Edelman, Lagos, Nicoletti, Kersner, and Groshaus (Chapter 19), members of the Psychological Assistance to the Mothers of Plaza de Mayo, give a historical account of torture and forced disappearances during the military dictatorship in Argentina between 1976 and 1983 – an account supported by detailed citations from a descriptive report by the Inter-American Human Rights Commission (CIDH) in 1979. The commission stated 'The people mentioned have been apprehended from their homes, from their places of work and from public places, depending on the case, by armed men who are *prima facie*, and always claiming, to be acting in the name of some manner of public authority ... the phenomena of the missing people affects professionals, students, labor leaders, draftees, businessmen, in other words, the better part of the many segments of Argentine society.' The authors point to the complicity of the justice system: 'Writs of habeas corpus were useless. Courts rejected attempts to free the missing people, claiming either that they had no information regarding the cases or that there were no legal grounds for action ... The news media did not report what was occurring.' Also presented in the chapter is a description of the other forms of torture widely used in Argentina during that period, their psychological effects and treatment.

Dowdall's chapter (Chapter 20) begins with an historical, social, and political account of apartheid, political repression and torture in South Africa and goes on to review the evidence on torture and the various methods practised. How have professions – law, medicine, and clinical psychology – coped with the challenge posed by torture? Dowdall replies: 'In each case a similar pattern has emerged: professionals employed by the state have tended to support the political *status quo* rather than human rights to a point that violates their own codes.' Also presented is a review of treatment and counselling methods for ex-detainees, some of which are tailored according to the realities of the South African situation. The chapter ends with two conclusions from the South African experience: 'Tyrannical regimes seem to be strangely thin-skinned when faced with rejection and international attack on their internal policies. The stands made by principled individuals do have a cumulative effect, and in the end they do bring changes ... therapeutic practice with torture survivors within a repressive country differs substantially from rehabilitation in a host country ... the political conflicts within the country permeate the operation of the professions and the judgment and modus operandi of the individual professional.'

Mahboob Mehdi (Chapter 21) from the Rehabilitation and Health Aid Centre for Torture Victims (RAHAT) in Islamabad reviews the historical background of torture in Pakistan. 'The Police department, established during the colonial period by the Police Act of 1861, continued unchanged and the legacy of torture from the past was inherited by the new state.' Among the prevalent forms of torture reviewed in the chapter is whipping as a method of punishment. The author questions the role of doctors in the execution of this punishment. He urges the doctors to refuse involvement in the execution of punishments such as whipping or amputation of limbs, in cover-up activities such as '... providing false death certificates and false clinical records', and in examinations to confirm certain offences such as 'drinking, "illicit" sexual relations and pregnancy out of wedlock for which severe and cruel punishments may be imposed'. Also reviewed in the chapter are the activities of Voice Against Torture (VAT) and RAHAT in the struggle against torture and in caring for tortured individuals. The author concludes by pointing out that those helping torture survivors are themselves at risk and that this risk may be reduced by support from the public, wide media coverage, and recognition and support from human rights organizations abroad.

Parong, Pagaduan-Lopez, Estrada-Claudio, Protacio-Marcelino, and Cabildo (Chapter 22) from the Medical Action Group in Manila also give an account of the historical and political context of torture in their country. Important lessons are derived from the experience of the Medical Action Group (MAG) and the Philippine Action Concerning Torture (PACT) in rehabilitation of torture survivors: 'Under conditions of continuing repression where even the physical security of the survivors and the health workers were not assured, the center-based approach was not very effective since the center can serve as a fixed point for military surveillance or re-arrest . . . [the treatment approach] . . . must be problem-oriented and action-oriented . . . comprehensive and systematic but flexible . . . individual, family and community oriented . . . must assist the survivor to regain independence and to go back to the mainstream of life . . . must consider the social, political and cultural situation of the country.' The chapter also provides a detailed account of the health care services for torture survivors in the Philippines.

PART VII: MODERN ETHICS AND INTERNATIONAL LAW

In the closing section of the book Sørensen (Chapter 23) traces the development of international law, starting with the Universal Declaration of Human Rights in 1948. The author also reviews the measures taken to implement the aims of the declarations and conventions adopted by the United Nations and the Council of Europe. Also discussed in this chapter are the principles of medical ethics in relation to the role and duties of doctors and other health personnel in the face of human rights violations. The author concludes that 'Possibilities of eliminating torture must be considered to exist.'

REFERENCES

Amnesty International Report (1991). Amnesty International Publications.
Peters, E. (1985). *Torture*. Basil Blackwell.

Part I

TORTURE AND ITS CONSEQUENCES

1
THE PREVENTION OF TORTURE AND THE CLINICAL CARE OF SURVIVORS: A FIELD IN NEED OF A NEW SCIENCE
Richard F. Mollica

INTRODUCTION

The health care of torture survivors has emerged as a new medical specialty. In less than two decades, health and mental health practitioners who care for torture survivors have generated considerable interest in their patients and their work. Many clinical programs worldwide specializing in this area, through their advocacy, have developed local and national constituencies capable of supporting clinical care and of increasing the access of survivors to medical and psychiatric services. Paradoxically, medicine's recent discovery of the torture survivor as patient has led to a fundamental clash between two opposing world views (Mollica, 1989). One world view argues that torture is an extraordinary life experience capable of causing in any individual a wide range of physical and psychological suffering and related disability. Therefore, a universal need for medical care for all torture survivors exist. The other world view, although acknowledging the injuries inflicted by torture, argues that since these injuries and psychological reactions are normal responses to abnormal life threatening experiences, the torture survivor should not be stigmatized by medical and psychiatric diagnoses and treatment. Furthermore, this viewpoint argues that, by medicalizing the sequelae of basic human responses to political oppression and human cruelty, the focus is shifted away from human rights and the prevention of torture to the objectifying and politically neutral diagnostic categories of modern medicine. Both viewpoints acknowledge, however, the problems inherent in medicine and psychiatry's traditional relationship to emarginated social groups. Barriers to access, inequities in treatment and quality of care, cultural insensitivity and increased social ostracization are well-documented aspects of Western medicine's care of poor, minority and seriously disabled patients (Mollica, 1983). Consequently, health practitioners working with torture survivors have consciously directed their efforts at avoiding those traditional aspects of medical care which further demean and diminish the self-esteem of individuals who have survived the degradation of torture.

Exposing torture survivors to medical research appears to many of its critics to expose the survivor to an impersonal doctor–patient relationship which has none of the protecting influences of the caring clinician. The scientific method is said to lack compassion as it extracts information from the survivor and intrudes into the privacy of his life experiences – but for what purpose? Memories of the use of science and technology throughout the centuries to perfect new instruments of torture (D'Arno, 1983), the twentieth century's experiment with psychological methods of torture and the Nazi medical experiments create a legitimate apprehension of any clinical system which seeks to transform torture survivors into research subjects. Furthermore, recent trends in the biomedical sciences have pushed scientific investigations further away from addressing meaningful and important social problems. The latter are crucial areas of investigation for this field's new science and include issues related to prevention, medicine's role in torture, and an empirical understanding of torturers and the organizations and societies from which they emerge.

Over the past 50 years, social scientists and public policy-makers have struggled with the lack of useful scientific knowledge for implementing social policies and mental health programs. Recently, Italian society enacted a radical psychiatric reform aimed at minimizing this gap (Bollini & Mollica, 1989). The late Franco Basaglia, leader of the Italian reform movement, in describing the relationship between psychiatric knowledge and the old Italian mental hospital system summarized this problem by stating (Mollica, 1985):

> And so we have, on the one hand, a science ideologically committed to quest for the origins of an illness it acknowledges to be 'incomprehensible' and, on the other, a patient who, because of his presumed 'incomprehensibility', has been oppressed, mortified, and destroyed by an asylum system that, instead of serving him in its protective role of therapeutic institution, has, on the contrary, contributed to the gradual and often irreversible disintegration of his identify.

Can similar clinical realities be avoided as we seek to develop an empirical research tradition for our new medical field?

The medical and psychiatric care and prevention of torture has arrived at a cross-road. Whether a political therapy is chosen for the torture survivor or a medical therapy (and who is to make these choices?), an advance in knowledge consistent with each theoretical position still needs to occur. The current clash in theoretical positions between opposing treatment approaches partially reflects the struggles of each group to achieve recognition and legitimacy within mainstream medicine. Unfortunately, successful advocacy on behalf of torture survivors has resulted in a lack of expression by the survivors of their political, social and personal needs. Similar to most oppressed and marginalized populations, the voice of the torture survivor is a whisper (Foucault, 1973). Where this voice can be heard is in the literature of survivors, i.e. in their art, poems, stories and biographies – and not in the medical literature. Of course, the medical practitioners pioneering this field cannot be faulted for emphasizing advocacy and establishing clinical programs. Yet, in spite of enormous energy expended on clinical services for torture survivors, the effectiveness of available treatment programs remain unproven. Clinical practitioners are ambivalent about whether they should investigate the survivor's illnesses; they hesitate to establish valid and reliable methods for clinical investigations. The latter has led to a scientific doughnut specific to the torture experience and an expanding ring of evidence derived from the study of other traumatized populations. Torture survivors and their health practitioners no longer need to borrow from the scientific efforts of others. They are in a unique position to identify new knowledge capable of producing effective interventions and prevention programs.

This chapter will focus on the principles and methods of scientific investigations and interpretations capable of advancing the goals of this embryonic medical specialty. The potential benefits of a research agenda can occur in spite of the acknowledged dangers of medical science if the basic commitment of patients and practitioners remains directed at protecting human rights and eliminating torture. The analysis that follows will proceed along a pathway moving from the development of theory and the formulation of hypothesis, through the validation of causal mechanisms, and the interpretation of results. Finally, a few concluding remarks will focus on those human attitudes which prevent the generation of new knowledge and strategies capable of understanding torture and eliminating its occurrence.

GOALS OF RESEARCH

Research that focuses on torture must be socially useful. The terms *social* and *useful* indicate that specific set of clinical attitudes and behaviors that affect the individual survivor as well as help mediate against society's production of new patients. Because of the extreme victimization and exploitation of the torture survivor, it is ethically correct to assume, as top priority, a research position which protects the patient from further exploitation and harm as well as provides the patient with the maximum benefits of the research process (Hellman & Hellman, 1991). Of course, many supporters of science would state that this position is shortsighted since such seemingly distal scientific experiments as those in molecular biology might have the greatest potential of elucidating the physical impact of torture and lead to effective biological interventions. In spite of the potential accuracy of this argument, the relationship between the torture survivor and investigator mitigates against any scientific situation in which the survivor becomes a passive participant to the observation and intrusive studies of social and biological sciences. Protection of the survivor from further victimization demands that the investigator forms a working partnership with the survivor, as well as a contract to share any new knowledge discovered. Unfortunately, recent trends in modern science have diminished the importance and respectability of *applied* research and have limited access of the research subject and his community to the findings obtained by scientific investigations. Any research generated in this new field must, therefore, properly answer the following question – 'Who benefits from this research?' If it is not the torture survivor, and if the benefits are not well defined and useful, then these studies should not be permitted.

Initial emphasis on socially useful research implies that studies should be directed at determining:

1 Why governments and institutions and/or individuals torture and what can be done to prevent it?
2 What factors can be introduced, manipulated and/or transformed in order to change the social, physical and psychological outcome of torture?

Scientific analysis of these two major areas – prevention and clinical treatment – should proceed through the proper stages of scientific investigations. Good intentions should not be allowed to replace good science. However, the research standards and methods of mainstream scientific approaches must be adapted to the problems and obstacles unique to the torture experience.

THEORY CONSTRUCTION

In spite of the paucity of modern social theories and their almost total lack of use in the investigations of medical and psychiatric practice, the elaboration and testing of grand theories still have considerable aesthetic appeal. Theoretical explanations of torture and its medical consequences should be readily forthcoming, especially because of the extensive literature already generated this century on political oppression and the social consequences of totalitarian societies and modern genocides (Chalk and Jonassohn, 1982). Yet, controversy exists in the philosophy of science, especially as applied to the medical sciences, as to the relative merits of deductive and inductive approaches in generating scientific paradigms (Harre, 1970). *Inductive* methods are those methods by which inferences pass from singular statements, to universal statements, such as hypotheses or theories. In contrast, theories are termed *deductive* which restrict their conclusions to premises and the conclusions drawn necessarily from these premises. This method is distinguished by deriving *outcomes* or *effects* as end products of a succession of steps, each of which represents the application of prior accepted principles.

In recent years, the deductive method has assumed ascendancy in the medical sciences and has become closely associated with testing and the experimental method (Popper, 1968; Buck, 1975). In the discussion that follows, the relative scientific validity of deduction and induction will not be emphasized but a closer inspection of the *norms* that guide the development of scientific investigation. The philosopher Frederick Will (1988) defines *norms* as those variety of patterns or procedures that serve as guides or standards of thoughts or actions in various fields. He states that norms are an archetype or model of instances of thought or action that serve to guide our scientific performance. Norms are considered to be templates that are thought to reside in individual minds, in symbolic systems, in some special realm of platonic forms, or even in external nature. Norms are the building blocks of scientific theory. Yet, as the late French philosopher Michel Foucault has demonstrated, these norms are also an essential aspect of what he describes as society's discursive formation (Mollica, 1987). Foucault, for example, uses psychiatry to illustrate his definition of a discursive formation. He first claims that psychiatry is a social practice. Like all social practices, it is constituted by power and serves as a 'setting' through which power is exercised and invested. Psychiatry is also a *discursive formation* because it consists of an interconnected pattern of historically contingent relationships. It is a *formation* because it has a history; how it came into being as a practice in the economy of power. And it is *discursive* because it not only came into being, but is also reproduced through the medium of language, practices and behavior.

The norms – archetypes, templates, platonic forms – of theory construction, therefore, constitute an historically based system that is complete unto itself. The use of grand theories and/or principles and the *deduction* of hypotheses from the latter are all part of a social value system with its categories, practices, routines and rules that are representative of a given culture and historical period.

Foucault, of course, was also interested in extending his insights to reveal the 'positive unconsciousness of science', i.e. those epistemological levels of theory that give the scientific approach its method, but that at the same time, generate assumptions that elude the consciousness of the scientist; although they are still part of the scientific discourse. Unfortunately, the uncritical use of norms in clinical and services research has led to the generation of investigations and findings which are self-fulfilling prophecies, i.e. the norms which have generated the initial hypotheses are in effect those very same norms which have already predetermined the social outcomes revealed by the researcher, as well as the meaning given to these findings. This quandary has been thoughtfully described by Quentin Skinner (Will, 1988 p. 9)

> How can we possibly hope, by using (as we are bound to) our own local assumptions and canons of evidence, to construct a theory which is then employed to criticize those precise assumptions and canons of evidence? How, in short, can we, through the legitimate employment of norms, develop further norms that, since they can be used to criticize the originals, must also transcend and sometimes negate them?

Skinner is essentially asking the investigator how we might be able to get behind the discursive formation and reveal its true nature.

Society's historically constituted relationship to the torture survivor (Peters, 1985) and the torture experience must also constitute elements of its discursive formation and have generated an interactive relationship between torture and the general medical and scientific definitions of disease and treatment (Levin, 1987). It can be assumed *a priori* that those norms which affect the scientific process must also be affected by socio-historical and cultural norms which affect the torture experience. How then can the scientific investigator generate new definitions, criticisms and reconstructions useful to ameliorating the problem of torture and its sequelae?

I suggest that the following four methods are capable of generating new scientific insights by revealing the discursive formation. They include:

1 Studying 'hard clinical cases', i.e. cases that do not provide unequivocal answers; unusual examples which challenge generally accepted norms and customs.
2 Collecting the life histories of torture survivors who have had the values of their social world threatened with collapse.
3 Conducting simple phenomenological descriptions of concrete clinical and socio-political practices.
4 Generating and testing hypotheses based upon radical theories.

Many case studies have been presented describing the treatment of torture survivors. Unfortunately, these studies usually illustrate specific treatment methods and are not directed at challenging medical and psychiatric norms or medical outcomes. The case study is not used as a scientific device to demonstrate new findings or clinical efficacy, but is given as evidence to support the clinician's belief system related to treatment. In other words, the case study declares its intentions by stating, 'I have evaluated the patient and found what I am looking for, and now I will discuss with you the results.' The accuracy of reporting and the hermeneutical value of most case studies in the torture field must be seriously questioned. Greater attention needs to be devoted to elucidating the meaning of the most difficult and refractory cases. These cases challenge our standard clinical approaches and attitudes.

Collecting the life histories (often called oral histories or testimonies) of torture survivors can reveal considerable knowledge of the changing influence of torture on the life experience of individuals, families and communities. The cross-sectional analyses of most medical and psychiatric approaches provide little information on the torture experience as it relates to the survivor's past, present and future life. In particular, modern methods of medical and psychiatric diagnosis use taxonomies which place survivors into static illness categories with no regard for the cultural and social meaning of the traumatizing event or the wide individual variations in psychosocial responses to the torture experience.

The systematic documentation of medical practices in medical and mental health clinics in countries where torture is occurring (e.g. prison health centers), and the contrasting documentation of practices in community programs (e.g. church groups) and treatment centers caring for survivors, if conducted cross-nationally could reveal crucial information on the differential relationships of medical organizations and health professionals to torture survivors. Analysis of innovative local responses to torture survivors and their families could provide considerable insights into the therapeutic aspects of cultural, religious and community-based interventions.

Torture treatment advocates have failed to critique their own clinical services through well conducted evaluation research. Established centers in Europe, the United States and elsewhere are in need of valid evaluation research in order to separate the advocacy claims of these centers from accurate measurements of their relative degree of success and failure in ameliorating the medical and psychiatric consequences of torture.

Finally, testable hypotheses should be generated from radical theories and the urgent necessities of responding to torture's aftermath. For example, Argentina needed to identify those victims of political oppression buried in mass graves while the Grandmothers of the Plaza de Mayo needed to identify the parental background of their grandchildren who had been taken from their tortured and murdered parents and given up for adoption (sometimes to the torturer's family). Both Argentine efforts achieved major advances in anthropologic labeling and forensic medicine (Chelsia, 1986; Joyce & Stover, 1991).

Original insights from these four methods, and others, can help elucidate hypotheses capable of scientific evaluation through experimentation.

EXPERIMENTATION

The theories and principles emerging from the above approaches may not need experimental testing. Yet, the crucial next step for theory construction consists in generating testable hypotheses capable of producing changes in our social systems. This human desire to 'fix' the system inevitably leads to the problem of experimentation and causality. Without causal explanations the desired improvements in the medical treatment of torture survivors or the elimination of torture cannot be achieved.

As Cook and Campbell (1979) state:

> What policy makers and individual citizens seem to want from the sciences are recipes that can be followed and that usually lead to desired positive effects, even if understanding of the ... process is only partial and the positive effects are not invariably brought about.

Testable hypotheses, therefore, will involve the scientific community in manipulating the medical system, and ultimately society, in order to produce desirable outcomes.

This commitment to intervention demands two processes that will have far-reaching impact on the interpretation of experimental results. The first process includes the clarification and recognition of the level at which the system will be studied, i.e. everything from the macro to the micro level of mediation. Although it is generally considered that one level of mediation does not have greater intrinsic value over another, in recent years, the molecular or biological level has been given greater value than social or political levels. This priority, of course, reflects current discursive norms which strive to negate the complexity and meaning of modern social life. As Knight (Will, 1988) ironically stated: 'The best minds of our race have decided that since natural objects are not like men, men must be like natural objects.'

Knight's statement leads to a brief explication of the second and most crucial process necessary for experimentation, i.e. the reduction of human practices and behaviors to simple abstractions that can provide measures of intervention and outcome. In a sense, the complex substance of human social existence reflected abstractly in our prevailing norms and theories are further *deflated* and *distilled* to usable *measures* and/or *constructs*.

Whether or not experiments prove causality they at least provide a rich opportunity for probing the relationship between specific interventions and outcomes (Bebbington, 1980; Cook, 1980; Harre, 1980). Popper's (1968) concept of 'falsification' shifted the focus from 'proof' to 'disproof' of causal theories and premises through experimentation. Popper indicated that the best we can do is demonstrate that a theory and its causal relationships have never been disproven (Buck, 1975).

In generating socially useful research capable of serving torture survivors, scientific investigations must emphasize not only what factors A caused B but also how B can be transformed into C, D, E, etc. This process reflects a radical shift away from causal mechanisms to establishing the successful achievement of outcomes. If B represents the torturing society or the medical disability caused by torture, our new field must give more consideration to achieving C, D, E and other outcomes (i.e. the transformation of the torturing society to a non-torturing society or the rehabilitation of the survivor) than to elucidating those factors which cause B. This shift, however, should occur without abandoning Popper's radical emphasis on ongoing falsification.

Greater value, therefore, is placed on those theories or aspects of a theory that can be translated into testable hypotheses and are tied to achievable outcomes. In contrast, any theory that is formulated in which nothing can be done to change the outcome, although interesting, is not considered a legitimate domain for research. The latter restriction is especially important for the scientific investigation of medical and psychiatric systems because while many studies explore the failures of the system, few provide insights and/or guidelines for reversing these failures. Empirical investigations which emphasize system failure, unfortunately, are also most likely driven by those norms that are ineffectual and are partially responsible for producing these failures. These investigations constitute an apologia or serve as rationalizations to help facilitate our accommodation to these practices and systems. Again, it is essential to state, therefore, according to this model, that research must be primarily committed to generating *achievable outcomes*. Achievable outcomes require theory construction, hypothesis building and experimentation capable of producing new, different and better outcomes.

METHODS FOR CAUSALITY AND EVALUATION RESEARCH

Methods and techniques for establishing causal relationships and for conducting evaluation of clinical practices have advanced dramatically over the past decade (Rothman, 1986). Furthermore, cross-cultural instrument development allows for cross-national studies that previously were not capable of occurring (Flaherty *et al.*, 1988). Until recently, the collection of information on torture survivors has been descriptive; few clinical outcome studies exist (Mollica *et al.*, 1990); no cohort and cross-national studies and few case-controlled studies have been conducted (Petersen, 1989). Many methodological issues specific to conducting scientific research related to social problems such as torture, including the basic issues of internal and external validity, have been extensively addressed by authors such as Cook and Campbell (1979). They address methods for research in which extreme limitations exist to the testing and the deliberate manipulation (e.g. randomization) of patient groups, community populations and exposure/treatment effects (Hellman & Hellman, 1991). The need for reliable and valid scientific research is, of course, essential to the generation of improved medical and psychiatric care for the torture survivor and for the elaboration of prevention programs.

INTERPRETATION

As we all know, the results of many of the above scientific methods often lead to trivial and/or inane results. Unfortunately, a review of the literature reveals an almost complete lack of sophistication as to the proper methods for the interpretation of experimental results. As Popper indicated, the investigator must be cautious in easily drawing conclusions as to the relative validity of a theory based upon a single experiment. The entire range of experimental results that might 'falsify' a given theory and outcome must be considered. In spite of Popper's emphasis on deductive methods, our earlier discussion indicates how inductive methods can also be used to challenge norms. In the simplest terms, the entire spectrum of *quantitative* and *qualitative* approaches should be used to validate the accuracy of a theory. Central to the latter assessment is the central question of how close to a description of reality are our theoretical norms.

The use of norms for theory construction and the reduction of these norms to experimental measures leads to major problems in interpreting the meaning of research.

Abstraction vs. reality

The general methods of scientific investigation briefly described in this chapter reveal the important shifts that are necessary for transforming the concrete practices of everyday life into abstractions called norms, outcomes, effects and measures. This fixation of reality into abstractions that can be used within a system of experimental rules and procedures although creating a method of understanding the world can also be seriously divorced from reality. Norms and measures can only partially replicate the essential inter-connectedness of human society as well as the embeddedness of individuals within their own unique, cultural, political, social and family environments. In addition, individuals are in a continuous relationship with their *life history* from childhood to adulthood and death. Institutions and institutional practices also have an organically emerging developmental history which creates an institutional memory. As Dollard (1935) states:

> Some writers treat life history material as if it were a series of incoordinated, unrelated events without sequence or necessary relationship. If they wish to study the religious behavior of adolescents, for instance, they will simply drop a statistical bucket into the well of adolescent experience and draw it out;

they will view their bucket full of data as self-explanatory and not as part of an individual unified life.

Interpretation of scientific results, therefore, demands an analysis of these findings within the wider life of the community, and the life history of the individual and the corporate memory of the institution. Again, this cross-checking of scientific abstractions with reality extends Popper's ideas beyond his limited reliance upon experimentally derived data to information that is both inductive and intuitively based.

Contradiction with custom

What happens when results 'fly in the face of custom' and 'just do not make common sense?' For example, it has been said, 'all you need to do is just define your terms and proceed faithfully according to the definitions' (Will, 1988). Unfortunately, the scientific confidence in this remark is often not a fair picture of everyday reality. Furthermore, the voice of custom is not always audible, or clear or univocal (Will, 1988). History has demonstrated that many inarticulate and unheeded customs are arising that may eventually transform our entire social world.

Finally, the scientific premises that are employed to guide investigations can also be powerfully influenced by the results themselves. Scientific experiments must also be seen as transforming processes in which the process of generating conclusions changes the initial premises.

Atomization

The process of shifting from the norms of grand theories to testable hypotheses requires a reduction process that 'atomizes' the integrated web of human life and social behavior. Scientific premises are related to life and must come as close as possible to approximating the complex components which constitute human existence. Whether or not it is truly possible scientifically to validate individual aspects of human behavior such as 'habits', 'attitudes' and 'aggression' is debatable. On the other hand, due to our commitment to achievable outcomes, the question must be asked whether or not our abstract norms and reductive processes have resulted in silly caricatures of real life experiences as illustrated by the following limerick provided by Will (1988):

There once was a man who said, 'Damn'.
It is borne in upon me I am
An engine that moves
In predestinate grooves;
I'm not even a bus, I'm a tram.

CONCLUSION

Science should be able to help societies prevent torture as well as heal and rehabilitate those who have been already damaged by political oppression and violence. Pilz and Tauth suggest that the Italian novelist Italo Calvino in describing his character Mr Palomar summarizes in a literary 'nutshell' a simple model for conceptualizing scientific research:

> In the life of Mr Palomar, there was a time when he obeyed the following rule: first, to construct a model in his mind, as perfect, logical, geometrical as possible; second, to prove whether the model fits the cases of practical, observational experience, and third and last, to make the necessary corrections in order to bring model and reality in accordance (Calvino, 1986).

Yet, almost all clinicians and health providers caring for torture survivors will immediately acknowledge that something is wrong with Mr Palomar's picture of the world, i.e. he has not indicated a mechanism for changing reality. A science for this new field must not only serve a heuristic value in describing, understanding and explaining torture and its consequences, it must also provide effective strategies for eradicating torture. Yet, the general social and political neglect of scientific findings and their description of causal relationships and processes is well known. Clearly, the inherent weaknesses of scientific methods cannot be totally faulted for the ineffectiveness of medical and psychiatric research in achieving new outcomes for torture survivors. Innate human and societal resistances or 'auto-protective' functions (Blankenburg, unpublished observations) have consistently and successfully worked – and they have worked all too well – to keep the horrors of torture, war and political oppression from personal and public awareness. It is clear that all persons know that torture is a horrible and 'uncivilized' form of human behavior. Yet, these resistances allow societies to accommodate themselves to torture, rationalize and accept the torturer and his behavior, and silence the pain of the tortured. Scientific investigations are in fact crucial elements of an integrated triad of *advocacy, clinical care* and *applied research* necessary to eliminate torture and successfully treat its victims. The overall process is actually a very difficult one because it entails the process of 'making the obvious, obvious,' i.e. rendering torture visible and subjecting it to reflection and study (Blankenburg, unpublished observations). This process of clarifying the obvious unfairness of torture and its unjustified infliction of suffering on others, forces citizens and their communities to reject their passive acceptance of cruel and inhuman behavior, especially when it is officially sanctioned. What is also clear, if we are to achieve the latter, is our new field's urgent need for the infusion of concreteness, practicality and originality into all aspects of its clinical and scientific efforts. Only in this way, do we have any real hope of influencing the real world around us.

REFERENCES

Bebbington, P. (1980). Causal models and logical inference in epidemiological psychiatry. *British Journal of Psychiatry*, **136**, 317–25.

Bollini, P. & Mollica, R. F. (1989). Surviving without the asylum: an overview of the studies on the Italian reform movement. *Journal of Nervous and Mental Disease*, **177**, 607–15.

Buck, C. (1975). Popper's philosophy for epidemiologists. *International Journal of Epidemiology*, **4**, 159–68.

Calvino, I. (1986). *Paloman*. New York: Harcourt, Brace and Jovanovich.

Chalk, F. & Jonassohn, K. (1982). The history and sociology of genocide. J. N. Porter ed., *Genocide and Human Rights – Part I.* New Haven, CT: Yale University Press.

Chelsia, C. A. (1986). Grandmothers of the 'disappeared'. *The Christian Science Monitor*.

Cook, D. J. (1980). Causal modeling with contingency tables. *British Journal of Psychiatry*, **137**, 582–584.

Cook, T. D. & Campbell, D. T. (1979). *Quasi-Experimentation: Design and Analysis Issues for Field Settings.* Boston: Houghton Mifflin Co.

D'Arno, Q. (ed.). (1983). *A Bilingual Guide to Exhibition of Torture Instruments, from the Middle Ages to the Industrial Period.* Firenze: Coste delle Rampa.

Dollard, J. (1935). *Criteria for the Life History.* New Haven: Yale University Press.

Flaherty, J. A., Gaviria, F. M., Pathak, D., Mitchell, T., Wintrob, R., Richman, J. A. & Birz, S. (1988). Developing instruments for cross-cultural psychiatric research. *Journal of Nervous and Mental Disease*, **176(5)**, 257–63.

Foucault, M. (1973). *Madness and Civilization: Its History of Insanity in the Age of Reason.* Translated by R. Howard. New York: Vintage, Random House.

Harre, R. (1970). *The Principles of Scientific Thinking.* Chicago: University of Chicago Press.

Harre, R. (1980). The notion of causality. *British Journal of Psychiatry*, **137**, 578–85.

Hellman, S. & Hellman, D. S. (1991). Of mice but not men: Problems of the randomized clinical trial. *New England Journal of Medicine*, **324(22)**, 1585–9.

Joyce, C. & Stover, E. (1991). *Witnesses from the Grave: The Stories Bones Tell.* Boston: Little Brown.

Levin, D. M. (1987). *Pathologies of the Modern Self: Postmodern Studies on Narcissism, Schizophrenia, and Depression.* New York: New York Universities Press.

Mollica, R. F. (1983). From asylum to community: The threatened disintegration of public psychiatry. *New England Journal of Medicine,* **308,** 367–73.

Mollica, R. F. (ed.). (1985). The unfinished revolution in Italian psychiatry: An international perspective. *International Journal of Mental Health,* **14,** 1–212.

Mollica, R. F. (1987). Upside-down psychiatry: A genealogy of mental health services. In: D. M. Levin, ed., *Pathologies of the Modern Self: Postmodern Studies on Narcissism, Schizophrenia, and Depression.* New York: New York Universities Press.

Mollica, R. F. (1989). What is a Case? In: M. Abbott (ed.), *Refugee Resettlement and Wellbeing.* Auckland, New Zealand: Mental Health Foundation of New Zealand.

Mollica, R. F., Wyshak, G., Lavelle, J., Truong, T., Tor, S. & Yang, T. (1990). Assessing symptom change in Southeast Asian refugee survivors of mass violence and torture. *American Journal of Psychiatry,* **147,** 83–8.

Peters, E. (1985). *Torture.* Oxford: Basil Blackwell.

Petersen, H. D. (1989). The controlled study of torture victims: Epidemiologic considerations and some future aspects. *Scandinavian Journal of the Society of Medicine,* **17,** 13–20.

Pilz, L. & Tauth, P. (1988). Causality and validation of mathematical models. *Methods of Information in Medicine,* **27,** 153–4.

Popper, K. R. (1968). *The Logic of Scientific Discovery.* New York: Harper & Row Publishers.

Rothman, K. J. (1986). *Modern Epidemiology.* Boston: Little Brown.

Will, F. L. (1988). *Beyond Deduction: Ampliative Aspects of Philosophical Reflection.* Routledge, New York.

2
THE PHYSICAL SEQUELAE OF TORTURE
Grethe Skylv

By torturing the body, the torturer's aim is to destroy his victim's mind. The physical injuries, sometimes present for life, have the effect of continuing the torture long after the detention. Pain, scars, and deformities will be a continuous reminder of the torture.

Torture is always aimed at the victim's vulnerable points, both physical and psychological. If it is at all possible to attempt an overall description of the sequelae of torture, it is because these vulnerable points are on the whole the same in people of all societies. Differences in types of injury following torture are therefore small between different parts of the world. However, particular forms of torture may predominate in certain cultures if there is a tradition of using these forms as 'ordinary' punishment, for instance in the bringing up of children or in the punishment of criminals.

Whether a form of maltreatment is considered to be torture depends on the context. What we in Scandinavia define as torture may in other parts of the world be considered 'justified punishment' or a normal procedure in connection with any imprisonment. We cannot therefore always expect a person to give a spontaneous account of all the forms of maltreatment to which he has been exposed, even if they have caused physical sequelae of importance for his later performance. Thus, it is not always sufficient to base our physical examination on information from the victim about the torture he has been exposed to. Another problem in this connection is the suppression, in the victim's memory, of certain forms of torture.

Specialities such as traumatology, sports medicine, forensic medicine, and rheumatology provide the basis for charting the injuries which may be caused by physical torture. Treatment principles may also be borrowed from those specialities, though it is obvious that some adaptation is necessary to suit the conditions required for treating torture victims. These principles may be summarized as follows:

1 All examination and treatment situations should resemble the torture situation as little as possible.

2 All painful procedures should be avoided.
3 All experimental situations should be avoided.

Therapists in the countries of exile only see the late sequelae of torture. The early sequelae, however, have been fully described in the reports of Amnesty International and in a thesis by Rasmussen (1990).

The sequelae that we see are characterized by being mainly in the musculoskeletal system (Juhler, 1990, unpublished observations; Rasmussen, 1990). Careful medical examination rarely shows signs of organ involvement, despite numerous subjective complaints. This may be because injury to vital organs caused the early death of the victim, or because medical treatment was given shortly after the torture. It should also be remembered that escaping to a country of exile requires a surplus of physical and mental strength, difficult to mobilize for a person with a severe organ condition following torture (Juhler, 1990). It is therefore possible that torture victims in exile are those who have suffered the least. A possible explanation for the many symptoms will be discussed below.

THE SEQUELAE OF BLUNT VIOLENCE

Almost all torture victims will have experienced blows to most parts of the body (from fists or boots or special instruments) or falls from heights, etc. The structural and functional sequelae, and the associated signs and symptoms, are similar to those that follow traumas such as assaults, and traffic accidents. These include healed fractures with or without deformities, ostitis, periostitis, nerve and vessel injury, fibrosis in muscles, fasciae, and connective tissue, injury to tendons and ligaments, distorsions and scars. The treatment follows the same principle as for treatment of other traumas.

FALANGA

Violence to certain parts of the body causes specific injuries, depending on the type of the tissues and their function. A typical example is falanga.

Falanga, or bastinado, is the beating of the soles of the feet with cables, iron rods, sticks or other instruments of wood or metal. The victim is usually fixed with his feet raised.

Falanga can be given to the naked soles, or with shoes or boots on, or the victim may be forced to put on his shoes as soon as the torture is over.

After the torture, he may be forced to walk on, for example pebbles, broken glass or on a wet floor. He may be forced to jump on the same spot carrying a heavy burden, such as the torturer. All these variations greatly increase the pain, and influence the extent and degree of the sequelae.

The late falanga symptoms include pain in the legs and feet, mainly deep in the tibial region and near the joints. It is described as jabbing, cutting or burning. It may be constant, but is usually intermittent. It increases during the day, does not necessarily diminish during rest, but may even increase during the night because of the warmth of the bed. The victim may experience short-lived relief when he gets up and walks on the cold floor. There is often a direct relationship between the pain and walking and running, especially up and down stairs, but also from standing for a long time. The rate of walking is slow and the distance limited. Now and then the victim has to stop and sit down before continuing. He cannot sit with crossed legs or squat. The pain is worse in cold, damp, windy weather.

The pain may be accompanied by tingling and pins and needles in the calves and even in the feet. There may be sensations of tiredness and heaviness in the thighs and legs, and of looseness in the knees and ankles, as if they are falling apart. The victim has often noticed that his gait has changed, he cannot move his feet freely, cannot roll over on them properly, he puts extra pressure on the lateral edges of the feet, etc.

Cramp is rare in the calves and feet, but it can be provoked by exertion and resemble the closed compartment syndrome (see below). There is often an increased tendency to lower back pain when standing or, more particularly, walking, but there are no typical radiating pains. There is no, or only limited, tendency to swelling of ankles or feet.

On inspection, the balls of the heels and the medial and lateral balls of the forefeet may be 'smashed', a sign of severe oedema immediately after the torture, in which the vertical connective tissue trabeculae from the skin to the bones, between the fat pockets, have been torn. In this way, the balls of the feet have lost their springiness and thus their function as buffers when the feet hit the ground in walking. As a result, this pressure will be transmitted unimpeded through the long bones and the joints to the spine, causing an increased tendency to lower back pain when walking.

'Smashed' heels can be diagnosed in two ways: 1) With the patient standing on a hard stool or low table, or with the examiner kneeling behind him, the heel is inspected directly from behind. A normal heel will have a rounded contour, but a 'smashed' heel is broad, flat, and compressed. 2) On palpation, with no weight on the heel, the normal elasticity has gone. With finger pressure on the heel at right angles to the lower side of the tuber calcanei, the prominence can easily be felt through the skin, and the elastic resistance from the fat pockets of the heel balls is completely or partly lacking. This condition is similar to one seen in long distance runners (Jørgensen, 1985), in whom only the balls of the *heels* are injured. Injury of the balls of the *forefeet* should be considered pathognomonic for falanga. However, I must stress that absence of injury of the balls of the feet does not necessarily exclude falanga. The degree of injury seems to depend on the extent of the post-traumatic oedema, which the torturers can control (as part of the torture) by putting boots on the victim immediately after the torture, or by cooling down the feet, for example.

The skin of the soles often shows hard, rough scars. These lead to a pathological gait, adopted to give relief. Dysaesthesiae are common and correspond to parts of the soles or the whole foot, without segmentary pattern. The symptoms may resemble reflex sympathetic dystrophy (RSD). There is often an increased tendency to sweating of the feet and to alternating hot and cold feet, but other signs of RSD are missing, i.e. reduced hair growth, nail growth disturbances, pointed toes, etc. We have not yet had the opportunity to perform thermography of the legs of falanga victims, but would expect pathological changes, either in a hot or a cold direction, depending on the degree of injury (Hobbins, 1984).

The arterial pulsation is normal in the feet, and there is no increased tendency to varicose veins.

On palpation, the whole length of the plantar aponeurosis is tender, not only at its posterior attachment, and it feels rough, as in a tendinitis caused by over-exercise. The distal attachments of the aponeurosis have often been torn, partly at the base of the proximal falanges, partly at the skin, and consequently the aponeurosis cannot be tightened as in normal walking. Its function as support of the longitudinal arch has thus disappeared. Walking is difficult and muscle fatigue follows, particularly of flexor digitorum accessorium (quadratus plantae) and peroneus longus. Passive extension of the big toe will reveal whether the aponeurosis has been torn. If it is intact, one should feel the start of tension in the aponeurosis on palpation when the toe is bent backwards 20 degrees; the maximum normal extension is 70 degrees. Higher values suggest injury of the attachments of the aponeurosis (Boisen-Møller & Flagstad, 1976).

At the dissection of the feet of six torture victims, and through experimental injections, Bro-Rasmussen and Rasmussen showed that the muscle compartments of the soles become tight and inelastic

following falanga, increasing the risk of developing closed compartment syndrome (Bro-Rasmussen & Rasmussen, 1978). A case of aseptic
necrosis of the bone of a toe has been described, probably following a
falanga-provoked closed compartment syndrome (Bro-Rasmussen
et al., 1982).

Passive movements of the small joints of the feet usually show
abnormal joint play, stiffness and decreased movements in many of
them. However, treatment often reveals underlying hypermobility of
several joints, resulting from injury to ligaments and capsules during
torture.

During falanga, as in a hard landing on the heels, the talus is forced
up against the tibia. This trauma and the accompanying oedema result
in overstretching of the stabilizing ligaments round the ankle, so that
the normal buffer and stabilizing function of the connection between
the tibia and fibula is compromised. In a falanga victim, the normal
tightening of the interosseous membrane does not occur when the foot
is placed on the ground in walking, and the tibialis posterior is not
activated; this muscle is the only one that supports this tightening
because it is attached to both the tibia and the fibula, and to the
membrane between them. Clinical examination reveals tenderness of
both the superior and the inferior tibio-fibular joints, and there is
indirect tenderness of these joints when pressure is put on the tuber
calcanei from below. There is a varying imbalance of the leg musculature, dependent on which compensatory way of walking the victim
has adopted, but a prominent feature is increased tension and active
trigger points of the tibialis anterior, biceps femoris, and the ilio-tibial
tract (Travell & Simons, 1983), as well as inactivity (but not paresis) of
the tibialis posterior and popliteus. The fasciae surrounding all the
muscle bundles feel tight at palpation. This muscular dysbalance can
result in musculo-tendinous inflammatory conditions in keeping with
'the medial tibial stress-syndrome' (Sub-Committee Classification of
Sports Injuries Committee, 1966), but with various localizations
depending on which muscles are overstrained during the compensatory way of walking (Slocum, 1967; Michael & Lawrence, 1985;
Mubarak *et al.*, 1982).

Sequelae of fractures of the bones of the feet have been described
following falanga torture (Rasmussen *et al.*, 1977; Meier & Andersen,
1985), but we see them rarely, probably because the structure of the feet
makes it possible to absorb the force to which the feet are exposed at
falanga. In the few cases of fracture sequelae we have seen, the victim
has been exposed to other forms of torture to the feet as well, for
instance, crushing the foot against the ground with the heel of a boot.

Since muscles, joints, ligaments, and skin are affected in the sequelae of falanga, exteroceptors and proprioceptors are disturbed, with consequent impairment of balance and space orientation (Carpenter, 1990; Stein, 1982). I shall return to this later.

It is satisfying to treat the sequelae of falanga torture. Most of the survivors can become symptom-free or can improve considerably with traditional physiotherapy, supplemented with supportive footware, elastic bandages, sports-tape, etc.

SUSPENSION

Suspension is a common form of torture, either alone or combined with other forms, such as beating or electrical torture. The victim is usually suspended by his arms stretched above his head or by the arms tied behind his back, but also by the hands tied together (one pointing forwards, the other backwards), by one arm and one leg, by both legs, by the arms tied together around the bent knees so that a stick can be introduced between the hollow of the knees and the elbows (*la barra* = the chicken = the wheel of Buddha), or by the hair. An unpublished account of late sequelae in the musculoskeletal system following torture (Skylv, 1990, unpublished observations) showed a close relationship between joint pain and previous suspension, but there was no relationship between back pain and suspension, as was indicated by Rasmussen (1990). Furthermore, the symptoms are compatible with a mild degree of RSD: burning and cutting pains diffusely in one or more extremities without segmental distribution, a sensation of tiredness and heaviness, hyperalgesia and hyperaesthesia, especially distally in the extremities, sometimes also vasomotor and sudomotor changes (Bonica, 1990).

The torture survivor often indicates that there was a symptom-free period, lasting months or years, between the torture and the occurrence of the symptoms. In connection with RSD, it is common for the patient gradually to develop psychological and emotional disturbances, which remit when the RSD is treated. Whether the torture victim's mental condition is further aggravated by the presence of RSD is not clear, but such a connection should be considered and result in simultaneous physio- and psychotherapy for all victims who may have RSD.

The clinical examination only reveals modest changes that can be ascribed to the suspension without doubt. It is rarely possible to demonstrate hypermobility in the exposed joints, except perhaps in the acromio-clavicular and sterno-clavicular joints after suspension by the arms tied behind the back. Furthermore, suspension by the tied wrists, so that one hand points forward and the other backward (Palestinian suspension), results in straining the upper and middle costo-vertebral and costo-transverse joints, causing pain and dysfunction, sometimes in the form of hypermobility. The torture survivor often interprets this pain as cardiac, but it disappears with physiotherapy. Tendinitis near the joints is common, particularly near the shoulders, but we have only once seen a tendency to luxation of a shoulder after suspension by the arms tied behind the back. However, the victims often perceive their joints as being loose, probably because of 'wrong' information from the afferent mechanoreceptors of the joint capsules and ligaments. Proprioceptive stimulation, combined with specific stabilization of the joint, reduces or removes this perception, so that bandaging can be avoided.

Only once have we seen a partial lesion of the brachial plexus with corresponding objective neurological signs following suspension by the arms. In contrast, subjective symptoms are common in the form of pain or paraesthesiae corresponding to the course of specific nerves, with aggravation following provocation tests in accordance with Adverse Mechanical Tension (Brieg, 1978; Butler, 1989). We have a theory that the symptoms may be caused by fibrosis following bleeding in the connective tissue surrounding the relevant nerve during the violent suspension stretching. This connective tissue compromises the ability of the nerve structure to adapt freely to the pulls and pressures of normal movements of the body. In such cases, physiotherapy directed to the changes in the connective tissue has a good effect.

Following suspension, active trigger points are often found in the musculature of the shoulder, giving characteristic patterns of referred pain, which to some extent can simulate radicular pain and paraesthesiae (Travell & Simons, 1983; Sola, 1984). These symptoms respond well to physiotherapy directed to muscles and trigger points.

Suspension by long hair can cause complete or partial loosening of the galea, a sort of scalping from within. The galea is usually moderately displaceable in relation to the periosteum, from which it is separated by a loose layer of connective tissue. In connection with this supension, bleeding can occur in the torn bundles of connective tissue and consequently cause fibrosis which will tie the galea to the periosteum in places. Both conditions cause pain and dysaesthesiae on touching the hair or scalp. Physiotherapy to the galea can make it regain its normal ability to be displaced in relation to the periosteum.

SEQUELAE FROM STRAPPING

As a form of torture in itself, or as part of another form, the victim is fixed with rope, straps, handcuffs, etc, round his body, neck or extremities. Tight strapping may leave pressure injuries in the underlying tissue. The sequelae may be regular nerve injury with loss of sensory and motor function (Rasmussen, 1990), but it is usually a question of subjective complaints of pain and paraesthesiae in the whole area peripheral to the strapping, without corresponding objective neurological impairment. Clinical examination shows that the structures under the skin in the affected area (muscles, tendons, fasciae, vessels, and nerve sheaths) do not slide freely in relation to each other, but are soldered together by irregular bundles of connective tissue. These can be treated by massage to re-establish the normal sliding of the tissues and thus reduce the subjective symptoms.

THE SEQUELAE OF ELECTRICAL TORTURE

Electrical torture can be performed with electrodes placed at different, usually very sensitive, areas of the body, with a mobile electrode, such as a shock baton, and a fixed electrode, such as an iron bed.

Characteristic skin changes following electrical torture have often been described (Danielsen & Berger, 1981; Danielsen, 1982; Thomsen, 1984; Karlsmark, 1990). There are no studies of possible changes in other tissues, but myoglobin is liberated in blood and urine after electrical accidents as a sign of damage to the muscle fibres. It is known from the descriptions of the victims that electrical torture results in violent muscular contractions which may well give lesions of the muscle fibres, especially when the victim is suspended. On palpation, muscle consistency is changed in large areas because of firm, fibrous connective tissue bundles, resulting from previous muscular lesion. The changes are the same as those seen after direct blunt traumas and blows, and the principles of the physiotherapy treatment are the same – muscle and fascia techniques followed by training.

FOREIGN BODIES (BROKEN GLASS, BULLETS, ETC.)

Various forms of torture may leave foreign bodies encapsulated in the connective tissue of the victim. These are usually bullets, but the victim may also have been forced to walk on broken glass or sharp gravel. If these foreign bodies gave discomfort, they will usually have been removed before the victim reaches his country of exile, but sometimes there are indications of removal of foreign bodies which do not cause any trouble. The awareness of their presence may be a great mental strain, giving a constant reminder of the torture.

SCARS

Many forms of torture, such as cuts, burns, corrosions with acid, can leave skin scars. The reasons for removing them are mainly psychological, since they are constant reminders of the torture, but if they are near joints, they may impair function so much that treatment is required. This is usually physiotherapy with massage and stretching of the scar tissue, sometimes supplemented with ultrasound. In this way, the connective tissue can be reorganized so that surgery is seldom necessary. The treatment can also have a psychological effect, since it will change the attitude to the scar during the intensive work on it.

TORTURE OF THE TEETH – TEMPORO-MANDIBULAR JOINT PROBLEMS

Torture of the teeth is common in the form of drilling or extraction of teeth, electrical torture, or blows to the face resulting in broken teeth or a broken jaw (Clavel, 1973; Rasmussen, 1990). Furthermore, insufficient food and poor dental hygiene during the detention, which increase the occurrence of gingivitis and caries, could be regarded as a form of torture of the teeth. Dental examination and treatment are therefore a natural part of the programme for an exiled torture survivor. Furthermore, all our clients at the RCT in Copenhagen are examined, and most are treated, for pain in, and dysfunction of, the temporo-mandibular joints, tension and active trigger points in the chewing muscles, bruxism, tongue pressure, mal-occlusion, and so on (Travell & Simons, 1983; Walther, 1983). Apart from a reconstruction of the teeth, many are treated with a pressure-relieving occlusal splint which may improve sleep. The most important treatment efforts, however, rest with the physiotherapist, who restores the normal balance of the musculature of the face and the chewing mechanism by treatment of the soft tissues, and by correcting the carriage of the head (and thus the whole body) and by various exercises. In this way, attention is paid to the great importance of the chewing apparatus for proprioception, and thus to the victim's sense of posture and space orientation, to which I shall return later.

SEQUELAE FROM FORCED POSITIONS

Several different forms of torture are directed towards the back, which can be strained in many ways. The victim may be exposed to kicks, blows, and punches to the whole back or to special parts of the spine, possibly while fixed or suspended. He may be forced to carry heavy weights or to stay for a long time in abnormal, incorrect positions. He may have been kept in a cell so small that he has not been able to stretch his body completely, neither standing nor lying down, or he may have been fixed standing, sitting, or lying, without being able to change position. These forced positions almost always result in the spine being bent forwards.

One might expect such abnormal strained positions, often with additional blows to the kyphosed back, to provoke prolapse of the discs, but it happens rarely. Instead, this maltreatment causes over-stretching of the stabilizing ligaments and joint capsules of the spine, giving segmentary instability and other segmentary dysfunctions. These lead not only to back pain, but, in accordance with our onto-genic development, may also give a sensation of pain corresponding to the dermatome, myotome, or sclerotome of the strained segment(s), as well as affecting the vessels and viscera belonging to the correspond-ing segment (Dvorak & Dvorak, 1984; Carpenter, 1990). The visceral symptoms, caused by the irritation of afferent sympathetic nerves going from the truncus sympathicus via the dorsal root-ganglion to the dorsal root, may simulate cardiac disease, gastrointestinal, genital or other conditions, depending on which spinal segment the dysfunction is localized to.

These symptoms are often interpreted wrongly by the torture survi-vor – and by many therapists – as injury to specific organs, and in this way they can lead to extensive medical and surgical examination pro-cedures. When these reveal normal function of the organ(s) in question, the survivor feels a discrepancy between his subjective perception of the symptoms and the interpretation of the therapists. He is easily labelled neurotic, the organic complaints being considered a part of the mental state following torture. The explanation to the survivor may be phrased as follows: 'The torturers have made you believe that they have destroyed the function of this or that organ inside you. Our exam-inations have shown that this is not true, and from now on you may ignore your subjective symptoms. They are just part of the psychologi-cal torture imposed by the torturers.' The survivor, who may continue to have the same perception of his symptoms, will rarely have the strength to consider himself as incorrectly diagnosed and therefore he will accept this explanation – but he will probably not be able to suppress his very real somatic symptoms. If he is not lucky enough to find a therapist with a good understanding of this complex of symptoms, this prolonged part of his torture will continue.

However, physiotherapy of the causal dysfunction in the spine, consisting of stabilization of the hypermobile segments and mobilization of the hypomobile segments, will normalize the condition and remove the 'inexplicable' organ symptoms.

SEQUELAE IN THE MUSCULOSKELETAL SYSTEM AFTER STRESS

It is not only the specific physical forms of torture that give somatic symptoms and signs from the musculoskeletal system. The situation of pain and stress, in which a torture survivor constantly finds himself as a consequence of the torture as a whole, results in several changes of the musculoskeletal system, also known in patients with chronic pain, and well described in the literature (Merskey Pain, 1986; Wall & Melzack, 1984).

On examination of the posture we find the classical depressed pattern with drooping head, increased cervical lordosis, raised shoulders, increased thoracic kyphosis and lumbar lordosis, changed pelvic inclination and a dysharmonic musculature, as described by Janda, with shortened, tight, painful postural muscles in the shoulder girdle, the pectorals, the thoraco-lumbar back-stretchers, the flexors of the hips, the muscles of the hollows of the knee and the calves, combined with flat, hypoactive phasic muscles between the scapulae, the abdominal muscles, the gluteal muscles and the knee extensors (Janda, 1983).

This anomaly of posture, combined with the unharmonic muscular pattern, increases the physiologically conditioned tendency of certain sections of the spine to be the site of hypo- and hypermobility: hypomobility corresponding to C1–C2, C4–T3, T6–T10, and L1–L4; hypermobility corresponding to C3–C4, T4–T5, T11–T12, and L5–sacrum (Grieve, 1981, 1986).

These changes are registered by specific examination of the passive movements of individual segments, and this method will also reveal the above-mentioned hyper/hypomobile areas caused by direct blows or strain to the back (Geden, 1985). All these data are considered in a physiotherapeutic treatment programme in which the posture is corrected, the harmony of the musculature restored, and the segments of the spine regain their normal stability and pattern of movements.

There is not room here for a description of all the symptom complexes that can be provoked by dysharmony of the function of the spine – symptoms that can be mistaken for those caused by specific forms of torture. I shall only mention a single example and otherwise refer to the abundant literature of physical medicine on this subject: A common late sequela of torture is vertigo. It can be caused by the repeated head injuries to which the survivor is usually exposed, and it is therefore justified to make a careful neurological and audio-vestibular examination. However, it is worth remembering the relationship between dysfunction of the cervical spine on one side, and headache and vertigo on the other, probably due to the cervical nucleus of the trigeminal nerve (Bogduk, 1986). The re-establishment of normal function of the cervical spine can remove the parts of the headache and the vertigo that originate in the cervical spine.

MUSCULAR TENSIONS AND THE MUSCULAR TENSION INDEX

The torture survivor's chronic pain and stress situation influences the overall tension of the musculature. With respect to the nomenclature, there has been considerable confusion during the past years concerning muscular tension in patients with chronic pain: fibrositis, fibromyalgia, myofascial pain, for example (Smythe, 1986; Simons & Simons, 1988). This must be seen as a result of disagreement on the aetiology and on the explanation models. We do not take part in this discussion, but at the clinical examination we register the tension of the voluntary musculature – not the tenderness, because as a principle we do not want to provoke pain during examinations. The tension of the back muscles is registered in eight regions, on the front of the body in four regions, and on the head in eight regions. The muscular tension in each region is evaluated arbitrarily and given scores ranging from 0 to 3. The muscular tension index (MTI) is thus the sum of the scores on the back (maximum 24), the front (maximum 12), and the head (maximum 24).

If we allow ourselves to consider the muscular tension as an expression of the torture victim's immediate stress situation, we can evaluate the effect of the combined physiotherapy and psychotherapy by measuring the MTI at the start and end of therapy. In this way, we have found out that most torture survivors have a very high MTI at the start of therapy, but that it falls to a level corresponding to that of healthy working adults by the end of treatment (Skylv et al., 1990).

By palpation we sometimes find a single muscle or a section of muscles with very low tone, with a consistency like dough. The sensitivity of the skin in the same area may be diminished or absent to an extent which does not correspond with neuro-anatomical conditions. It usually transpires that the victim has been exposed to a particularly painful or humiliating torture at this very area. In these cases, it is important to obtain quick treatment results by closely combining physio- and psychotherapy.

THE SEQUELAE OF SEXUAL TORTURE

All forms of torture include an overtone of sexual humiliation, but physical sexual torture comprises direct maltreatment of the genitals and the anal region in the form of homo- or heterosexual rape, electrical torture, or maltreatment with various tools.

Sexual torture may also leave traces in the musculoskeletal system, as both structural injury and functional disturbances.

Victims who have been exposed to sexual torture rarely tell about it spontaneously because of fear of losing the respect of the family (Lunde, 1981; Agger, 1986). They often have uncharacteristic low lumbar pain, sometimes radiating to the pelvis or gluteal region. Many have difficulty in standing or sitting for long periods. They complain of pain in both the external and the internal genitalia, of menstrual disturbances, urination and defaecation problems, and sexual problems.

Apart from visible injury of the genitalia and scars from lesions around the anus and the vagina (which will not be described here), there are sequelae in the form of dysfunction of the pelvic joints: sacro-iliac, sacro-coccygeal, and the pubic symphysis.

The dysfunctions of the sacro-iliac joint and symphysis are revealed during posture examinations, when the extent and direction of movements of the joints are registered at special function tests (Grieve, 1976).

At the same time, pronounced dysharmony of the musculature of the pelvis is seen, corresponding to the above pattern: shortening and tightness of the psoas major, the thoracolumbar back-stretchers, piriformis and hamstrings, combined with weak abdominal and gluteal muscles. The torture victim will completely lack the ability to move the pelvis actively in relation to the lumbar spine, since it requires a combined work by the pelvic muscles, a combination that has been suppressed.

The importance of restoring normal function to the pelvic joints should be seen not only in connection with the functions relevant to posture and to sexuality, but also to a high degree in the light of their functions as buffers while walking. The pelvis is part of the series of buffers between the feet and the brain that also includes the balls of the heels, the arches of the feet, the knee joints, and the intervertebral discs. These structures dampen the forces that are released when the body collides with the ground, so that the brain is protected. If the torture victim has been exposed to falanga and has dysfunction of the joints of the pelvis as well, it is extremely important to re-establish the spring-function of the pelvis.

Dysfunction of the sacro-coccygeal joint can be difficult to diagnose, because a rectal examination is required, and this procedure will in most cases be too strong a reminder of the torture itself. At RCT, this examination is therefore only performed under anaesthesia in connection with other interventions (and naturally only with the permission of the patient). At this examination, which takes place as a bimanual palpation with the patient lying prone or on his side, the position of the coccyx is noted and passive movements are tested. If there is displacement or the mobility is decreased, which is a common cause of difficulty when sitting down, the bone is carefully mobilized by bimanual traction until free mobility has been achieved. At the same intervention the sacro-tuberous ligaments are palpated, and shortening of any of the ligaments is corrected by stretching. Such a shortening may have occurred from a wrong position of the sacro-iliac joint which will consequently be locked in a forwardly rotated position.

The physiotherapist also works with the survivor's changed picture of himself that has been caused by the sexual torture – and torture in general. Through exercises, he learns to be able to like his own body, to use it actively, and to like to be touched.

INCREASED SYMPATHETIC ACTIVITY AND SYMPATHETIC REFLEX DYSTROPHY

When there is pain from changes in the neurological, myofascial, circulatory, or skeletal system, the skin temperature changes as a sign of autonomic nervous system involvement. This can be demonstrated by using thermography (Hobbins, 1984). The pattern of the thermographic changes supplements the clinical signs and can help in the differential diagnosis of complicated or uncharacteristic symptoms such as headache of mixed origin, the thoracic outlet syndrome or lumbo-sacral neuralgia (Le Roy & Filasky, 1991). Torture victims, in particular, present many symptoms and signs from the musculoskeletal system. These may be difficult to characterize because the tissues have been exposed to several different forms of torture directed at the same parts of the body, leaving many correspondingly different injuries. It has not been possible for us to include thermography in our diagnostic procedures, but with experience from pain clinics the world over it can strongly be recommended whenever possible.

Thermography also has a place during treatment to follow possible improvements and thus encourage both the patient and the therapists. It should also be possible to restrict treatment to the injuries with the best prognosis, i.e. the patho-physiological processes that give 'warm' thermograms. Wasteful treatment efforts can be avoided in injuries that give 'cold' thermograms, which are known to have a poor prognosis (Goodman et al., 1985).

SPACE ORIENTATION AND SENSORY–MOTOR TRAINING

Our orientation in space and continuous adjustment of posture for equilibrium depend on afferent impulses. not only from the eyes and the vestibulary apparatus of the inner ear, but also from proprioceptors in muscles, tendons, joints, and skin. These impulses are transmitted to the cerebellum.

Particularly important impulses come from the muscles of the neck, the joints between the ribs and the spine, and the weight-carrying parts of the soles. Wrong information from the proprioceptors of the body because of tissue injury, shortened muscles, changed carriage, etc, is coded into the central nervous system, which in this way 'accepts' the new posture and the new pattern of movements.

In connection with the physiotherapeutic correction of the many dysfunctions after torture, it is extremely important to change the 'code' of the central nervous system so that after treatment the afferent information will again release normal efferent impulses. This is done most purposefully by using exercises for tactile, proprioceptive, vestibulary, and kinaesthetic stimulation, such as are also used in sensory integration therapy.

CONCLUSION

It is the very nature of torture that makes it so difficult to classify the sequelae: the various forms of torture are followed by both structural injury and disturbed function, each type of torture giving many different sequelae in different tissues. More than one form of torture has usually been applied, causing overlapping injuries. It is therefore impossible, even with the most careful history taking and physical examination, to define the symptoms and signs that have been caused by a particular form of torture in an individual victim. Though unpleasant to live with, a thorough understanding of the principles of the various forms is necessary to categorize the symptoms and signs. This enables us to plan the treatment, but above all to give the survivor, little by little, some understanding of the connection between his pains and the vulnerable points towards which the torturers directed their torture. This understanding is the first and most important step in physiotherapy.

REFERENCES

Agger, I. (1986). Seksuel tortur af kvindelige, ideologiske fanger. *Nordisk seksologi*, **4**, 147–61.

Bogduk, N. (1986). Cervical causes of headache and dizziness. In G. P. Grieve, ed. *Modern Manual Therapy of the Vertebral Column*, pp. 289–302, London: Churchill & Livingstone.

Boisen-Møller, F. & Flagstad, K. E. (1976). *Journal of Anatomy*, **121**, 599–611.

Bonica, J. J., ed. (1990). *The Management of Pain*, 2nd edn, pp. 220–41, Philadelphia: Lea and Fibiger.

Brieg, A., ed. (1978). *Adverse Mechanical Tension in the Central Nervous System*, pp. 1–182, Stockholm: Almqvist & Wiksell.

Bro-Rasmussen, F., Henriksen, O. B., Rasmussen, O. V. & Sakellariades, P. D. (1982). Aseptic necrosis of bone following phalanga torture. *Ugeskrift for Laeger*, **144**, 1165–6.

Bro-Rasmussen, F. & Rasmussen, O. V. (1978). Are the sequelae of falanga torture due to the closed compartment syndrome in the feet and is this a common clinical picture? *Ugeskrift for Laeger*, **140**, 3197–202.

Butler, D. S. (1989). The concept of adverse mechanical tension in the nervous system. *Physiotherapy*, **75(11)**, 622–9.

Carpenter, R. H. S., ed. (1990). *Neurophysiology*, 2nd edn, pp. 87–123 and 189–90, London: Edward Arnold.

Clavel, J-P. (1973). Doctors who torture. *World Medicine*, **14**, 15–31.

Danielsen, L. (1982). Torture sequelae in the skin. *Månedsskrift for praktisk Laegegerning*, **111**, 193–209.

Danielsen, L. & Berger, P. (1981). Torture located to the skin. *Acta Dermatologica*, **61**, 43–6.

Dvorak, J. & Dvorak, V. eds. (1984). *Manual Medicine, Diagnostics*, pp. 27–46, Stuttgart: Thieme.

Geden, L. G. (1985). A biomechanic rationale for osteopathic-type manipulative technique in the restoration of normal physiological function in the lumbar and cervical spine. In R. M. Idczak, E. F. Glasgow, L. T. Twomey, E. R. Scull and A. M. Kleynhans, eds. *Aspects of Manipulative Therapy*, pp. 48–51, Melbourne: Churchill Livingstone.

Goodman, P. *et al.* (1985). Stress fracture diagnosis by computer assisted thermography. *Physical Sportsmedicine*, 13, 114.

Grieve, G. P., ed. (1986). *Modern Manual Therapy of the Vertebral Column*, pp. 3–898, London: Churchill & Livingstone.

Grieve, G. P., ed. (1981). *Common Vertebral Joint Problems*, pp. 1–576, London: Churchill & Livingstone.

Grieve, G. P. (1976). The sacroiliac joint. *Physiotherapy*, 62, 384–401.

Hobbins, W. M. (1984). Differential diagnosis of pain using thermography. In E. F. Ring & B. Phillips, eds. *Recent Advances in Medical Thermology*, pp. 503–6, New York: Plenum Press.

Janda, V. (1983). On the concept of postural muscles and posture. *Australian Journal of Physiotherapy*, 29, 83.

Jørgensen, U. (1985). *American Journal of Sports Medicine*, 13(2), 128–32.

Karlsmark, T. (1990). Electrically induced dermal changes. (Thesis). Copenhagen: The Danish Medical Association.

Le Roy, P. L. & Filasky, R. (1991). Thermography. In J. J. Bonica, ed. *The Management of Pain*, pp. 610–21, Philadelphia: Lea & Fibiger.

Lunde, I. (1981). *Les Agressions Sexuelles et la Torture*. Lille: 20. Cong. Francais de Criminologie.

Meier, J. & Andersen, J. G. (1985). Sclerosing of calcaneus following phalanga torture. *Ugeskrift for Laeger*, 147, 4206–7.

Merskey Pain, H., ed. (1986). *International Association for the Study of Pain: Classification of Chronic Pain Syndromes and Definition of Pain States*. Suppl. 3, 51.

Michael, R. H. & Lawrence, E. H. (1985). The soleus syndrome. *American Journal of Sports Medicine*, 13, 87–94.

Mubarak, S. J., Gould, R. N., Lee, Y. F., Schmidt, D. A. & Hargens, A. R. (1982). The medial tibial stress syndrome. *American Journal of Sports Medicine*, 10(4), 201–5.

Rasmussen, O. V. (1990). Medical Aspects of Torture. (Thesis). Copenhagen: The Danish Medical Association.

Rasmussen, O. V., Dam, A. M. & Nielsen, I. L. (1977). Tortur. *Ugeskrift for Laeger*, 139, 1049.

Simons, D. G. & Simons, L. (1988). Chronic myofascial pain syndrome. In C. D. Tollison, ed. *Handbook of chronic pain management*, pp. 509–29, Baltimore: Williams & Wilkins.

Skylv, G., Bloch, I. & Høhne, L. (1990). Muscle tension and articular dysfunction in torture victims. *Journal of Manual Medicine*, 5, 158–61.

Slocum, D. B. (1967). The shin splint syndrome. *American Journal of Surgery*, 114, 875–81.

Smythe, H. (1986). Tender points: evolution of concepts of the fibrositis/fibromyalgia syndrome. *American Journal of Medicine*, 81(3A), 2–6.

Sola, E. (1984). Treatment of myofascial pain syndromes. In E. Benedetti *et al.*, eds. *Recent Advances in Pain Research and Therapy*, vol. 7, pp. 467–85, NY: Raven Press.

Stein, J. F. ed. (1982). *An introduction to neurophysiology*, pp. 171–6, Blackwell.

(1966). *Sub-Committee Classification of Sports Injuries Committee on the Medical Aspects of Sports. Standard nomenclature of athletic injuries.*. Chicago: American Medical Association.

Thomsen, H. K. (1984). Electrically induced epidermal changes. (Thesis). Copenhagen: The Danish Medical Association.

Travell, J. G. & Simons, D. G. eds. (1983). *Myofascial Pain and Dysfunction*, pp. 24–37, 46–50, 59–63 and 219–272, Baltimore: Williams & Wilkins.

Wall, P. Q. & Melzack, R., eds. (1984). *Textbook of Pain*, pp. 1–866, London: Churchill & Livingstone.

Walther, D. S., ed. (1983). *Applied Kinesiology*, vol. 2, pp. 401–38, Colorado: SDC.

3
PSYCHO-SOCIAL CONSEQUENCES OF TORTURE: CURRENT KNOWLEDGE AND EVIDENCE

Finn Somnier, Peter Vesti, Marianne Kastrup, Inge Kemp Genefke

INTRODUCTION

During the first part of the twentieth century the long-lasting psychological effects of trauma were conceptualized mainly within a genetic or psychoanalytic framework. Consequently, individuals with long-term sequelae of trauma were considered as suffering from an inborn weakness of the central nervous system or from psychological injury during particularly vulnerable periods of early childhood. An exception to this is the neuroses observed during World War I.

After World War II many concentration camp survivors suffered from long-term sequelae due to organized violence during the Holocaust (Eitinger, 1980). Psychological consequences of long-term warfare stress were also observed in other survivors, such as war sailors (Askevold, 1980; Sørensen, Hansen & Worm-Petersen, 1983). The demonstration of such sequelae in previously well-adapted adults seriously challenged the dogma of classical German psychiatry alleging that life experiences can never by themselves cause lasting mental symptoms. Trautman (1964) proposed that prolonged existential stress, fear and anxiety might result in long-term psychological consequences. Evidence in favour of this view has gradually accumulated from studies of other groups exposed to prolonged traumatic stress, such as acts of war, rape, and hostage taking (Eitinger & Strøm, 1973; Kieler, 1980). The consequences of natural disasters such as earthquakes and volcanic eruptions have also been studied (Figley, 1985).

Initially, attempts were made to identify key features of the effects of various types of trauma which were subsumed under headings such as battered child syndrome, torture syndrome, and so on. However, with the introduction of the *Diagnostical and Statistical Manual of Mental Disorders* (DSM–III) published by the American Psychiatric Association (APA) in 1980, a generic theory unifying the single stress approaches was proposed. According to this theory different types of trauma may provoke similar symptomatology. A weakness of this theory is the fact that essential symptoms may be overlooked in a process of ascertaining the criteria for the diagnosis of posttraumatic stress disorder (PTSD, code 309.89), since the interviewee's answers may be biased by the semi-structured questions posed. Furthermore, torture is a unique form of trauma in being a deliberate attack aimed at destroying the individual's identity. Thus, we will adopt a single stress approach in discussing various issues in this chapter.

DEFINITION OF TORTURE

There is, as yet, no comprehensive definition of torture, an issue dealt with by Mollica and Caspi-Yavin in this volume. For the purposes of this chapter, we will use the definitions stated in the Tokyo Declaration of the World Medical Association and in United Nations declarations. We see torture as a dynamic process beginning with arrest, involving a sequence of traumatic events that may take place at different times and places, and ending with the release or demise of the victim.

CLASSIFICATION OF TORTURE SEQUELAE

Various phenomenological and diagnostic descriptions of torture sequelae so far have been reported.

Rather than falling into distinct syndromes, symptoms following different traumatic experiences show considerable overlap. Human response to various stressors thus appears to be confined to somewhat restricted psychological pathways (Rasmussen, 1990).

Thorvaldsen (1986) concluded that no particular constellations of symptoms could be specifically related to torture since a causal relationship between a 'torture syndrome' and previous exposure to torture could not be demonstrated. The concept of 'torture syndrome' thus appears to be unsubstantiated and possibly consists of a list of common symptoms observed in torture survivors. This raises the question whether these symptoms really constitute a specific syndrome qualitatively different from other stress response syndromes (Rasmussen, 1990; Turner & Gorst-Unsworth, 1990).

As noted earlier, the DSM–III diagnosis PTSD was introduced in an attempt to unify the various stress response syndromes. An underlying assumption in this diagnostic category is the existence of a final common psychophysiological pathway by which different types of traumatic experiences are processed. Many researchers have raised questions concerning the usefulness of the diagnosis of PTSD particularly in relation to the classification of torture sequelae. Many symptoms seen in torture survivors are, no doubt, in agreement with the DSM–III criteria for PTSD, and some torture survivors may well be diagnosed as having PTSD. On the other hand, the current version of the criteria for PTSD (DSM–III–R, APA 1987) has certainly important shortcomings such as the exclusion of 'changed identity or personality', the allowance for a rather insufficient length of time between the occurrence of the trauma to the onset of symptoms, and the failure of the syndrome to account for the chronically traumatized individual (Lansen, 1988). Furthermore, PTSD reduces complex political and historical problems into symptoms at the individual psychological level (Punamaki, 1989), and also appears exclusively to apply to adults (Lansen, 1988).

STUDY OF TORTURE SURVIVORS: SELECTION FACTORS AND METHODOLOGICAL PROBLEMS

Most studies of torture survivors appear to be biased by complex selection factors which are often impossible to elucidate. Some survivors may choose not to tell about their torture experiences and their effects on them. Most surveys are conducted on exiled torture survivors, and only a few studies have been carried out in the country where the torture actually took place. Often torture survivors from different ethnic backgrounds are included for study. Structured interviews or other systematic procedures are only occasionally used, and usually no detailed information about the methods of examination is given. Psychometric methods, such as standardized neuropsychological tests or rating scales are rarely employed. Most reports do not present a balanced assessment of the relative importance of the various aspects of the trauma such as torture, other stressful experiences and difficulties during imprisonment, and additional stress factors after release (e.g. further persecution or exile). Furthermore, many studies do not report adequate information about the time of onset of various symptoms following the traumatic experience.

The paucity of controlled studies and of follow-up surveys precludes definitive conclusions concerning the long-term effects of torture (see below). Reports of various sequelae after torture may thus have limited generalizability to the 'population' of torture survivors. Future research will need to overcome such methodological problems to allow better study of torture sequelae.

Another methodological limitation concerns the occasional failure to take into account the possible relationship between torture and other mental diseases such as major depression, paranoia, and anxiety states. It is often difficult to demonstrate a cause-and-effect relationship between torture and late sequelae since torture is usually carried out as a clandestine activity almost always denied by the perpetrators. Unless the physical sequelae of torture are evident, formal proof in most cases must be based on testimonies of survivors. The time lapse between the trauma of torture and the point of assessment is also of importance due to difficulties in recall and the likelihood of new traumatic events. Başoğlu & Marks (1988) and Petersen (1989) have emphasized the need for controlled evaluation. In addition to providing a detailed discussion of the methodological problems in assessing torture survivors, Petersen (1989) has also suggested that longitudinal studies are needed to investigate the specific diagnostic features of post-torture psychological problems.

Choice of mental symptoms to monitor in torture survivors

Despite the methodological shortcomings, the published studies of the effects of torture do suggest a correlation between torture and the observed sequelae. However, the variability in terminology used in the various studies prompted the RCT to set up an academic, multidisciplinary group (a consensus group: CG) in 1990 with a view to defining a more uniform and clear terminology, applicable on an international scale and also allowing direct comparisons between studies. The experience of the RCT during the last decade and the results of an epidemiological survey (Lunde *et al.*, 1988) indicated that it was possible to categorize the most frequently occurring torture-related symptoms and signs under a limited number of headings. After carefully examining the available nosological systems, the CG decided that a grouping of the psychological symptoms in accordance with DSM–III–R would be appropriate (see Table 3.1). Groups I (Activity), III (Appearance), VI (Eating disturbance), and XV (Thought content) were omitted. In addition, multiple occurrences of symptoms were reduced to only one group, and a few symptoms were omitted or transferred to more relevant groups.

REVIEW OF LITERATURE

In February 1991, a literature search through the major data bases (Medline, Psychinfo) yielded approximately 150 references concerning the psycho-social consequences of torture. It is evident from these reports that the sequelae of torture comprise a wide range of cognitive

Table 3.1. *Symptom groups according to the Diagnostic and Statistical Manual of Mental Disorders (DSM–III–R pages 521–523 and pages 290–296) modified with particular focus on torture sequelae*

II **Anxiety symptoms**
    Also included: anxiety; Excluded: depersonalization or derealization
IV **Behaviour**
    Only following symptoms are included: aggression or rage, antisocial behaviour, disorganized behaviour, feigning of symptoms, reckless activity, and suicide attempts
V   **Cognition/memory/attention**
    Excluded: aphasia
VII **Energy**
VIII **Form and amount of thought/speech**
    Excluded: abnormalities in the production of speech, impressionistic speech, racing of thoughts, slurred speech
IX **Mood/affect disturbance**
X   **Occupational and social impairment**
XI **Perceptual disturbance**
XII **Personality traits**
    Also included: assumption of a new identity (transferred from group IV). Excluded: grandiosity
XIII **Physical signs and symptoms** (when not applied elsewhere)
    Only following symptoms included: chest pain, dizziness or lightheadedness, dry mouth, flushes or chills, sweating, pupillary constriction, pupillary dilation, tachycardia
XIV **Sleep disturbance**
    Also included: nightmares
Code 302.7x
    Sexual dysfunctions

and emotional symptoms in addition to a variety of social consequences. We have limited our review to reports published in English or providing an English abstract and focused particularly on studies of torture survivors. Case histories, reports exclusively referring to others' work, and studies not distinguishing torture sequelae from the general problems of traumatized refugees have been excluded from our survey. This screening procedure yielded 46 references which will be reviewed in this chapter.

Uncontrolled studies

Torture survivors

Studies of exiled survivors A pilot study by Cathcart, Berger & Knazan (1979) showed that anxiety and sleeping difficulties were common in torture survivors. In 1980, a special issue of the *Danish Medical Bulletin* published the results of an Amnesty International Seminar (December, 1979) on the documentation of physical and mental sequelae of torture. In addition to various physical sequelae, Warmenhoven *et al.* (1981) reported a clustering of psychological symptoms attributable to previous torture. These findings were confirmed by an early Canadian study (Allodi & Cowgill, 1982). Cerebral atrophy in young torture survivors has been reported (Jensen *et al.*, 1982; Somnier *et al.*, 1982), implicating torture as a possible aetiological factor. However, computerized tomography of the brain in a larger group of torture survivors failed to confirm the results of these studies (Somnier *et al.*, unpublished data). Furthermore, there is so far no evidence of dementia or progressive cognitive impairment in torture survivors (Somnier & Genefke, 1986). Domovitch *et al.* (1984), in a study of 104 torture survivors, observed the following mental symptoms in descending order of frequency: anxiety, insomnia, nightmares, depression, withdrawal, irritability, loss of concentration, sexual dysfunction, memory disturbance, fatigue, emotional lability, aggressiveness, impulsiveness, and hypersensitivity to noise. Some of these early studies were reviewed by Goldfeld *et al.* (1988).

In a study of the long-term neuropsychological complaints of torture survivors (Somnier & Genefke, 1986), the most common symptoms, in decreasing order of frequency, were sleep disturbances with nightmares, headaches, impaired memory and concentration, fatigue, fear/anxiety, social withdrawal, vertigo, and sexual disturbances. The three key features were chronic anxiety, depression, and the subjective sense of a changed identity, and no spontaneous recovery was noted. Polysomnography revealed abnormal sleep patterns in previously healthy torture survivors compaired with normal age – and sex-matched controls (Åstrøm *et al.*, 1989). 70% of the 148 torture survivors treated at the RCT from 1984 to 1987 showed symptoms and signs of a changed identity (Ortmann & Lunde, 1988), chronic anxiety, poor self-esteem, and depression. Somatization may be a characteristic feature of South-East Asian torture survivors (Mollica, Wyshak & Lavelle, 1987). A recent follow-up study of female torture survivors (Fornazzari & Freire, 1990) suggested that *indirect* torture (e.g. threats

Table 3.2. Studies reporting symptoms in modified DSM–IIIR symptom groups in Table 3.1

Studies	II Anxiety symptoms	IV Behaviour	V Cognition/memory/attention	VII Energy	VIII Form & amount of thought/speech	IX Mood/affect disturbance	X Occupational/social impairment	XI Perceptual	XII Personality traits	XII Physical signs and symptoms	XIV Sleep disturbance	Sexual dysfunctions Code 302.7x
Cathcart et al., 1979	x		x			x	x				x	x
Daly, 1980						x	x				x	
Lunde et al., 1980												x
Rasmussen & Lunde, 1980	x		x							x	x	x
Warmenhoven et al., 1981	x		x	x		x					x	x
Allodi & Cowgill, 1982	x	x	x			x				x	x	x
Wallach & Rasmussen, 1983	x	x	x	x		x					x	x
Domovitch et al., 1984	x	x	x	x		x				x	x	x
Petersen et al., 1985a	x		x	x		x					x	x
Petersen & Jacobsen, 1985b	x		x			x					x	x
Randall et al., 1985	x		x	x		x			x	x		
Sonnier & Genefke, 1986	x	x	x	x		x			x	x	x	
Foster, 1987	x	x	x	x		x	x			x	x	
Mollica et al., 1987											x	
Pagaduan-Lopez, 1987	x		x	x		x			x	x	x	x
Arenas, 1987	x		x			x				x	x	x
Deutsch, 1987	x		x	x		x					x	
Hougen et al., 1988	x		x	x		x					x	
Jaffe, 1988	x	x	x			x					x	
Kordon et al., 1988	x		x			x					x	x
Lunde et al., 1988	x	x	x	x		x	x		x			x
Comite de Defensa, 1989	x	x					x		x		x	
Weisaeth, 1989	x	x				x			x		x	
Åstrom et al., 1989	x		x			x					x	
Fischman & Rose, 1990	x	x	x	x		x			x	x	x	x
Fornazzari & Freire, 1990	x		x						x	x	x	
Gonsalves, 1990	x						x		x			
Rasmussen, 1990	x	x	x	x		x	x		x		x	x
Chester, 1990	x		x			x			x		x	x
Lunde & Ortmann, 1990	x		x			x					x	x

of death) relative to *direct* (e.g. physical or more definite psychological) forms of torture might have less serious long-term effects. However, the authors recognized that somewhat subjective measures were used for the assessment of recovery rates. The distinction between indirect and direct torture may be spurious in view of the fact that all torture, whether physical or not, has a psychological impact on the individual.

Studies of non-exiled torture survivors A study of Greek torture survivors (Lunde *et al.*, 1980) found sexual dysfunctions including libido and erectile difficulties in 30% of the individuals. Torture-related sexual problems in both exiled and non-exiled torture survivors have also been reported by other investigators (see Table 3.2). Sexually tortured survivors were more likely to have sexual difficulties than were non-sexually tortured individuals (Lunde & Ortmann, 1990).

Abildgaard *et al.* (1984) and Petersen *et al.* (1985*a*) examined the state of health in 22 Greek torture survivors 10–14 years after the torture and conducted a follow-up assessment one year later. These surveys were carried out in Greece, so the results were not confounded by exile status. No improvement in the survivors' health was noted since the first assessment. Eight of the survivors (36%) fulfilled the criteria for chronic organic psycho-syndrome (COP). The survivors suffering from psycho-syndrome had been exposed to torture for significantly longer periods of time than those without COD. The severity of the symptoms was evidenced by significant impairment in both family life and work adjustment. The COP could not, however, be related to any head trauma, loss of consciousness, age, or to the time interval between the torture and the examination. The authors compared the symptoms to those of concentration camp survivors and also to the sequelae of diffuse brain damage of different aetiology. The psychological sequelae were more persistent and troublesome than the physical disability. Wallach & Rasmussen (1983), in a study of Chilean torture survivors living in Chile, found that the frequency of sequelae was of the same magnitude as that reported for exiled survivors. This finding was consistent with those of other studies (Foster, 1987; Pagaduan-Lopez, 1987; Kordon *et al.*, 1988). Among South-African survivors, blacks were more severely affected than whites, and women were more distressed than men (Foster, 1987). Dr Pedro Marin coordinated a study of the physical and psychological morbidity of political prisoners during the two years he himself was a detainee in a prison in Santiago (Jadresic, 1990). The most commonly observed complaints were tension headaches, anxiety or depressive symptoms, and sleep disturbance.

A particularly disturbing effect of torture is the compulsive and repetitive recall of the traumatic events (Somnier & Genefke, 1986: Deutsche, 1987). Recently, similar symptoms were observed in the crew of a Norwegian ship who were tortured abroad and later examined in their home country (Weisæth, 1989).

Study of exiled and non-exiled survivors Rasmussen (1990) compared the symptoms of 111 torture survivors in exile with those of 89 survivors residing in their native countries. The author found that the sequelae did not differ significantly between the two groups, though impaired memory and concentration, nightmares, and depression were more frequent in survivors living in exile.

Children and spouses of torture survivors

In a study of 75 Chilean children of exiled torture survivors living in Denmark, Cohn *et al.* (1980, 1985) found that more than one-third of the children were anxious and hypersensitive to noise, suffered from insomnia and frequent nightmares, and 23% had a regular nocturnal enuresis. Similar studies by Allodi (1989*a*) suggested that emotional distress in children was related to previous traumatization of the parents and the coping style of the latter; parental absence as a stress factor was associated with events surrounding torture. These conclusions are in agreement with reports from specialized health care groups dealing with children suffering from the effects of organized violence (e.g. Children's Rehabilitation Center in the Philippines (Protacio-Marcelino, 1989; Acuña, 1989) and Foundation for the Protection of Infancy damaged by Emergency States (PIDEE) in Chile). The Philippino group (Acuña, 1989) has confirmed the common occurrence of sleep disturbances reported by Cohn *et al.* (1980, 1985). Furthermore, Acuña (1989) noted that withdrawal, depression, irritability, aggressiveness, generalized fear, excessive clinging and dependence on the parents were common characteristics of children of torture survivors. Also observed in these children were a deterioration in school performance and distortions in the way they conceptualized a family. A commentary concerning these features has recently been published (Weile *et al.*, 1990). The latter study reported the results of re-examination of 76% of the children in the Cohn studies (1980, 1985). The children of traumatized families were fragile, vulnerable, and had more psychosomatic problems than age-matched native school children.

Allodi *et al.* (1989*b*) noted symptoms in the relatives of the 'disappeared' in Honduras which fulfilled the DSM–III–R criteria for PTSD. Family organization may suffer (Comité de Defensa, 1989). The experience of torture appears to remain unresolved longer among men than among women and among older than younger men (Comité de Defensa, 1989). Behavioural traits, due to previous experience of torture, included introversion, withdrawal, isolation, and excessive stubbornness. Another characteristic feature concerned an authoritarian attitude aiming at regaining status and control in the family with a tendency to suppress the differences of opinion among family members rather than seriously trying to resolve the conflicts (Comité de Defensa, 1989). Torture survivors are often stigmatized as terrorists, a source of serious social problems for their families already under great strain due to unemployment and poverty (Daly, 1980). Social and/or political activities do not seem to protect survivors from psychological consequences of torture (Fornazzari & Freire, 1990). This latter finding has not been confirmed by other groups.

Controlled studies

In collaboration with Spanish physicians, Petersen & Jacobsen (1985b) examined ten torture survivors and ten non-tortured individuals from the same region of Spain. The torture survivors showed depression, anxiety, impaired memory, and difficulty in concentration while none of these symptoms was present in the control group. In a study of 105 Latin American refugees in Denmark (Thorvaldsen, 1986), 44 (42%) tortured refugees were compared with those without a history of torture. In contrast to controls, the tortured group showed a higher incidence of headaches, fatigue, sleep disorders, nightmares and concentration problems. The differences between the two groups were statistically significant. Though health problems were common in the entire sample, torture survivors tended to have more symptoms than did the non-tortured refugees. For example, 73% of the tortured versus 51% of the non-tortured refugees reported one or more symptoms, such as fatigue, sleep disorders, nightmares, impaired memory and concentration difficulties.

Hougen et al. (1988) and Hougen (1988) compared exiled torture survivors from Turkey and Lebanon with non-tortured immigrants from the same countries, both groups residing in Denmark at the time of the examination. These studies suggest that torture plus exile status has a more deteriorating effect on the health status than being expelled alone. Yüksel, Paker & Paker (1990) compared tortured prisoners ($n = 196$) with non-tortured individuals ($n = 30$) living in the same prison in Turkey. The authors used Symptoms Checklist-90 (SCL-90) to assess the prisoners' psychological profile. Though the same prison conditions applied to both groups (other than the one group having been tortured), the tortured group scored significantly higher on the following subscales of SCL–90: obsession–compulsion, inter-personal sensitivity, depression, anxiety, anger, hostility, phobia, and paranoid ideation. The two groups were not matched for sex, age, marital status, and duration of stay in the prison but multiple regression analysis controlling for these variables revealed an independent effect of torture (see Paker *et al.*, this volume, for more details of this study).

DISCUSSION

The complexity of torture and its consequences cannot be adequately captured in a brief review written solely from a medical perspective. However, a multidimensional approach dealing with all aspects of torture is clearly beyond the scope of this chapter. Studies providing only limited evidence for a causal relationship between torture and reported sequelae have been excluded from this review, even though they may be of interest in other aspects. So far, most topics have been insufficiently studied, in particular the broader psychological effects on the survivor's family and community. There is a paucity of information concerning important issues such as survivors' guilt, shame and repentance.

As noted earlier, despite the methodological shortcomings of the studies reviewed so far, there is sufficient evidence to suggest a relationship between torture and subsequent psychological sequelae. The results of the early studies of torture survivors appear to be consistent with the outcome of more recently published surveys. Furthermore, the conclusions drawn by groups of rather different observance are in agreement. The consistency of symptoms is also evident across different groups of torture survivors, such as exiled and non-exiled survivors and tortured prisoners.

The most characteristic features of post-torture psychological sequelae appear to be sleep disturbances with frequent nightmares, affective symptoms (chronic anxiety, depression), cognitive impairment (memory defects, loss of concentration) and changes in identity (Somnier & Genefke, 1986). The psychological symptoms have been described in detail and grouped into categories (Table 3.2) which may have implications for the choice of treatment (see Chapter 18 by Başoğlu, this volume). Some of the important psychodynamic reactions of an individual submitted to psychological torture have been pointed out by, among others, Somnier & Genefke (1986) and Turner & Gorst-Unsworth (1990). The Latin American Collective of Psychosocial Work (COLAT) in Belgium has published several papers on the changed identity of political refugees due to torture and exile status (Barudy, 1989). Animal studies suggest that uncontrollable and unpredictable stress are major predictors of post-traumatic symptoms (for a review see Başoğlu & Mineka, this volume). Learned helplessness is a characteristic consequence of certain methods of torture (Somnier & Genefke, 1986).

Individual modifying factors may play a role in determining post-torture psychological problems. Not yet resolved is the extent to which trauma interacts with concomitant factors such as the inherent vulnerability of the individual. Presumably, factors such as age, sex, firmness of political belief system, and cultural background may affect the long-term outcome. Psychological processes, such as the defence mechanisms and coping strategies used under stress, appear to play a significant role in symptom formation (Somnier & Genefke, 1986). External factors such as the prison conditions, being subjected to indoctrination, and an environment run by arbitrary rules all seem to determine the chances for psychological survival (see also Chapter 9 by Başoğlu and Mineka, this volume).

Most torture survivors reside in their native country after release from detention or prison. Most physical symptoms and signs of torture rapidly disappear. The persistent physical and mental sequelae are not easily recognized by medical personnel unless they are specially trained. As noted earlier, several aspects of psychological functioning may continue to be impaired in the long-term. The survivor and his/her family may have to mobilize all available energy and resources for mere survival. We know from survivors who resume struggle against the oppressive regime after their release that both psychological and physical symptoms may be suppressed for some time. Rejoining the struggle, however, may also add to the distress of the family. In such cases, the relatives may have to go on living in eternal dread with a serious risk of being themselves arrested, interrogated, or perhaps even tortured.

For those survivors who manage to escape to other countries or who are sent into exile, symptoms and signs may assume a new social meaning. They may be required to prove that they have been tortured in order to obtain asylum. Failure to produce evidence of torture may mean being repatriated against their will. The problems related to forced exile often aggravate the psychological symptoms outlined earlier. The refugee's cultural background seems to influence the way he/she copes with the sequelae of torture and also determines the chances for successful integration into the new society. Although no systematic investigation of these aspects has been carried out, it has been observed that refugees may be better off psychologically living in a host culture similar to their own than in a new society of a very different cultural orientation. Most torture survivors, particularly those who have been sexually tortured, avoid discussing their past experiences with their families in detail. The survivor may be blamed for all the hardship the family has to face as refugees.

The special health care needs of torture survivors require specialized health care facilities. Past experience has shown that traditional health care services do not adequately meet the needs of torture survivors. Rehabilitation centres for torture survivors have therefore been set up in several countries around the world. In addition, survivors of torture must be afforded social programmes to facilitate integration into the new society. Vitally important for the achievement of these objectives is properly to inform the public about the aims, methods and consequences of torture and the fact that spontaneous recovery from torture-related disability is unlikely to occur unless help is provided. We have come to agree with Trautman (1964) that psychological sequelae of torture should be seen as meaningful conditional reactions for a sound and forceful constitution that make survival possible in a very pathological situation.

REFERENCES

Abilgaard, U., Daugaard, G., Marcussen, H., Jess, P., Petersen, H. D. & Wallach, M. (1984). Chronic organic psycho-syndrome in Greek torture victims. *Danish Medical Bulletin*, **31**, 239–42.

Acuña, J. E. (1989). *Children of the Storm*. Children's Rehabilitation Center: Philippines.

Allodi, F. & Cowgill, G. (1982). Ethical and psychiatric aspects of torture: a Canadian study. *Canadian Journal of Psychiatry*, **27**, 98–102.

Allodi, F. (1989a). The children of victims of political persecution and torture: a psychological study of a Latin American refugee community. *International Journal of Mental Health*, **18**, 3–15.

Allodi, F., Pereira, W. & Rousseau, C. (1989b). The trauma of forced disappearance in the families of victims as post traumatic stress disorder. *Society for Post Traumatic Stress Studies*: San Francisco.

Arenas, J. G. (1987). Flygtninge, eksil og psykiske kriser (Refugees, exile, and psychological crises). In J. G. Arenas, P. Steen, V. Jacobsen, U.S. Thomsen, eds. *Flygtningens Psykiske Kriser* (Psychological crises of refugees), Chap. 4, Dansk psykologisk Forlag: Copenhagen, Denmark.

Askevold, F. (1980). The war sailor syndrome. *Danish Medical Bulletin*, **27**, 220–3.
Åstrøm, C., Lunde, I., Ortmann, J. & Boysen, G. (1989). Sleep disturbances in torture survivors. *Acta Neurologica Scandinavica*, **79**, 150–4.
Barudy, J. (1989). A programme of mental health for political refugees: dealing with the invisible pain of political exile. *Social Science and Medicine*, **28**, 715–27.
Başoğlu, M. & Marks, I. (1988). Torture. Research needed into how to help those who have been tortured. *British Medical Journal*, **297**, 1423–4.
Cathcart, I. M. Berger, P. & Knazan, B. (1979). Medical examination of torture victims applying for refugee status. *Canadian Medical Association Journal*, **121**, 179–84.
Chester, B. (1990). Because mercy has a human heart: centers for victims of torture. In P. Suedfeld, ed., *Psychology and Torture*. pp. 165–69, Hemisphere Publishing Co.
Cohn, J., Holzer, K., Koch, L. & Severin, B. (1980). Children and torture. An investigation of Chilean immigrant's children in Denmark. *Danish Medical Bulletin*, **27**, 238–9.
Cohn, J., Danielsen, L., Koch, L. *et al.* (1985). A study of Chilean refugee children in Denmark. *Lancet*, ii, 437–8.
Comité de Defensa de los Derechos del Pueblo (Codepu, Chile), (1989). The effects of torture and political repression in a sample of Chilean families. *Social Science and Medicine*, **28**, 735–40.
Daly, R. J. (1980). Compensation and rehabilitation of victims of torture. An example of preventive psychiatry. *Danish Medical Bulletin*, **27**, 245–8.
Deutsch, A. (1987). The psychological effects of torture. Symposium: 'Working with Victims of Violence and Torture'. April 23–26, 67th Annual Convention of the Western Psychological Association: Long Beach, California.
Domovitch, E., Berger, P. B., Wawer, M. J., Etlin, D. D. & Marshall, J. C. (1984). Human torture: description and sequelae of 104 cases. *Canadian Family Physician*, **30**, 827–30.
Eitinger, L. & Strøm, A. (1973). *Mortality and Morbidity after Excessive Stress*. Universitetsforlaget: Oslo.
Eitinger, l. (1980). Jewish concentration camp survivors in the post-war world. *Danish Medical Bulletin*, **27**, 232–5.
Figley, C. (1985). *Trauma and Its Wake*. New York: Brunner Mazel.
Fischman, Y. & Ross, J. (1990). Group treatment of exiled survivors of torture. *American Journal of Orthopsychiatry*, **60**, 135–42.
Fornazzari, X. & Freire, M. (1990). Women as victims of torture. *Acta Psychiatrica Scandinavica*, **82**, 257–60.
Foster, D. (1987). *Detention & Torture in South Africa. Psychological, Legal, and Historical Aspects*. David Phillip: Cape Town & Johannesburg.
Goldfeld, A. E., Mollica, R. D., Pesavento, B. H. & Faraone, S. V. (1988). The physical and psychological sequelae to torture. Symptomatology and diagnosis. *Journal of American Medical Association*, **259**, 2725–9.
Gonsalves, C. J. (1990). The psychological effects of political repression on Chilean exiles in the US. *American Journal of Orthopsychiatry*, **60**, 143–53.
Hougen, H. P., Kelstrup, J., Peterson, H. D. & Rasmussen, O. V. (1988).

Sequelae to torture. A controlled study of torture victims living in exile. *Forensic Science International*, 36, 153–60.

Hougen, H. P. (1988). Physical and psychological sequelae to torture. A controlled clinical study of exiled asylum applicants. *Forensic Science International*, 39, 5–11.

Jadresic, D. (1990). Medical, psychological and social aspects of torture: prevention and treatment. *Medicine and War*, 6, 197–203.

Jaffé, H. (1988). 46 cas de refugies turcs – Sévices et plaintes. Personal Communication: *HAVRE*, Paris.

Jensen, T. S. Genefke, I. K., Hyldebrandt, N., Pedersen, H., Petersen, H. D. & Weile, B. (1982). Cerebral atrophy in young torture victims. *New England Journal of Medicine*, 307, 1341.

Kieler, J. (1980). Immediate reactions to capture and deportation. *Danish Medical Bulletin*, 27, 217–20.

Kordon, D., Edelman, L. I. Nicoletti, E., Lagos, D. M., Bozzolo, R. C. & Kandel, E. (1988). Torture in Argentina. In Group of Psychological Assistance to Mothers of 'Plaza de Mayo' (eds.) *Psychological Effects of Political Repression.* pp. 95–107, Sudamericana/Planeta Publishing Company: Buenos Aires, Argentina.

Lansen, N. A. (1988). A critical view of the concept PTSD. Paper presented at *WHO workshop on health situation of refugees and victims of organized violence*, August 26–27: Gothenburg, Sweden.

Lunde, I., Rasmussen, O. V., Lindholm, J. & Wagner, G. (1980). Gonadal and sexual functions in tortured Greek men. *Danish Medical Bulletin*, 27, 243–5.

Lunde, I., Foldspang, A. Hansen, A. H. & Ortmann, J. (1988). Monitoring the Health of Torture Victims. A pilot study. Paper presented at *WHO workshop on health situation of refugees and victims of organized violence*, August 26–27: Gothenburg, Sweden.

Lunde, I. & Ortmann, J. (1990). Prevalence and sequelae of sexual torture. *Lancet*, 336, 289–91.

Mollica, R. F., Wyshak, G. & Lavelle, J. (1987). The psychosocial impact of war trauma and torture on Southeast Asian refugees. *American Journal of Psychiatry*, 144, 1567–72.

Ortmann, J. & Lunde, I. (1988). Changed identity, low self-esteem, depression, and anxiety in 148 torture victims treated at the RCT. Relation to sexual torture. Paper presented at *WHO workshop on health situation of refugees and victims of organized violence*, August 26–27: Gothenburg, Sweden.

Pagaduan-Lopez, J. C. (1987). *Torture Survivors. What can we do for them?* Medical Action Group, Inc.: Manila, Philipines.

Petersen, H. D., Abildgaard, U., Daugaard, G., Jess, P., Marcussen, H. & Wallach, M. (1985a). Psychological and physical long-term effects of torture. A follow-up examination of 22 Greek persons exposed to torture 1967–1974. *Scandinavian Journal of Social Medicine*, 13, 89–93.

Petersen, H. D. & Jacobsen, P. (1985b). Psychological and physical symptoms after torture. A prospective controlled study. *Forensic Science International*, 29, 179–89.

Petersen, H. D. (1989). The controlled study of torture victims. Epidemiological considerations and some future aspects. *Scandinavian Journal of Social Medicine,* **17**, 13–20.

Protacio-Marcelino, E. (1989). Children of political detainees in the Philippines: sources of stress and coping patterns. *International Journal of Mental Health,* **18**, 71–86.

Punamaki, R. L. (1989). Political violence and mental health. *International Journal of Mental Health,* **17**, 3–15.

Randall, G. R., Lutz, E. L. Quiroga, J., Zunzunegui, M. V., Kollf, C. A., Deutsch, A. *et al.* (1985). Physical and psychiatric effects of torture. In: E. Stover, E. O. Nightingale, eds., *The Breaking of Bodies and Minds: Torture, Psychiatric Abuse and the Health Professions.* W. H. Freeman and Company: New York.

Rasmussen, O. V. & Lunde, I. (1980). Evaluation of investigation of 200 torture victims. *Danish Medical Bulletin,* **27**, 241–3.

Rasmussen. O. V. (1990) Medical aspects of torture. (Thesis). *Danish Medical Bulletin,* **37**, 1–88.

Somnier, F. E., Jensen, T. S., Pedersen, H., Bruhn, P., Salinas, P. & Genefke, I. K. (1982). Cerebral atrophy in young torture victims. *Acta Neurologica Scandinavica,* **65**, 321–2.

Somnier, F. E. & Genefke, I. K. (1986). Psychotherapy for victims of torture. *British Journal of Psychiatry,* **149**, 323–9.

Sørensen, H., Hansen, O. E. & Worm-Petersen, J. (1983). Krigssejlere 40 år efter. (War sailors forty years after). *Ugeskrift for Laeger,* **145**, 3685–8.

Thorvaldsen, P. (1986). Torturfølger blandt latinamerikanske flygtninge i Danmark. (Torture Sequelae among Latin American Refugees in Denmark). (Thesis). Laegeforeningens Forlag: Copenhagen, Denmark.

Trautman, E. G. (1964). Fear and panic in Nazi concentration camps: a biosocial evaluation of the chronic anxiety syndrome. *International Journal of Social Medicine,* **10**, 134–41.

Turner, S. & Gorst-Unsworth, C. (1990). Psychological sequelae of torture: a descriptive model. *British Journal of Psychiatry,* **157**, 475–80.

Wallach, M. & Rasmussen, O. V. (1983). Tortur i Chile (Torture in Chile). *Ugeskrift for Laeger,* **145**, 2349–52.

Warmenhoven, C., van Slooten, H., Lachinsky, N., de Hoog, M. I. & Smeulers, J. (1981). The medical after-effects of torture. An investigation among refugees in the Netherlands. *Nederlands Tijdschrift voor Geneeskunde,* **125**, 104–8.

Weile, B., Wingender, L. B., Bach-Mortensen, N. & Busch, P. (1990). Behavioral problems in children of torture victims: a sequel to cultural maladaptation or to parental torture? *Journal of Developmental & Behavioral Pediatrics,* **11**, 79–80.

Weisæth, L. (1989). Torture of a Norwegian ship's crew. The torture, stress reactions and psychiatric after-affects. *Acta Psychiatrica Scandinavica,* **80**, 63–72.

Yüksel, Ş., Paker, M. & Paker, Ö. (1990). Torture in Turkey. Psychological consequences and treatment. Presented at the *Second European Conference on Traumatic Stress:* Amsterdam, Holland.

4
PSYCHOLOGICAL EFFECTS OF TORTURE: AN EMPIRICAL STUDY OF TORTURED AND NON-TORTURED NON-POLITICAL PRISONERS
Murat Paker, Özgün Paker and Şahika Yüksel

INTRODUCTION

Although much has been written about the psychological effects of torture, there are few controlled studies of its psychological impact (Goldfeld *et al.*, 1988; Başoğlu & Marks, 1988). While most studies concur about the nature of the psychological problems in the short and long term following torture (e.g. Rasmussen & Lunde, 1980; Kjaersgaard & Genefke, 1977; Cathcart *et al.*, 1979; Lunde *et al.*, 1980; Abilgaard *et al.*, 1984; Domovitch *et al.*, 1984; Petersen *et al.*, 1985; Petersen & Jacobsen, 1985; Allodi *et al.*, 1985; Allodi & Cowgill, 1982; Hougen *et al.*, 1988; Goldfeld *et al.*, 1988; see also Somnier *et al.*, this volume), the question whether these problems are independent of other confounding variables such as other associated traumatic events before and after torture has thus not been fully resolved.

Much of our knowledge about the effects of torture stems from work with tortured political activists or other individuals tortured for political reasons. As is extensively discussed in this volume, torture is only one of the many forms of organized violence suffered by the survivors. Persecution and harassment by the authorities, detention, imprisonment, disrupted ties with loved ones, forced uprooting, and refugee status are but a few examples of the associated traumatic situations. Thus study of the effects of torture *per se* would need to take into account the additional effect of these factors.

A controlled study (Hougen *et al.*, 1988) showed that a group of tortured Turkish political refugees living in exile had more severe psychological symptoms compared to non-tortured controls who otherwise had similar experiences. Although the findings of this study have important implications, certain methodological problems such as inadequate matching of controls, screening biases in sample selection, and a relatively small sample size ($n = 28$) preclude definitive conclusions.

Another recent controlled study on exiled Latin Americans reported more symptoms among tortured people than among controls (Thorvaldsen, 1985, cited in Hougen *et al.*, 1988). The differences were significant despite several controls having been imprisoned and ill treated (but not tortured) in their countries.

A prospective controlled study (Petersen & Jacobsen, 1985) found that tortured individuals were in a worse state of health compared with their controls, showing symptoms of depression, anxiety, emotional lability, sleep disturbance, nightmares, and memory and concentration difficulties. The controls, however, were not adequately matched and the sample size ($n = 10$) was too small for statistical analysis of the association between severity of torture and psychological sequelae.

In the study that will be presented here, we have attempted to overcome some of the methodological problems discussed above. First, we have systematically investigated the effects of torture in a sample of 246 prisoners (38 of whom were not tortured) in a prison for non-political prisoners, thus controlling for the effects of imprisonment. Secondly, since the subjects had been living in more or less the same prison conditions (e.g. physical environment, rules and regulations, staff, etc), the sample was relatively homogenous with respect to adverse circumstances affecting psychological functioning. Thirdly, as we were able to study the entire prison population satisfying our selection criteria, our sample was not biased by factors such as unavailability of subjects or refusal to participate in the study. Finally, we obtained data on a sizeable sample which afforded the opportunity for multivariate analyses. As the prison circumstances would not allow a controlled study, multivariate analyses were required to control for some of the intervening variables in examining the effects of torture. Our study, however, has some limitations which will be reviewed in the discussion. We hypothesized that a history of torture would predict higher levels of psychopathology among prisoners.

PROCEDURES

The study was conducted in 1988 at Tekirdag prison, an institution for non-political prisoners, by the first author (M.P.) during his employment there as a general practitioner. Only prisoners who were literate, between 18 and 60 years of age, and imprisoned for at least 6 months were selected for the study. Of the 383, 246 (64%) inmates fulfilled these inclusion criteria and all volunteered for the study.

D

Assessment

The study was conducted in difficult prison conditions. The prison authorities were informed about the study which was designed to 'better understand the general psychological problems of the prisoners', but, for obvious reasons, they were not given specific details about the questions included in the interview. The necessarily secretive nature of the project limited the amount of data that could be collected for the study of relevant variables.

A semi-structured interview form was used to obtain information on demographic characteristics, type of prison (closed or open), time so far served in prison, expected duration of imprisonment, the nature of the crime committed, and the details of prison history including the nature of ill-treatment and torture suffered during imprisonment.

The World Medical Association defined torture as '... deliberate, systematic or wanton infliction of physical or mental suffering by one or more persons acting alone or on the orders of any authority, to force another person to yield information, to make a confession, or for any other reason' (Tokyo Declaration, 1975). This definition of torture was adopted for the purposes of this study. Relatively mild forms of ill-treatment such as swearing, slapping on the face, and solitary confinement for brief periods (e.g. one day) were regarded as torture.

Prisoners who claimed to have been tortured at some stage during their imprisonment were medically examined for any signs of physical sequelae. No further laboratory investigations could be performed due to limited facilities in the prison. In most cases, the nature of the physical sequelae seemed related to the method of torture reported by the subjects (e.g. falanga and scarred and/or enlarged feet, hanging and habitual luxation of the shoulder).

A translated and standardized (Dağ, 1991) version of Symptom Check List-90 (SCL-90, Derogatis, Lipmon & Covi, 1973) was used to obtain data on the psychological profile of the prisoners. This scale consists of nine factors: somatization, obsessive–compulsive symptoms, interpersonal sensitivity, depression, anxiety, anger–hostility, phobias, paranoid ideation, and psychoticism. In addition, it provides total scores of General Symptom Index (GSI-mean score of all items), Positive Symptom Distress Level (PSDL-mean score of positive items), and Positive Symptom Total (PST-number of positive items). Symptom ratings range from 0 (not at all) to 4 (extremely severe).

The subjects were also screened for post-traumatic stress disorder (PTSD) symptoms using the DSM-IIIR criteria.

Table 4.1. *Sample characteristics* (n = 246)

Sex:		
Male	226	(92%)
Female	20	(8%)
Mean age	34	(SD 7.6)
Education:		
Literate	23	(9%)
Primary school	174	(71%)
Secondary school	34	(14%)
High school	15	(6%)
Marital status:		
Single	165	(67%)
Married	81	(33%)
Social class:		
Lower	135	(55%)
Middle	39	(16%)
Upper middle	72	(29%)
Type of prison sentence being served:		
Closed	193	(79%)
Open	53	(21%)
Expected duration of imprisonment (yrs)	17.1	(SD 6.2)
Mean time served in prison (yrs)	7.4	(4.5)
Physical sequelae due to torture	82	(33%)
History of torture:		
Tortured	208	(85%)
Non-tortured	38	(15%)
Mean SCL-90 scores:		
GSI	1.24	(SD .65)
PSDL	2.08	(SD .60)
PST	51.6	(SD 19.4)

RESULTS

Sample characteristics (Table 4.1)

Only 8% of the subjects were female. Mean age was 34 (SD 7.6). Of the subjects, 87% had employment before imprisonment. The types of crime committed were murder (41%), smuggling (32%), physical assaults and causing bodily harm (29%), robbery (18%), and others (26%). 26% had committed more than one crime. The mean duration of the sentences being served was 17.1 (SD 6.2) years. The mean duration of time already spent in prison was 7.4 (SD 4.5) years. Of the inmates 78% were kept in the closed section of the prison while 22% were living in the open section.

Types of torture

Only 15.4% of the prisoners reported no form of torture. Of the subjects 84.6% reported having experienced a mean of 5 (SD 2) different types of torture (range 1–11). The most commonly reported methods were psychological torture (threats, swearing, being forced to witness others being tortured; 94%), beating (with or without a stick or baton; 86%), falanga (beating of the soles of the feet with a stick; 73%), solitary confinement (71%), electrical torture (33%), hanging by the arms (28%), and cold water showers (22%), and being beaten by a group of wardens (4%). Other less common forms of torture included putting a hot egg under the armpit, cutting a wound with a knife and applying salt on it or inflicting pain by inserting a pin into the wound, applying weight on the testicles, removing the nails with pincers, burning with cigarettes, beating with a sandbag, and food deprivation.

Physical sequelae

Of the tortured subjects (n = 208) 39% had physical sequelae. The most common physical signs and complaints were:

1   scars in the soles of the feet (11%)
2   muscle and joint disorders (e.g. myalgia, arthralgia) (10%)
3   scars in parts of body (7%)
4   chronic pain due to faulty healing of bone fractures (5%)
5   peripheral nerve damage (4%)
6   scars of burns (4%)
7   enlarged feet (3%)
8   hearing loss (3%)
9   broken or missing nails (3%)
10   habitual luxation of the shoulder or knee (2%)
11   broken or missing teeth (2%)
12   nasal septum deviation due to blows on the nose (1.4%)
13   others (5%)

The physical signs and complaints correlated with the forms of torture reported by the subjects. For example, the sequelae numbered 1, 2, 3, 4, 7, 10 (knee) were associated with falanga; 2, 3, 4, 8, 11 and 12 with beating with a heavy stick or baton, 5 and 10 (shoulder) with hanging by the arms, 2 with solitary confinement (in a wet cell), and 6 with burning with cigarettes.

Incidence of PTSD

PTSD was diagnosed in 39% (81) of the 208 tortured prisoners. None of the non-tortured prisoners had PTSD. Among the prisoners who had PTSD, the condition was severe in 8% (6), moderate in 49% (40), and mild in 43% (35). There was no significant sex difference in the incidence of PTSD. Among the tortured prisoners, 71% (58) of the 82 subjects who had physical sequelae met the criteria for PTSD as opposed to only 18% (23) among those who did not have any physical sequelae (X2 = 55.4, p = .0000).

Predictors of psychopathology: multiple regression analyses

Multiple regression analyses were performed to examine the predictors of psychopathology in the entire sample. The independent variables were history of torture (0 = not tortured 1 = tortured), sex (0 = female, 1 = male), type of prison (0 = closed, 1 = open), marital status (0 = married, 1 = single), education (1 = literate, 2 = primary school, 3 = secondary school, 4 = higher), social class (0 = lower, 1 = middle, 2 = upper middle), age, expected duration of imprisonment, time already served in prison. Separate multiple regression analyses were performed using the 9 SCL-90 sub-scale scores, General Symptom Index (GSI), Positive Symptom Distress Level (PSDL), and Positive Symptom Total (PST) as the dependent variables. The independent variables were entered into the regression equation in a stepwise fashion. The results are shown in Table 4.2.

A positive history of torture predicted higher scores on anxiety, obsessive compulsive symptoms, depression, interpersonal sensitivity, paranoid ideation, anger–hostility, phobias and on the GSI, PSDL and PST. Female sex predicted higher scores on somatization, anxiety, obsessive–compulsive symptoms, depression, paranoid ideation, phobias, PSDL, and GSI. Lower education correlated with higher scores of anxiety, depression, phobias, and symptom distress. Living in the closed section of the prison predicted higher scores on obsessive–compulsive symptoms (intrusive thoughts, difficulty remembering things, slowness, and checking), phobias (discomfort in crowded places), and PST. The amount of variance explained by the independent variables was quite low, ranging from 2% to 7%.

Table 4.2. *Predictors of psychopathology in 246 non-political prisoners (multiple regression analysis)**

	Beta	R2 change	p(t)
Total SCL-90 score:			
Type of prison	−.24	.06	.0002
Torture	.15	.02	.02
General Symp. Index:			
Sex (female/male)	−.21	.03	.001
Torture	.19	.03	.004
Symp. Distress Level:			
Sex	−.29	.07	.0000
Torture	.19	.03	.003
Education	−.17	.03	.006
Anxiety:			
Torture	.22	.03	.0004
Sex	−.20	.04	.002
Education	−.15	.03	.02
Obsessive–compulsive			
Type of prison	−.15	.03	.02
Torture	.18	.02	.005
Sex	−.17	.03	.008
Depression:			
Sex	−.24	.05	.0002
Torture	.16	.02	.02
Education	−.12	.02	.05
Interpersonal sens.:			
Torture	.14	.02	.03
Paranoid ideation:			
Torture	.20	.03	.002
Sex	−.16	.03	.02
Social class	.11	.02	.04
Anger–hostility:			
Torture	.20	.04	.002
Phobias:			
Sex	−.23	.06	.0002
Education	−.19	.03	.002
Type of prison	−.16	.03	.009
Torture	.14	.02	.03

*Significant predictor variables shown under each dependent variable.

Further regression analyses examined whether the presence of physical sequelae predicted greater psychopathology among the tortured prisoners ($n = 208$). All previous independent variables were included in the analyses. GSI, PSDL, and PST were used as dependent variables. Physical sequelae explained 8% of the variance in GSI (Beta = .30, p = .0000), 9% of the variance in PSDL (Beta = .29, p = .0000), and 3% of the variance in PST (Beta = .16, p = .02). Female sex again predicted higher scores on GSI (Beta = $-$.20, R2 change = .04, p = .003) and PSDL ($-$.30, R2 change = .08, p = .0000). Being kept in the closed section of the prison predicted higher scores on PST (Beta = $-$.21, R2 change = .05, p = 003).

DISCUSSION

This study has several limitations. First, the time since torture last took place was not taken into account. The mean time served in prison was 7.4 years (SD 4.5), which possibly means a long time gap between the assessment of psychological problems and the last experience of torture for many subjects. A long stay in prison after the experience of torture can help recovery from the effects of uncontrollable stress, especially in a predictable and emotionally supportive environment (Başoğlu & Mineka, this volume). The solidarity among the inmates may have provided sufficient emotional support for the tortured prisoners. Had duration since torture experience been taken into account, subjects with a more recent history of torture might have been found to have greater psychopathology. The effect of time might explain a) the relatively low total SCL-90 scores for both the tortured (53, SD = 19) and the non-tortured (44.1, SD = 20) prisoners, and b) the relatively low percentage of variance in the dependent variables accounted for by the history of torture. It should also be borne in mind that SCL-90 is a measure of general psychopathology and may thus have missed certain PTSD symptoms. The fact that 39% of the tortured prisoners met the criteria for PTSD suggests that other scales specifically designed to tap PTSD symptoms might have revealed higher psychopathology scores.

Another limitation of the study concerns the definition of torture. The use of categorical variables (tortured/not tortured) in this study might have led to loss of information concerning the subjective meaning of the experience which is critical in determining the severity of the trauma (Yüksel, 1991). A subjectively graded measure of trauma severity might have been a stronger predictor of psychological functioning. Certain forms of ill-treatment such as swearing or slapping in the face, although classified as torture in this study, might have been perceived as a relatively mild form of trauma by some subjects. Unfortunately, lack of more detailed information precluded more refined analyses.

The relationship of physical sequelae with higher levels of psychopathology, however, can be seen as indirect evidence supporting the role of the intensity of the stressor in post-traumatic stress. It seems reasonable to assume that more severe torture is more likely to produce physical sequelae. For example, a form of torture called Palestinian hanging (hanging by the wrists tied at the back) is extremely painful and cannot be tolerated for more than 15–20 minutes. It also involves a risk of serious physical damage and even threat to life. Thus having peripheral nerve damage as a consequence of this form of torture would possibly indicate (all other factors being equal) an experience of greater overall traumatic stress, relative to someone who was not subjected to this form of torture. Although this association cannot be generalized to all forms of torture, the correlation between physical sequelae and higher long-term psychopathology is suggestive of greater traumatic stress involved in procedures causing physical sequelae.

It is also conceivable that the physical sequelae *per se* may account, at least in part, for subsequent psychopathology. This seems, however, unlikely to have played a significant role in our sample since the physical signs detected in our subjects had not involved physical disability severe enough to cause permanent impairment of daily functioning in an already restricted prison life. The presence of physical sequelae though may have served as a constant reminder of the traumatic experience and thereby helped maintain feelings of helplessness experienced during torture. It would have been informative to compare the psychological profile of prisoners who had torture-related physical sequelae with that of those who had similar physical sequelae due to other reasons (e.g. accidents), but unfortunately information on the latter could not be obtained because of the restrictions in conducting the study.

Being kept in the closed rather than the open section of the prison correlated with higher scores on phobia and O-C factors and greater overall psychopathology. In fact, this was a more important predictor of total SCL-90 scores than a positive history of torture. This may be due to the differences between the living conditions in the two sections. Life in the open section of the prison was much less stressful than in the closed section as the inmates were allowed to work in the prison workshop, have longer time in open air, and go out of the prison twice every year on leave for a week. Newcomers to the prison were first placed in the closed section and those who 'behaved well' became entitled to a transfer only two years before the end of their term. Having nearly served their term may also have affected the psychological status of open section inmates. However, those 'well-behaved' inmates might also have had less psychological disturbance before their transfer to the open section. This potential confound precludes definitive conclusions on the effects of the closed section.

It is not clear from available data why women had greater psychopathology independent of torture and the other predictor variables. The women may have experienced greater stress in the prison than men since all of them were kept in the closed section. Furthermore, three of the women were caring for their children (one to four years old) in prison. However, in the absence of more detailed information about their experience and a control group, it is difficult to reach a definitive conclusion on this issue.

In conclusion, our findings are suggestive of a long-term psychological effect of torture and is thus consistent with similar findings in the literature (e.g. Hougen *et al.*, 1988; Petersen & Jacobsen, 1985). Although our study was not controlled, we tried to examine the effect of torture on long-term psychological functioning, controlling for some of the relevant confounding variables by multiple regression analyses. As noted earlier, the predictor effects, though statistically significant, are relatively weak but nevertheless present, despite the confounds posed by the problems in defining torture, the time factor, and a retrospective study design. These results are further supported by the finding that 39% of the tortured prisoners had PTSD whereas none of the non-tortured prisoners did.

REFERENCES

Abildgaard, U., Daugaard, G., Marcussen, H. *et al.* (1984). Chronic organic psycho-syndrome in Greek torture victims. *Danish Medical Bulletin*, **31**, 239–41.

Allodi, F. & Cowgill, G. (1982). Ethical and psychiatric aspects of torture: A Canadian study. *Canadian Journal of Psychiatry*, **27**, 98–102.

Allodi, F., Randall, G. R., Lutz, E. L. *et al.* (1985). Physical and psychiatric effects of torture: two medical studies. In E. Stover and E. O. Nightingale, eds., *The Breaking of Bodies and Minds*. New York: W. H. Freeman and Company.

Başoğlu, M. & Marks, I. M. (1988). Torture. Research needed into how to help those who have been tortured. *British Medical Journal*, **297**, 1423–4.

Cathcart, L. M., Beger, P. & Knazan, B. (1979). Medical examination of torture victims applying for refugee status. *Canadian Medical Association Journal*, 121, 179–84.

Dağ, I. (1991). Symptom Check List (SCL-90): a reliability and validity study. *Turkish Journal of Psychiatry*, 2(1), 5–12.

Derogatis, L. R., Lipmon, R. S. & Covi, L. (1973). SCL-90: An outpatient psychiatric scale – preliminary report. *Psychopharmacological Bulletin*, 9, 13–28.

Domovitch, E., Berger, P. B., Wawer, M. J. *et al.* (1984). Human torture: description and sequelae of 104 cases. *Canadian Family Physician*, 30, 827–30.

Goldfeld, A. E., Mollica, R. F., Pesavento, B. H. & Faraone, S. V. (1988). The physical and psychological sequelae of torture: Symptomatology and diagnosis. *Journal of American Medical Association*, 259, 2725–9.

Hougen, H. P., Kelstrup, J., Petersen, H. D. & Rasmussen, O. V. (1988). Sequelae to torture. A controlled study of torture victims living in exile. *Forensic Science International*, 36, 153–60.

Kjaersgaard, A. R. & Genefke, I. K. (1977). Victims of torture in Uruguay and Argentina: case studies. In *Evidence of Torture: Studies of the Amnesty International Danish Medical Group*. London: Amnesty International Publications.

Lunde, I., Rasmussen, O. V., Lindholm, J. & Wagner, G. (1980). Gonadal and sexual functions in tortured Greek men. *Danish Medical Bulletin*, 27, 243–5.

Ortmann, J., Genefke, I. K., Jakobsen, L. & Lunde, I. (1987). Rehabilitation of torture victims: an interdisciplinary treatment model. *American Journal of Social Psychiatry*, 4, 161–7.

Petersen, H. D. & Jacobsen, P. (1985). Psychical and physical symptoms after torture. A prospective controlled study. *Forensic Science International*, 29, 179–89.

Petersen, H. D., Abildgaard, U., Daugaard, G. *et al.* (1985). Psychological and physical long-term effects of torture. A follow-up examination of 22 Greek persons exposed to torture 1967–1974. *Scandinavian Journal of Social Medicine*, 13, 89–93.

Rasmussen, O. V. & Lunde, I. (1980). Evaluation of investigations of 200 torture victims. *Danish Medical Bulletin*, 27, 241–3.

Somnier, F. E. & Genefke, I. K. (1986). Psychotherapy for victims of torture. *British Journal of Psychiatry*, 149, 323–9.

Thorvaldsen, P. (1985). Torturefolger blandt latinamerikanske flygtninge i Danmark. Laegeforeningens forlag, Kobenhavn.

Yüksel, Ş. (1991). Therapy of sexual torture. Paper presented in the 11th World Congress of Sexology, Amsterdam.

5

PSYCHOSOCIAL CONSEQUENCES FOR TORTURED REFUGEES SEEKING ASYLUM AND REFUGEE STATUS IN EUROPE

Ron Baker

INTRODUCTION

In a range of generally informative material on refugees and situations that create them such as war, political instability and genocidal threat the special needs and experiences of the tortured refugee is rarely discussed (Vernant, 1953; Tabori, 1972; UNHCR, 1979; De Souza, 1981; Kuper, 1982; Simmonds, 1984; Harrell-Bond, 1984; Nettleton, 1989). This represents serious neglect of a substantial proportion of the world's refugees. Refugee statistics are notoriously unreliable. Much depends on the way they are collected, who collects them and whether they include or exclude forcibly uprooted people inside or outside their own country's boundaries. Legally speaking, a refugee can only be so defined when outside the country of origin (UN 1951, 1967), whilst the term 'internal displacement' refers to a person who feels forced to move but who stays within his or her own country. Current estimates of the world's refugee population is around fourteen million people of whom 95% are in the underprivileged world (Refugee Council, 1989). It is not known with any degree of accuracy how many of this number have been, and continue to be, tortured, though it can be said that all refugees will have intense feelings to cope with associated forced uprooting and loss (Crisp, 1990). Before discussing what may be called the 'triple trauma paradigm of the tortured refugee', a few cautionary comments about refugees in general seem warranted. First the term 'refugee' is in danger of being used as a stereotype. The image of a depressed, powerless, unskilled and poverty stricken person comes readily to mind and is often promoted by the media. Such a picture is both naive and usually untrue. The label 'refugee' really says nothing about how a particular person has reacted to forced migration. The way any individual copes with severe trauma and stress will be influenced by a range of factors including the family and community support that is available, the intensity of the trauma, its duration, the age, sex, personality and social class of the person, and the political, religious and cultural affiliations held. The point is that refugees can, in no way, be regarded as a homogeneous group. Very broadly speaking, what they have in common is the experience of forced uprooting, but their reactions to this are not necessarily similar or totally predictable. Some refugees have highly developed occupational skills, tertiary levels of training and education and given the smallest of chances will quickly demonstrate their ability to resettle positively and make a useful contribution as a new citizen in the host country. Others are, or become, depressed, lack the skills, training and intelligence to be able to make a quick adaption to a new and alien country, yet are no less committed to positive resettlement in time.

Secondly, it needs to be remembered that not every person who is forced to uproot is necessarily traumatized by the experience, though there is a strongly held view that the tortured refugee remains tortured, a view which warrants research. Experience of working with refugees suggests that some individuals grow through their traumas and as a consequence become more humane and maturer human beings. It is as if the experience has actually enabled the psychological and social self to gain in strength and the insights derived provide a base for a successful occupational and personal life (Movschenson, 1988; Gill, 1988). For some, creative writing becomes an important outlet to express strong feelings and to explore the complexities of being a survivor (Aberbach, 1989; Gershon, 1989). However, it is not known from Holocaust and other genocide survivors studies what proportion of survivors might be seen as 'successful' survivors. The danger of any stereotype is that it can take hold in negative ways influencing policy and relationships in a detrimental way. Keeping in mind these cautionary comments, generalizations can nevertheless be useful in promoting thought and in encouraging empathy for refugees in general, and tortured refugees in particular. What then of the tortured refugee? Some immediate and obvious questions come to mind. How many are there? Where do they come from? What is the long-term effect of being a refugee and a torture victim? How can they be assisted? Regrettably there are as yet no definitive answers to these questions. It is only in the last 10 years or so that serious and specific attention has been paid to this category of refugee and then primarily in the western world where in recent years refugees have been trying to enter in increasing numbers. Some tentative estimates of the numbers of tortured refugees there are can be derived from secondary source data. Amnesty International refers to almost 100 current governments that practise, support or turn a blind eye to state induced torture (AI, 1984). It is suggested that, in at least 63 of the world's nations, citizens are unable to freely and openly disagree with their own governments, though these figures may now need to be revised in the light of recent developments in Eastern Europe and Central America. Imprisonment, disappearance, torture or even death may result if they do. The World Human Rights Guide estimates the world's population around four billion people with only one-fifth of this number 'enjoying lives consistent with modern ideas of what constitutes human rights' (Humana, 1983). It is a sobering and chilling fact that only 800 million people, a privileged minority, can speak out without severe reprisals by their own governing body. Though it needs to be remembered that, even amongst this privileged minority, control and punishment of 'deviant' people can occur by governments and other power holders in overt and covert ways which may be acceptable to the majority, yet, in fact, is cruel, dehumanising and borders on torturous treatment, e.g. racist attacks on ethnic minorities, negative attitudes to homosexuals, conditions for prison inmates, etc. It becomes clearer then that the majority of tortured refugees come primarily from the 3.2 billion people in the Middle East, Latin America, Africa and Asia, and one can only hazard guesses as to the actual number who have been systematically and individually tortured in these regions. Even in the developed world, the percentage figure is likely to be inaccurate partly because the definition of torture varies in different countries and because it is well established that people who have been tortured are often reluctant to admit that they have had such an experience (Jepson, 1988). Nevertheless, some figures can be extrapolated from the information that is available. Drawing from the reports of 12 centres in western countries that specialize in assisting torture survivors, a range of 5% to 35% represents the number of tortured refugees of their total refugee population (Horvarth-Lindberg, 1988; Reid & Strong, 1987; Oasis, 1989). Using the lowest figure of 5% of the world's 14 million refugees, one arrives at a figure of 700,000 people who have been tortured. Based on 35%, 4.9 million people would have had single or multiple torture experiences. Whichever is the truer figure, there is no doubt that what we have here is an appalling yet neglected man-made human rights problem. The fact that it is only in the last decade or so that serious attention has been paid to it by way of research and specialist rehabilitative services is in itself a massive indictment of a practice that goes back into antiquity (Peters, 1985). There is no doubt that torture has been used throughout the ages to terrorize people and force them to conform to one ideology or another. Denial of this has led to a lack of serious concern about this practice until very recently. At last, however, a small number of committed clinical researchers have developed specialist centres for the assistance of victims of torture and trauma and their publications are now increasingly appearing in the professional care literature (Allodi, 1980, 1982; Genefke & Aalund, 1983; Mollica, 1987; Reid & Strong, 1987, 1988; Miserez, 1988; Landry, 1989; Viñar, 1989).

The approach taken in this chapter is psychosocial. That is, it is concerned with the complex interplay and the inextricable links between the inner world of feelings, values, assumptions and interpreted experiences and their effect on the external world of roles, relationships, ambitions and opinions. It is assumed therefore that the psychological, physical, social (and for some the spiritual) worlds of the individual constantly interpenetrate and influence each other in complex and not readily understood or researchable ways. Thus, refugee and torture experiences will affect the sense of identity, trust and security felt by the person which in turn will impact on roles of parent, spouse, employee, employer, citizen, etc. In turn, the obstacles and successes the individual meets in the environment will affect the psychological state, well-being and sense of identity being experienced. The psychosocial situation is dynamic with the present and past constantly intermingling and with shifts and changes evident in feelings and behaviour. To further understanding and insight into the world of the tortured refugee, a 'triple trauma paradigm' is offered in what follows. The exploration will focus on, in turn:

the nature of refugee experience and its long-term psychosocial implications;
the particular impact of torture on refugees; and
the further trauma of the tortured refugee who seeks asylum and refugee status in Western Europe, and in particular the UK.

A brief discussion of negative, adaptive and constructive survival behaviour following severe violence will end this chapter.

It needs to be acknowledged at the outset that most of the data drawn on here are derived from the published experience of assisting torture survivors in the western world (Schlapobersky & Bamber, 1988; Buus & Agger, 1988; Turner, 1989; Blackwell, 1990). In view of the fact that 95% of the world's refugees are in the underprivileged world such knowledge and expertise may be of only limited value to assisting tortured refugees elsewhere because of sociocultural, political, religious and economic differences. It also needs to be acknowledged that help systems have been developed within non-European oppressed communities which are reported on but rarely find their way into the western world's journals. Whatever the reason for this (problems with language, content, funding, racism, etc), such neglect leads to the lack of important information and editors should make intensive efforts to encourage the writing, translating and publishing of such material. With these qualifications in mind, it is hoped that the information and guiding principles that are emerging from torture assistance centres in the West will be a useful addition to the development of insights in helping torture survivors anywhere. At the very least, it can focus attention on a problem which power holders may not wish to acknowledge, where needed specialist services are virtually non-existent and stimulate concern and empathy for one of the most neglected and appalling human problems in the world today.

THE REFUGEE EXPERIENCE AND ITS LONG-TERM PSYCHOSOCIAL EFFECTS

The most significant emotional effect of being forcibly uprooted is the intense feeling of loss that is experienced. Elsewhere, the writer has described a relationship web which, in the normal course of events, constantly defines and confirms the individual as to who, where, and what he or she is (Baker, 1984, 1985). To be forcibly uprooted is to have this relationship web stripped away, an experience previously described as follows:

> Refugees are dominated by one feeling and that is a painful, traumatic and deep sense of loss. Loss of what is obvious and tangible and external such as possessions, a home, work, role, status, life style, a language, loved members of the family or other close relationships, and the loss that is less obvious, 'internal' and 'subjective' such as loss of trust in the self and others, loss of self esteem, self respect and personal identity (Baker, 1985).

Refugees themselves have vividly and frequently described how they felt following upheaval and this material provides important and valuable insight into the refugee experience (Munoz, 1980; Loizos, 1981; Hawthorne, 1982; Jonas, 1988; Gilad, 1989).

Students of the process of becoming a refugee seem agreed that a number of critical phases can be identified which usually (but not always) include a period of threat, the decision to flee, the flight itself, reaching a place of possible asylum, a phase when asylum and refugee status is sought and resettlement in the medium and long term (Baker, 1990). Each of these stages represents a potential crisis and trauma point much depending on how it is experienced, what support is available and the strength of the individual's coping capacities. We know very little about each of these phases apart from the testimonies of the refugees themselves. There is no comparative study or systematic analysis of how refugees in different refugee situations reacted to being uprooted and what generic elements, if any, can be identified. Why there is a lack of research on the refugee process cannot be explored here but warrants a book itself! What is worth reflecting on is that the apparent choice to flee, to decide to leave everything that has emotional, social, practical, cultural and perhaps spiritual significance is rarely a real choice at all. Usually, it is forced on a person by threatened or actual victimization, dehumanization or impending death either of oneself or one's loved ones. Thus it is in the service of survival that the person takes flight and the massive stress involved is for many a significant trauma in itself. The reality for refugees and those who assist them is captured by one writer in the following words:

> Most refugees have been exposed to violence one way or another. They or their families may have been victims of violence or they may have witnessed or heard about horrific events. Most of us who work with refugees have heard over and over again about terror, rape, physical abuse and other forms of humiliation. (Breyer, 1988).

A number of writers have likened the refugee experience and forced migration to a form of bereavement which has lifetime and intergenerational effects on the individual, the family and victim communities (Munoz, 1980; Baskuskias, 1981; Danieli, 1982; Davidson, 1985). There certainly seem to be strong connections and some similar emotional reactions which should be closely examined. Research into loss and mourning reactions has a long and well-established history. (Freud, 1917; Lindemann, 1944; Gorer, 1965; Kubler-Ross 1969; Marris, 1974; Robertson, 1971; Bowlby, 1980; Murray-Parkes, 1975; Raphael, 1984, 1986; Berger, 1988). From such research, much of it clinical but not exclusively so, we now know that it is important, for future healthy functioning of the person, to go through a mourning process. On average, this can take about two years and includes phases of shock, denial, bargaining, anger, grief, and eventually, re-integration. Let us now relate this process to the refugee experience. The reality is that he or she is likely to have been personally threatened or has experienced relatives and friends disappear, return as tortured people or be killed either in the country of origin or during flight. Frequently, the refugee was unable to protect the victim or intervene in any way for fear of being the next scapegoat to be picked on. Worse still, it is usually impossible to express normal emotional reactions of grief or anger because it may lead to exposure and personal danger. In consequence, the person is forced to dam up natural and powerful emotions, the expression of feelings becomes a threat to life itself and must be totally stifled. Vietnamese who have been raped and robbed by pirates on the South China Sea, and concentration camp inmates (Tu Khuong, 1988a, b; Bettelheim, 1980) are classic and horrendous examples of people caught in such harrowing emotional double bind situations. As such, they become powerless witnesses of appalling acts which can leave them angry, guilty and depressed for years. The emotional price paid for survival in such situations can be very high indeed. As one observer puts it:

> complete suppression of all negative emotional reactions was a
> necessary pre-requisite to survival (Sterba, 1967 p. 59).

We must ask what is the real cost of having to endure extreme acts of violence? What happens to the feelings of a person when they dare not be openly expressed? Clinical workers refer to the 'emotionally frozen' personality caught in a straightjacket of powerful and paralysing emotions. The inability to mourn appropriately is technically referred to as a delayed mourning reaction (Lindemann, 1944; Meerloo, 1967; Raphael, 1984) and the experience of working with refugees suggests that many are in such a state. Typically, they are 'locked' into the anger and grief stages of the process. The result is that they are either totally unable to express their feelings (often rationalized on the grounds that it would hurt others too much) or they are chronically depressed and angry. Either way, they find no relief or resolution to their emotional 'stuckness' with these forms of defensive coping. The result is that they are hindered in getting on with their lives effectively. They underfunction in a range of social roles and remain chronically unhappy and unfulfilled. Such defensive coping will be discussed further when different forms of survival are explored.

To summarize this section, the refugee experience represents for many (but not all) a range of traumatic losses of roots, culture, home, family, friends, role, status, language, religion, etc. In addition, threatened or experienced violence either before flight or during it compounds the trauma. If normal mourning processes cannot occur, the likelihood of a delayed mourning reaction taking hold is considerable. Experience of assisting refugees suggests that such a situation is quite common. When this happens, the person can remain in a state of anger and repressed grief for many years and the psychosocial effects are usually obvious. The person will be unable to function adequately as a parent, spouse, employee, employer and citizen and he or she is likely to experience a series of strained relationships. In addition, the degree of vulnerability to mental illness is significantly increased when compared with the general non-refugee population (Hitch & Rack, 1980; Eitinger, 1983).

THE TRAUMA OF THE TORTURED REFUGEE

Refugees are people who have survived intolerance, persecution, torture and fear of death (British Refugee Council, 1990).

The history of torture goes back into antiquity (Van Geuns, 1983; Peters, 1985). Its ultimate form is perhaps seen in genocide which takes the form of state organized murder of millions of people, and, 'a crime committed, encouraged and tolerated by heads of state' (Fein, 1979). Minority groups are the inevitable scapegoats and are at the receiving end of genocidal attacks (Kuper, 1981; Charny 1982, 1988). The most infamous examples of genocide in the twentieth century are the attacks mounted by German Nazis against European Jewry as well as on Gypsies, the Turkish genocide of the Armenians, the Pol Pot regime's murder of Cambodians and Stalin's annihilation of the Kulaks. Inevitably, torture and, by extension, the threatened or actual destruction of the family and community the person belonged to has been used to strike terror into people. Total control and dehumanization is the intended outcome. Despite the 1975 UN convention against the use of torture Amnesty International claims that its use is steadily increasing with over one-third of the world's countries engaged in it. It is therefore practised by some of the countries that are actually signatories to the convention – a nauseating contradiction! To acquaint oneself with the literature of torture is to enter a world of appalling inhumanity by the perpetrators and unbelievable suffering and courage among its victims. Personal and very poignant testimonies abound (Lengyel, 1972; Amnesty International, 1977; Leitner, 1978; Friedlander, 1980; Hart, 1981; Wiesel, 1981; Kielar, 1982; Bitton Jackson, 1984; Hillesum, 1985; Foster, 1986; Poltawska, 1987; Levi, 1987, 1988; Gill, 1988; Cohen, 1988; Pin Yathay, 1989). Again we are left with many relatively unresearched and unanswered questions. How does the personality survive such dreadful experiences; to what extent is the victim of torture psychologically scarred and crippled; what are the effects on family and other close relationships; is physical and psychological torture equally damaging or damaging in different ways; how are 'minority' communities affected when a number of its members have been tortured? Obviously, this is but a selection of important questions. Research done so far does provide some beginning insights and answers but it is not definitive. Essentially, information is gathered from victims seen in clinical settings. They are in a sense accidental and self-selected populations. It is well known that many people who have been subjected to torture do not readily speak about their experiences. The reasons seem to be many and varied; denial of their reality, guilt, fear of being labelled 'different' or 'ill', repression, use of the rationalisation that it would be too painful for others to hear, etc. The people who are not prepared to speak may represent a 'silent majority' and it needs to be kept in mind that the following summary of research-based data may only be partly or not at all relevant to them.

People who experienced violence in prisoner of war or concentration camps, or who have had refugee experience, are at greater psychiatric risk than the general population, particularly as they get older (Eitinger, 1983; Daly, 1983; Hitch & Rack, 1980).

Delayed psychological responses to torture are being confirmed by clinical researchers in various countries (Niederland, 1968; Harding, 1983; Abildgaard *et al.*, 1984; Allodi *et al.*, 1985; Cowgill & Doupe, 1985; Petersen & Jacobson, 1985; Reid & Strong, 1987).

Torture survivors can have difficulty in establishing satisfactory relationships with their children and transmit their problems of maladaptation to their offspring. The home is typically a depressive place where physical health is a constant preoccupation, where the independence of the growing child particularly in adolescence is interpreted as betrayal, where privacy is given little priority and where children are taught to mistrust others (Eitinger, 1983; Harding, 1983; Reid & Strong 1987; Horvath-Lindberg & Movschenson, 1988).

There are symptoms identifiable after different forms of organized violence (e.g. torture, rape, mugging, concentration camp, etc). All these symptoms (or perhaps more correctly termed behavioural reactions as the survivor is not 'ill' but having a 'normal' reaction to an abnormal experience), correspond closely to the post-traumatic stress syndrome. Some researchers claim that specific sequelae can be identified in those who have experienced torture (see discussion on this in

Reid & Strong, 1987, pp. 66–8) but others argue that the
differences seen reflect difference in personality, type and
intensity of the violence, the events associated with it and the
support available to the victim after the event.

A most thorough review of the western literature has been
undertaken by two Australian researchers, Reid and Strong
(1987, 1988), who analysed the publications of the twelve
rehabilitation centres in Western Europe and North America.
They conclude with the heartening comment that torturers
may inflict serious damage but they do not achieve their
ultimate goals and never destroy the person's identity totally.

Drawing from Reid and Strong's excellent work, several studies
are cited which suggest that as many as 90% of torture victims
do suffer from chronic psychological symptoms such as
emotional instability, depression, passivity, fatigue and disturbed sleep (Reid & Strong, 1987). What all these data clearly
point to is that for the majority of victims, torture leaves an
indelible and traumatic psychological mark in the long term.

To summarize this section, the experience of torture is the second
major trauma which is superimposed on to the refugee experience
itself. Massive loss has to be coped with along with what has been
described as 'paradoxical' or 'survivor's guilt' (Lifton, 1968). This takes
the form of an unanswerable question, 'why have I survived when so
many others have perished?' In the long term, clinical research
suggests that the majority of survivors have a range of physical and
psychological 'symptoms' which may be linked to the severe trauma
they have experienced or be complicated by the psychological state of
the person prior to becoming a survivor, collectively known as the
post-traumatic stress syndrome. Helpers of victims of torture have
observed that they can remain relatively 'symptom free' for months or
years during which time painful feelings can be denied or repressed.
However this can represent a trap for both the tortured refugee and
those who provide assistance. Asylum and refugee status is sought in
this 'symptom-free interval' and much energy is expended in achieving satisfactory initial resettlement if it is granted. It is all too easy to
assume that because there are no obvious symptoms there are no
psychological problems. These are likely to emerge in the medium and
long term when the relationship web has been partially re-spun, and
resettlement seems to have been achieved. Let me now move to the
third group of traumas that the tortured refugee will experience as
asylum and refugee status is sought.

THE TRAUMA OF THE TORTURED PERSON SEEKING REFUGEE STATUS IN W. EUROPE AND IN PARTICULAR IN THE UK

The task of achieving refugee status in what is called the pre-asylum period is a tortuous process in itself. The asylum seeker has to convince immigration officials that he or she is a genuine refugee with a well-founded fear of persecution. Beyond this, paperwork, interviews and negotiations with government departments are necessary for the request of refugee status to be formally considered. At the very minimum, it is a process of intense stress, involving physical, political, economic, psychological and cultural change (Berry, 1988). In recent years, the popularity of refugees has plummeted across Western Europe. Previously, applicants for refugee status were dealt with compassionately and more humanely. There was ready acceptance that they were victims of oppression and injustice. Today, alongside supposed economic instability in host countries, 'foreigners' are viewed with suspicion and they can be rejected in very insensitive ways. (Taviani, 1988; Exile, 1990a) With the advent in European political and economic union by 1992 a reappraisal as to who has the right of entry is actively under way. It has become clear that 'a clamping down', which is actively working against asylum seekers, is occurring in what has come to be called a fortress mentality in Europe. In practical terms, this can take the form of major obstacles and long delays when visas are sought in countries of persecution. On arrival in a potential country of asylum, the refugee has to prove his or her credibility with untrained immigration officials who are more concerned with how travel documents were secured than the reasons for taking flight. Further, they have to deal with an impersonal bureaucracy (the Home Office in the UK) and with sympathetic and well-motivated but chronically under-resourced non-government helpers (Shaw, 1988). Asylum seekers are interviewed, usually immediately on arrival, when they are tired, frightened and often confused. If they do not speak the language of the host country, there is the added complication of lack of properly trained interpreters. The whole situation is fraught and weighted against the asylum seeker. It is estimated that, by 1986, the refugee population in Europe reached 200 000, having tripled since 1983. Of this number, 50% have come from Asia with the rest predominantly from Africa and Latin America (Andreassen, 1988). Five strategies have been identified as being used increasingly to discourage refuges coming to Europe in the last five years.

1 Detention on arrival and severely limiting the right to work in the pre-asylum period. Minimal social benefits. Inhospitable group accommodation. No provision of advisory and counselling services.

2 Strict entry criteria. Immigration officials' refusal to allow asylum seeker in with no time given to appeal and no right of appeal against rejection.

3 Very tough visa requirements. Legal and economic sanctions against carriers of refugees who do not have the correct documentation.

4 Rigid application of the concept of the 'country of first asylum' which is used as a deterrent. Thus a country may refuse entry because the refugee came through another one which strictly speaking was the first country of asylum. The result is that the refugee is pushed out and becomes what has been called the 'orbit refugee' – a person constantly in flight whom no country will now accept.

5 Extremely tough procedures for determining refugee status. Can one imagine a scenario that could be much worse for the asylum seeker who has been tortured? He or she has been oppressed and brutalized. Flight is seen as the only road to physical and perhaps psychological survival. There may be little time to apply formally for a visa. There is also justifiable and deep mistrust of government departments and officials. How is such a person supposed to get the necessary papers quickly? Waiting or making a formal approach may mean drawing attention to oneself, arrest, further torture or even death. The psychological state of such a person, on reaching a place of possible asylum faced with the above, can be imagined readily! Depression, anger directed to officials, property or the self by way of suicide is not uncommon. To illustrate:

> 'Two Kurdish refugees who had been on hunger strike and faced deportation orders set fire yesterday to their room in a detention centre at Harmondsworth near Heathrow Airport. The two men in their twenties were described as suffering 20–30% burns to their bodies after breaking a window and climbing out of the blazing room ... the Home Office said they had been called into the detention centre [last] Wednesday, told they would be refused permission to stay in the country and then

detained.' A local counsellor who witnessed the above is reported as saying 'I believe these men would rather die than go back and live under persecution and torture in Turkey' (Bowcott, 1989).

A 22 year old Somalian jumped from a second floor window and killed himself having become lonely and depressed after being unable to find accommodation near the Somali London community (Exile, 1990b), and the inquiry into the circumstances of the Ugandan refugee who hanged himself in Pentonville Prison after being refused refugee status was 'suicide aggravated by official indifference and lack of care'.

One of the most articulate and knowledgeable voices on the precarious plight of asylum and refugee status seekers in Europe is that of Rudge, Secretary of the European Consultation on Refugees and Exiles (Rudge, 1988). He points to the discrepancy that exists between impressive national legislation which incorporates internationally accepted human rights principles and the denial of asylum to obvious victims of persecution and torture. This gap between accepted principle and what actually happens has widened significantly in recent years. Even if asylum is granted, which can take an average of 12 months, the mechanism of 'exceptional leave to remain' rather than refugee status is increasingly granted (Nettleton, 1989). In the UK, this is reviewed annually and if it is judged that the circumstances have improved in the country the refugee comes from he/she will be expected to return there. During the pre-asylum period the refugee is in a kind of economic, practical and social no-man's land, not deported but not allowed to work and denied the kind of assistance (accommodation, money, etc) which is desperately needed. The ongoing anxiety of knowing that if 'exceptional leave to remain' is granted it may be withdrawn at the end of the year increases insecurity and stress. Rudge draws attention to other important gaps and practices which work against asylum, and refugee status seekers. All Western European countries are signatories to the European Convention for the Protection of Human Rights and Fundamental Freedoms within the Asylum Policies of European States and the UN 1951 Convention and the 1967 Protocol on refugees. These statutes lay down refugee rights but there is nothing about the procedures which countries should use to determine refugee status. As Rudge points out, in reality, the 21 countries making up Western Europe have different attitudes to refugees and 'in principle each country is free to create its own procedures', despite advice and guidance by the UN High Commissioner for Refugees (UNHCR, 1979). The situation is rich in the potential for different interpretations. What represents human treatment is not standardized. This leaves refugees exposed, vulnerable and powerless which must affect their physical and mental health. What Rudge goes on to observe is that the deterrent policies do not actually reduce the total number of refugees but, because they are used indiscriminantly, they increase the misery and insecurity of the asylum seeker. Plans and policies are already far advanced to harmonize asylum seekers. Plans and policies are already far advanced to harmonize asylum law in the 12 member states of the EEC (see the Schengen treaty and Exile 1990c) but there is no effort whatsoever to standardize reception, assistance and resettlement approaches (ECRE, 1988, 1989). Negotiations and discussions have occurred and policies agreed behind the scenes by ministers and civil servants. Government representatives make decisions without others being involved in a democratic process. 'Under these circumstances, a public debate amongst well-informed people is not possible' (ECRE, 1988, p. 4). Where, it is asked:

> are the European standards which would prohibit prolonged detention in humiliating prison-like conditions, reduce excessive length of time it takes to determine refugee status, ensure adequate psychosocial as well as legal counselling services, ensure respect for deeply held cultural or religious principles, maintain the integrity of the family and bring about reunification of children with parents and partners with each other (Rudge, 1988, p. 66).

Rudge goes on to raise further significant and important questions: is there, he asks, 'growing racism and discrimination in the way we treat asylum seekers from non-European countries?' And why is there no charter of rights for people in the pre-asylum period? Why are there no counselling services for people whose application is rejected either to assist in their return home or to another possible host country? Should we not be developing laws that stop the criminalization of the asylum seeker? Why is there no appeal process to review and prevent errors of official judgement, and, perhaps most important of all, why is there such antagonism when there is incomplete documentation and an acknowledgement of the painful realities of the reasons for flight? These questions demand answers from privileged host countries! It all adds up to a very disturbing situation and creates a context for the asylum seeker in which physical and mental health is severely threatened. Article 5 of the UN Declaration of Human Rights states, 'no one shall be subjected to torture or to cruel inhuman or degrading treatment or punishment' (see also Brownlie, 1981, on 'The European convention on Human Rights'). It does not require too much stretch of the imagination to suggest that current ways in which asylum and refugee status seekers are handled border on what is inhuman and degrading, and constitute a breach of Article 5. For many, it is a form of torture in its own right! In view of this, it is surprising that no real criticism has been expressed by the international community or the United Nations towards these United Kingdom policies and practices.

The above then represent the 'triple trauma paradigm' of the tortured refugee. How does anyone survive such an experience? What is the psychosocial price of survival and are there different types of survival that can be identified? These are complex questions which I have found myself struggling with for a number of years. Different facets of survival following extreme experiences have captured the interest of a few researchers. Some have explored human survival in the nuclear age (Huddle, 1984), or the nature of survival following concentration camp experience (Gill, 1988), and others the long-term effects on personality following organized violence in one form or another (Krystal, 1968; Lifton, 1968, Amnesty International, 1977; Eitinger 1980; Dimsdale, 1980; Frederick, 1983; Davidson, 1985; Cohen, 1988; Turner, 1989). The following notes draw primarily from the last mentioned material and from my own experience of providing therapeutic counselling to people who continue to suffer long-term emotional disturbance and severe trauma following genocide, holocaust, refugee and torture experience.

NOTES ON LONG-TERM SURVIVAL PATTERNS OF BEHAVIOUR FOLLOWING THE EXPERIENCE OF ORGANIZED VIOLENCE: SOME TENTATIVE FORMULATIONS

Frederick (1983) has attempted to delineate distinguishing reactions following human and natural disaster. The long-term effect of human violence he suggests are depression, paranoid reactions, withdrawal and isolation, phobias, alcoholism and drug abuse. Daly (1983) finds 'a high level of physical and psychiatric morbidity which appeared to worsen over the years ... and a very high mortality rate of severely tortured people' (Daly, p. 63). Much of the writing on long-term effects has been done by clinical workers such as psychiatrists and clinical psychologists with the inevitable emphasis on identifying the link between psychiatric morbidity and torture and approaching the issue of rehabilitation from a pathology perspective. I would argue that victims of organized violence are not necessarily psychiatric cases though they may become so because of their experiences or their pre-torture personalities. Some survivors appear to recover 'spontaneously' though it is unclear what accounts for this or what the percentage might be. Yet another area in which research is needed! Crucial to the question of what kind of assistance should be available is skilled assessment with perhaps the determining factors being the excessively long time severely disturbed behaviour is evident and the nature of this. The trap for anyone involved is to take extreme positions of either: a) assuming that all tortured refugees require specialist psychiatric and clinical help, or b) that only initial advice, guidance and practical resources are needed to ensure satisfactory coping and resettlement. These are not 'either' 'or' options, both should be available and offered, based on ongoing assessment and need. My experience suggests that the struggle to adapt and resettle may be seen in some typical and repeating patterns of behaviour. Some of these behaviours serve the individual's psychosocial functioning whilst others do not. If there is a key task for the tortured refugee to undertake (and those who provide assistance if this proves necessary), it is to achieve constructive rather than adaptive or negative forms of coping reactions. This would seem to be the only genuine path to mental health in the long run. What I have found useful in therapeutic counselling of victims of organized violence are the conceptual tools of negative, adaptive and constructive survival. I share these ideas with readers cautiously, knowing they require further research and development or rejection if they prove to be unhelpful.

NEGATIVE SURVIVAL PATTERNS

The word 'negative' requires immediate qualification. Obviously, anything that enables a person to continue to eat, breath, sleep, etc, is positive for that person. By negative, I refer to the personal and social behaviour which restricts the individual and inhibits social functioning. Such behaviour locks the torture victim into the negative components of the trauma. Typically, it is reflected in extreme egotism with the experience colouring virtually every aspect of the person's life. The trauma may be held on to and constantly used to arouse sympathy, perhaps money or even 'fame'. Such a person can readily become a 'survivor bore'. Defensive coping is usually evident and seen in a range of behaviour. These include excessive talking about the experience, or making it a taboo subject never to be talked about. In the latter situation, those closely related to the survivor are aware of his/her suffering, a 'martyr' role may be adopted, but they have no clear idea what the person went through and therefore feel they cannot respond appropriately. Omnipotent and arrogant behaviour might also be to the fore with the message 'I survived and nothing that anyone says or does now can touch me'. I have also seen excessively obsequious behaviour, or the alternative of extreme aggression in personal relationships at home and/or work. These 'strategies', not on the whole consciously employed, neither dull nor relieve the emotional pain they are rooted to. As a result, virtually all relationships become severely strained and the person is left increasingly alone. The survivor suffers more hurt but is unable to draw lessons from the trauma nor has any insight into the link between past trauma and present functioning. Often s/he remains in the painful grip of the survivor syndrome with psychic numbing, flashbacks during the day or in dreams at night, guilt and mistrust constant and deeply troubling. Experience suggests that only skilled and intensive therapeutic counselling is likely to effect any kind of genuine change.

ADAPTIVE SURVIVAL PATTERNS

On first impressions, the adaptive survivor appears to have made a sound adjustment both personally and occupationally. Closer examination will reveal however the adaption is still essentially egocentric and self-serving. Real effort is made to respin the relationship web, but basically to re-create everything as closely as possible to what was lost. Numerous examples illustrate this. The way Irish and Chinese people settle around the world, the re-creation of the 'stetl' in New York or London by the Central European Jew, the West Indian, Pakistani and Chilean communities in the UK who are determined to reconstruct the lost world in the present one so that children can be wholly indoctrinated and socialized into it. Usually it is rationalized on the grounds of protection of the culture. Such adaption involves little thinking, acting or feeling beyond the trauma the individual, family or community experienced. Few questions are asked about why the victimization occurred and the part those who have suffered may have played in it, either consciously or unconsciously. What one sees is enormous energy being expended on anything to do with their own group via fund-raising, or massive concern when something happens in the country of origin. However, this concern is not apparent when other minority groups are being oppressed. Disinterest, silence and minimal involvement is the typical response. So, what one sees is an

apparently well-adjusted and successful person in personal and occupational roles but someone who has not been able to use their
traumatic experiences to develop general principles of sound human
relationships or a commitment to universal human rights. Nor have
universal empathies emerged for others being dehumanized and
disadvantaged. Few lessons are learned or taught to the next generation, beyond how to 'look after your own!'.

CONSTRUCTIVE SURVIVAL PATTERNS

As the term 'constructive' implies, this kind of survival response draws
lessons and insights from the trauma which positively serve the
person in all relationships. The individual is neither stuck in, nor
constrained by past painful experiences. Such people 'worked
through' their traumas and, as a result, develop deep levels of sensitivity, compassion, as well as remarkable understanding and empathy
for the human condition (Wiesel, 1981; Levi, 1987, 1989). This does not
mean that they 'forget' or repress their trauma. Rather, they use it to
learn and to teach the inhumanity that human beings can all be party
to in certain circumstances. Such survivors are genuinely in touch with
themselves and the realities of the external world. They tend to
become socially involved in many ways, depending on temperament,
through creative writing, art or direct political involvement. Constructive survivors may be described as 'other directed' people and they are
often found as active members of human rights organizations such as
Amnesty International and Greenpeace. They fit the description of
mental health as someone 'who is functioning at a high level of
behavioural and emotional adjustment and adaptiveness' (Reber, 1985,
p. 434). The fundamental difference between negative, adaptive and
constructive survival is that the individual uses his or her traumatic
experiences in ways that are not primarily defensive or self-seeking.
They seek to build bridges rather than put up barriers between
themselves and others whether they belong to their own group or not.
They are not in the paralysing grip of the survivor syndrome, or suffer
from the guilt of survival, or the constant need to find or justify their
existence. Obviously, there are no ideal types and these categories are
not mutually exclusive. Any survivor may demonstrate elements of all
the patterns of behaviour at different times. But the overall goal for
both survivor and helper is to achieve as near as possible a state of
constructive survival. This is the path to a fully functioning and
satisfying life as well as mental health. As one constructive survivor
beautifully puts it 'it is not just survival but the quality of survival that

is important: the question is did we survive without abandoning a sense of morality, ethics, humanity? If we survived by jettisoning that sense, one didn't survive at all' (Gill, 1988, p. 389).

SUMMARY

This chapter has explored a 'triple trauma paradigm' which the tortured refugee struggles to master as he or she seeks asylum and refugee status in another country. Anyone working with tortured refugees should have a thorough understanding of the refugee process and the significant losses associated with forced uprooting, as well as the psychosocial effects of torture and the present procedural and socio-political barriers facing refugees in Europe.

From his experience of therapeutic counselling with survivors, the writer has become aware of the three repeating behavioural coping patterns. These are tentatively described as negative, adaptive and constructive forms of survival in the long term. They have been found useful to the author in practice and now require further development and systematic research.

REFERENCES

Aberbach, D. (1989). Creativity and the survivor: the struggle for mastery. *International Review of Psychoanalysis*, **16**, 273–86.

Abildgaard, U., Daugaard, G., Marcusson, H. M., Jess, P., Petersen, H. D. & Wallach, M. (1984). Chronic organic psycho-syndrome in Greek torture victims. *Danish Medical Bulletin*, **31**, 229–32.

Allodi, F. (1980). The psychiatric effects of political persecution and torture in children and families of victims. *Danish Medical Bulletin*, **27**, 229–32.

Allodi, F. (1982). Psychiatric sequelae of torture and implications for treatment, *World Medical Journal*, **29**, 71–5.

Allodi, F., Randall, G. R., Lutz, E. L., Quiroga, J., Zunzunegui, M. V., Kolf, C. A., Deutsch, A. & Doan, R. (1985). Physical and psychiatric effects of torture. In *The Breaking of Bodies and Minds: Torture Psychiatric Abuse and the Health Professions*. E. Stover & E. O. Nightingale, eds., New York: Freeman & Co.

Amnesty International (1977). *Torture in Greece: The First Torturers' Trial 1975*. London: Amnesty International Publications.

Amnesty International (1984). *Torture in the Eighties*. London: Amnesty International and Robertson.

Amnesty International (1987). *Amnesty International Report*. London: Amnesty International Publications.

Andreassen, D. (1988). Refugees and asylum seekers coming to Europe today. In *Refugees – The Trauma of Exile*. D. Miserez, ed. Dordrecht: Martinus Nijhoff.

Baker, R. (1984). Parentless refugee children: the question of adoption. In *Adoption Essays in Social Policy, Law and Sociology*. P. Bean, ed. London: Tavistock.

Baker, R. (1985). *The Psychosocial Problems of Refugees*. London: British Refugee Council/European Consultation on Refugees & Exiles.

Baker, R. (1990). The refugee experience: communication and stress. *Journal of Refugee Studies*, **3**, (1).

Baskuskias, L. (1981). The Lithuanian refugee experience and grief, *International Migration Review*, **15**, (1), 276–91.

Berger, R. (1988). Learning to survive and cope with human loss, *Social Work Today*. 28 April.

Berry, J. W. (1988). Acculturation and psychological adaption among refugees. In *Refugees – The Trauma of Exile*. D. Miserez, ed., Dordrecht: Martinus Nijhoff.

Bettelheim, B. (1980). *Surviving and Other Essays*. New York: Vintage Books.

Bitton Jackson, L. E. (1984). *Elli*. London: Panther.

Blackwell, D. (1990). *Testimony and Psychotherapy, Refugee Participation Network*, 7 February, Oxford: Refugee Studies Programme.

Bowcott, O. (1989). Kurds set fire to their room in detention centre protest, *Guardian* 6 October.

Bowlby, J. (1980). Loss: sadness and depression. In *Attachment and Loss*, vol. 3, London: Hogarth Press.

Breyer (1988). Living in a vacuum: psychological problems of refugees and asylum seekers. In *Refugees – The Trauma of Exile*. D. Miserez, ed., Dordrecht: Martinus Nijhoff.

British Refugee Council (1990). Major Statement in Appeals Leaflet, 3 January.

Brownlie, I. (ed.) (1981). European institutions and conventions. In *Basic Documents of Human Rights*, pp. 242–320, Oxford: Clarendon Press.

Buus, S. & Agger, I. (1988). The testimony method: the use of therapy as a psychotherapeutic tool. In *The Treatment of Traumatised Refugees in Denmark*, Refugee Participation Network: 3 November, Oxford: Refugee Studies Programme.

Charny, I. (1982). *How Can We Commit The Unthinkable: Genocide: The Human Cancer*. Boulder: Westview Press.

Charny, I. (ed.) (1988). *Genocide: A Critical Bibliographic Review*. London: Mansell.

Cohen, E. A. (1988). *Human Behaviour in the Concentration Camp*. London: F. A. Books.

Cowgill, G. & Doupe, G. (1985). Recognising and helping victims of torture, *Canadian Nurse*, **81**, (11) 14–22.

Crisp, J. (1990). Caring in the community, refugees, **74**, April, *United Nations High Commissioner for Refugees, Geneva, Switzerland*.

Daly, R. J. (1983). Torture and other forms of inhuman and degrading treatment. In *Helping Victims of Violence*. Proceedings of a Working Group on the Psychosocial Consequences of Violence, Holland, Ministry of Health and Cultural Affairs, Government Publication Office, The Hague.

Danieli, Y. (1982). *Families of Survivors, in Stress and Anxiety.* S. Milgram, ed. pp. 405–21, New York: Hemisphere.

Davidson, S. (1985). The psychosocial aspects of Holocaust trauma in the life cycle of survivor refugees and their families. In *The Psychosocial Problems of Refugees.* R. Baker, ed., British Refugee Council/European Consultation on Refugees and Exiles.

De Souza, F. (1981). *The Refugee Dilemma.* **43**, London: Minority Rights Group.

Dimsdale, J. E. (ed.) (1980). *Survivors, Victims and Perpetrators: Essays on the Nazi Holocaust,* Washington: Hemisphere.

Eitinger, L. (1980). The concentration camp syndrome and its late sequelae. In *Survivors, Victims and Perpetrators.* J. Dimsdale, ed. Washington: Hemisphere Pub. Co.

Eitinger, L. (1981). Feeling at home: immigrants' psychological problems. In *Strangers in the World.* L. Eitinger & D. Schwarz, eds., Bern: Hans Huber.

Eitinger, L. (1983). *Psychological Consequences of War – Disturbances in Helping Victims of Violence.* The Hague, Holland: Government Publishing Office.

European Consultation on Refugees and Exiles (1988). *Towards Harmonisation of Refugee Policies in Europe?* A Contribution to the Discussion, London.

European Consultation on Refugees and Exiles (1989). Refugee Policy in a Unifying Europe. Report on Seminar held in Zeist, Holland. 5th–7th April 1989.

Exile (1990a). Better image needed. *The Refugee Council Newsletter,* February, No. 36.

Exile (1990b). Housing, a factor in suicide. *The Refugee Council Newsletter,* March, No. 37.

Exile (1990c). The common barrier. *The Refugee Council Newsletter,* June, No. 40.

Fein, H. (1979). *Accounting for Genocide.* New York: Free Press.

Foster, J. (1986). *Community of Fate.* Australia: Allen & Unwin.

Frederick, C. J. (1983). Violence and disaster: immediate and long term consequences. In *Helping Victims of Violence.* The Hague, Holland: Government Publishing Office.

Freud, S. (1917). Mourning and meloncholia. In *Sigmund Freud: Collected Papers,* vol. 4, New York: Basic Books.

Friedlander, S. (1980). *When Memory Comes.* New York: Discuss Books.

Genefke, I. K. & Aalund, O. (1983). Rehabilitation of torture victims, – research perspectives, *Manedsskrift for Praktish Laegegerning,* January.

Gershon, K. (1989). *We Came As Children.* London: Papermac.

Gilad, L. (1989). A Baha'i refugee story, *Journal of Refugee Studies,* **2**, 276–83.

Gill, A. (1988). *The Journey Back from Hell.* London: Grafton Books.

Gorer, G. (1965). *Death, Grief and Mourning in Contemporary Britain.* London: Cresset Press.

Harding, T. (1983). Summary and recommendations of the WHO Working Group on the psychosocial consequences of violence. In *Helping Victims of Violence,* pp. 61–69, The Hague, Holland: Government Publishing Office.

Harrell-Bond, B. (1984). *Imposing Aid: Emergency Assistance to Refugees.* Oxford: Oxford University Press.

Hart, K. (1981). *Return to Auschwitz*. London: Granada.

Hawthorne, L. (ed.) (1982). *Refugee: The Vietnamese Experience*, Melbourne: Oxford University Press.

Hillesum, E. (1985). *Etty*. London: Triad/Panther.

Hitch, P. & Rack, P. (1980). Mental illness among Polish and Russian refugees in Bradford. *British Journal of Psychiatry*, **37** (3), 206–11.

Horvath-Lindberg, J. (1988). Victims of torture – the Swedish experience. In *Refugees – The Trauma of Exile*. D. Miserez,. ed., Dordrecht: Martinus Nijhoff.

Huddle, N. (1984). *Surviving*. New York: Schoken Books.

Humana, C. (1983). *World Human Rights Guide*. London: Hutchinson.

Jepson, S. (1988). The general health of asylum seekers. In *Refugees – The Trauma of Exile*. D. Miserez, ed., Dordrecht: Martinus Nijhoff.

Jonas, M. (1988). An interview with Nuruddin Farah. *Journal of Refugee Studies*, **1** (1), 74.

Kielar, W. (1982). *Annus Mundi*. London: Penguin.

Keller, S. (1975). *Uprooting and Social Change*, Delhi: Manohar Book Service.

Krystal, H. (ed.) (1968). *Massive Psychic Trauma*. New York: International University Press.

Kubler-Ross, E. (1969). *On Death and Dying*. London: Tavistock.

Kuper, L. (1981). *Genocide*. London: Pelican.

Kuper, L. (1982). International action against genocide, *Minority Rights Group*, Report No. 53.

Landry, C. (1989). Psychotherapy with victims of organised violence: an overview, *British Journal of Psychotherapy*, **5**, (3), 349.

Leitner, I. (1978). *Fragments of Isabella*. London: New English Library.

Lengyel, O. (1972). *Five Chimneys*, London: Panther.

Levi, P. (1987). *If Not Now, When?* London: Sphere Books.

Levi, P. (1989). *The Drowned and The Saved*. London: Sphere Books.

Lifton, R. J. (1968). The survivors of the Hiroshima disaster and the survivors of Nazi persecution. In *Massive Psychic Trauma*, H. Krystal, ed. 168–201, New York: International Univesity Press.

Lindemann, E. (1944). Symptomatology and management of acute grief. *American Journal of Psychiatry*, **101**, 141–8.

Loizos, P. (1981). *The Heart Grown Bitter*. London: Cambridge University Press.

Marris, P. (1974). (Revised 1986) *Loss and Change*, Routledge: Kegan Paul.

Meerloo, J. A. M. (1967). Delayed mourning in victims of extermination camps. In *Massive Psychic Trauma*. H. Krystal, ed., pp. 8–22, New York: International University Press.

Miserez, D. (ed.) (1988). *Refugees – The Trauma of Exile*. Dordrecht: Martinus Nijhoff.

Mollica, R. F. (1987). The trauma story: the psychiatric care of refugee survivors of violence and torture. In *Post-Traumatic Therapy and Victims of Violence*. F. M. Ochberg, ed., New York: Brunner/Mazel.

Movschenson, P. (1988). Torture intends to destroy. In *Refugees – The Trauma of Exile* D. Miserez, ed. Dordrecht: Martinus Nijhoff.

Munoz, L. (1980). Exile as bereavement: social-psychological manifestations of Chilean exiles in Great Britain. *British Journal of Medical Psychology,* **53,** 227–32.

Murray-Parkes, C. (1975). *Bereavement: Studies of Grief in Adult Life,* Pelican.

Nettleton, C. (1989). Asylum seekers in the United Kingdom, essential statistics. London: British Refugee Council.

Niederland, W. G. (1968). 'The problem of the survivor' pp. 8–22. An interpretation of the psychological stresses and defenses in concentration-camplife and the late after effects pp. 51–60. In *Massive Psychic Trauma,* H. Krystal, ed., New York: International University Press.

Oasis (1989). *First One and a half years: A Report 1987–88,* Copenhagen, Denmark.

Peters, E. (1985). *Torture,* Oxford: Blackwell.

Petersen, H. D. & Jacobsen, P. (1985). Psychical and physical symptoms after torture. A prospective controlled study, *Forensic Science International* **29,** 179–89.

Poltawska, W. (1987). *And I am Afraid of My Dreams.* London: Hodder & Stoughton.

Raphael, B. (1984). *The Anatomy of Bereavement.* London: Hutchinson.

Raphael, B. (1986) *When Disaster Strikes.* London: Hutchinson.

Reber, A. S. (1985). *Dictionary of Psychology.* London: Penguin.

The Refugee Council (1989). *Annual Report, London.* British Refugee Council Publication.

Reid, J. & Strong, T. (1987) *Torture and Trauma: The Health Care Needs of Refugee Victims in New South Wales,* Sydney, Australia: Cumberland College of Health Sciences.

Reid, J. & Strong, T. (1988). Rehabilitation of refugee victims of torture and trauma. principles and service provision in New South Wales, *Medical Journal of Australia,* **148,** 4 April.

Robertson, J. (1971). Young children in brief separation: a fresh look. *Psychoanalytic Study of the Child,* **8,** 288–309.

Rudge, P. (1988). Reflections on the status of refugees and asylum seekers in Europe. In *Refugees – The Trauma of Exile.* D. Miserez, ed., Dordrecht: Martinus Nijhoff.

Schlapobersky, J. & Bamber, H. (1988). Rehabilitation work with victims of torture. In *Refugees – The Trauma of Exile.* D. Miserez, ed., Dordrecht: Martinus Nijhoff.

Shaw, J. (1988). UK rates of return, *Amnesty International,* Feb/March.

Simmonds, S. (1984). Refugees, health and development. *Transactions of the Royal Society of Tropical Medicine and Hygiene,* **78,** 726–33.

Sterba, E. (1967). The effect of persecution on adolescents. In *Massive Psychic Trauma.* H. Krystal, ed., pp. 51–60, New York: International University Press.

Tabori, J. (1972). *The Anatomy of Exile.* London: Harrap.

Taviani, H. (1988). Perspectives of a host country. In *Refugees – The Trauma of Exile.* D. Miserez, ed., Dordrecht: Martinus Nijhoff.

Tu Khuong, D. (1988a). Victims of violence in the South China Sea. In *Refugees – The Trauma of Exile.* D. Miserez, ed., Dordrecht: Martinus Nijhoff.

Tu Khuong, D. (1988b). Flight from Vietnam. In *Refugees – The Trauma of Exile*. D. Miserez, ed., Dordrecht: Martinus Nijhoff.

Turner, S. (1989). Working with survivors. *Psychiatric Bulletin*, 13, 173–6.

United Nations (1951). *Convention Relating to the Status of Refugees*. Geneva, Switzerland: Office of the United Nations High Commissioner for Refugees.

United Nations (1967). *Protocol Relating to the Status of Refugees*. Geneva, Switzerland: Office of the United Nations High Commissioner for Refugees.

United Nations High Commissioner for Refugees (1979). *Handbook on Procedures and Criteria for Determining Refugee Status*. Geneva, Switzerland: Office of United Nations High Commissioner for Refugees.

Van Geuns, H. A. (1983). Introduction. In *Helping Victims of Violence*, Proceedings of a Working Group on the Psycho-Social Consequences of Violence, The Hague, Holland: Government Publications Office.

Vernant, J. (1953). *The Refugee in the Post-War World*, Allen & Urwin.

Viñar, M. (1989). Pedro or the demolition: a psychoanalytic look at torture, *British Journal of Psychotherapy* 5 (3), p. 353.

Wiesel, E. (1981). *Night*. London: Penguin.

Yathay, Pin (1989). *Stay Alive, My Son*. London: Arrow Books.

6
LONG-TERM EFFECTS OF TORTURE IN FORMER PRISONERS OF WAR
Thomas W. Miller

INTRODUCTION

Considerable interest in the long-term effects of captivity on former prisoners of war has become the focus of several recent research investigations (Page & Engdahl, 1990, unpublished observations; Miller, 1989; Speed *et al.*, 1989; Stenger, 1988; Ursano, 1985). The National Academy of Sciences – National Research Council (Page, 1988) has been studying the physical and psychological health of former POWs since the early 1950s. Researchers Cohen and Cooper (1955) developed rosters of former prisoners of war of World War II and non-POW controls. These data were characterized for mortality, morbidity and disability post-captivity. Its uniqueness to clinical research was the focus on designing a study with a representative sample of former prisoners of war and a control group. The authors based their assumption for the need for control groups on the fact that whatever the consequences of imprisonment might have been, there would likely be marked similarities between prisoners of war and those individuals who experienced combat disease, malnutrition and other adverse experiences and who were not prisoners of war. The crucial issues, however, would be in severity and duration of the prisoner of war experience. Nefzger (1970) added to the roster of World War II prisoners of war Korean conflict prisoners and controls which provided a population of POWs under different wartime conditions and cultural diversity. Subsequent studies by Beebe (1975), Keehn (1980) and Page (1988, unpublished observations) have provided the basis for a careful assessment of the longitudinal effects of former prisoners of war in the twentieth century.

CAPTIVITY AS A STRESSFUL LIFE EVENT

Combat in, and of, itself is a stressful experience, but to be imprisoned as a result of failure in combat creates an additional burden on the prisoner of war. The impact of stressful life imprisonment for former prisoners of war of any era is manifested in the survival rate realized during their capture (Miller, 1989). Of Americans imprisoned during World War II by both Germany and Japan, 21 000 prisoners of war who were returned to American control in 1945 represented about 63% of all of those placed in captivity during this wartime experience. The survival rate for this period was slightly less than two thirds of the total prisoners of war taken. These individuals were generally of poor physical health and suffered prolonged stress and symptoms consistent with both anxiety and depression. In 1981, Public Law #97–37 defined prisoner of war status and established VA eligibility criteria for former prisoners of war. The Department of Veterans Affairs played a key role in evaluating the status of former prisoners of war since that time. It provided both psychological and medical evaluations of imprisonment and yielded profiles that raised the question as to the differences that may have existed between prisoners of war held under different conditions of captivity.

Recent studies (Arthur, 1982; Miller, Martin & Spiro, 1989; Speed *et al.*, 1989; Nelson, 1985) along with earlier studies by Cohen and Cooper (1955) and Wolf and Ripley (1947) have provided a substantial database to better understand the long-term effects of severe trauma and later life adjustment on former POWs. The POW endured not only malnutrition and incarceration, but torture and, as a result, represented severe, prolonged stress. Horowitz and Wilner (1980) suggested that some POWs have suffered long-term adaptive disability complicated by memories of guilt and anxiety that resulted from atrocities of both military and a civilian nature during their wartime experience. Polner (1986) cites several cases in which combat experiences disturbed individuals after they returned to civilian life. In such instances, the difficulties appear to center around guilt feelings related to fellow non-survivors. Studies on combat veterans who experienced post-military psychiatric disturbance concluded that this population demonstrated a high incidence of depression and of conflict in close interpersonal relationships as well as aggressive tendencies and suicidal threats that counterparts not subjected to captivity or prisoner of war status failed to show. Most prominent among the symptomatology were frequent nightmares and recurring thoughts of wartime experiences. In seeking to understand the etiology of post-traumatic stress disorder in long-term victims of captivity, clinical researchers have identified a variety of questions of interest such as the effects of genetic constitutional predisposition or the pre-existence of psychopathology (Ursano, 1985) as well as the role of specific elements of traumatic events in the genesis of post-traumatic stress disorder (Horowitz & Wilner, 1980).

Zeiss and Dickman (1989) studied 442 former prisoners of war of World War II assessing PTSD related symptoms and evaluating the incidence of serious difficulties with PTSD symptoms over a 40-year period. Of the POWs, 56% responding indicated serious difficulties with PTSD symptoms and suggest a complex interaction between situation and person in producing and maintaining the symptoms of PTSD. Subsequent to severe trauma such as a prisoner of war experience, residual difficulties are likely to occur as long as 40 years after the event. Rank at time of capture was a consistent and powerful predictor in this study as well as in earlier reports and accounts for the largest proportion of variance. In each case, those with higher rank at the time of capture noted less severe symptomatology than those of lower rank. Differential treatment of POWs by rank is not a complete explanation of these findings. The authors hypothesized that certain personal characteristics such as greater self-efficacy, emotional maturity, intelligence, interpersonal skill, educational level, commitment to the war effort, and locus of control may be mediating variables that resulted in both promotion in rank and the relative ease of adjustment to the stresses of captivity and subsequent repatriation. Retrospective reporting by former prisoners of war further suggests an interpretation that post-traumatic stress disorder must be viewed as a field and dynamic rather than a static or constant constellation of symptoms. The authors noted that a minority of respondents reported either always or never having difficulty with symptoms, and most noted changes in symptoms over the years though not in a uniform pattern. It is hypothesized that this may reflect a gradual diminution of symptoms but with increased vulnerability to re-emerge or exacerbation of symptoms when exposed to other life stressors.

While some of these studies have methodological limitations which include small sample size or imprecise sampling procedures, they help to clarify a consensus on the incidence of major symptoms related to post-traumatic stress disorder in former prisoners of war. Furthermore, they give greater strength to the observation that captivity and the multiplicity of experiences related thereto can clearly be defined as a severe stressor. Finally, they suggest key variables related to the severity of the experience and how it may be a predictor of current symptomatology some 40 years post-captivity.

Kluznik *et al.* (1986) retrospectively diagnosed psychiatric disorders among 188 World War II and Korean conflict former prisoners of war. Within 1 year of their release, 67% fulfilled the diagnostic criteria for post-traumatic stress disorder and more than half of those affected continued to have symptoms over 40 years post-captivity. Also noted were that general anxiety disorders and depression were frequent among this population. Depressive symptoms have been shown most consistently in research related to former prisoners of war (Tennant, Goulston & Dent, 1986a; Dent, Tennant & Goulston, 1987). Tennant's study of 170 former prisoners of war and comparable controls revealed that former prisoners of war were significantly more depressed than non-prisoner of war controls some 40 years post-repatriation. To explain the presence of depressive symptoms 40 years post-captivity, these clinical researchers suggested that anxiety might diminish over that period but depression would increase as a reaction to the chronic post-traumatic impairment. Dent *et al.* (1987), completing a regression analysis for the same population, showed the following variables to be predictive of present-day depressive symptoms: low education and socioeconomic status, being unemployed, retired, unmarried, and having experienced and documented an anxiety or depressive illness during World War II.

The psychiatric profession has endeavored to address the import-ance of stress in our life through the inclusion of evidence of stressful life experiences as they occur and with levels of severity noted on axis IV in the *Diagnostic and Statistical Manual* of the American Psychiatric Association (DSM–III) (1980). There appears to be an important devel-opment by health-related professionals to address the assessment of life stress as it affects the psychological and social adaptation of the individual and to evaluate its role in precipitating illness. To assess this, Speed *et al.* (1989) evaluated the relative contributions of trauma and premorbid disposition in the development and persistence of post-traumatic stress disorder symptoms in former prisoners of war. Half of the sample studied satisfied DSM–III–R criteria for PTSD in the year following repatriation. Of the sample, 29% continued to meet the criteria for PTSD 40 years after their captivity. Family history of mental illness and pre-existing psychopathology were at best only weakly correlated with persistent post-traumatic stress disorder symptoms. The strongest predictors of PTSD were the proportion of body weight lost and the experience of torture during captivity. The authors believe that the study demonstrated that former POWs frequently developed post-traumatic stress disorder and that for one half of those who developed the symptoms, there was the likelihood of persistence over a long-term 40-year period. Family risk factors and pre-existing psychopathology often are superseded by an overwhelming nature of the trauma. The persistence of the symptoms for a 40-year post-captivity period may well be a reflection of the severity of the trauma, according to the authors.

Severe weight loss has long been recognized as a determinant of psychological sequelae (Beebe, 1975; Eitinger, 1971). Thygesen, Hermann & Willanger (1970) studied more than 1600 survivors of the Danish resistance movement incarcerated by the Nazis during World War II. Many of them assessed on several occasions over a 20-year period following World War II showed strong correlations between weight loss and the degree of incapacity even 20 years after their repatriation. Kolb (1987) and others have suggested that weight loss has psychometric properties that enhance its value as a marker of trauma severity. Kolb hypothesized that excessive stimulation may cause permanent cortical changes that impair control mechanisms in post-traumatic stress disorder. Malnutrition may sensitize the brain to the effects of trauma and thus may give a clue to the biological mechanisms underlying psychiatric illness that may result due to imprisonment and long-term captivity. Such biological mechanisms of specific interest include neuroendocrine axes, cerebral blood metabolism and neuropathology. Watson, Hoffman & Wilson (1988) have emphasized, as has Kolb, the importance of the biological perspective in assessing post-traumatic stress disorder and its long-term impact. Among the recommendations called for is closer collaboration between learning theorists in behavioral psychology, neurochemistry and neurophysiology.

TRAUMATIC STRESS AND THE IMPACT OF TORTURE DURING CAPTIVITY

Torture of both a physical and psychological nature have long been associated with captivity and prisoner of war status. The deliberate infliction of pain and suffering on fellow human beings has long-term physical and psychological sequelae (Başoğlu & Marks, 1988). Allodi and Cowgill (1982) investigated the long-term physical and psychological effects of torture on political prisoners. From their study is generated a 'torture syndrome' which is characterized by psychosomatic, affective, behavioral and intellectual abnormalities. Within the torture syndrome, psychosomatic symptoms are most frequently characterized by headache, nightmares, insomnia, night terrors, dizziness, tremor, fainting, pain, diarrhea, and sweating. Affective dysfunction is most often manifested through anxiety, depression, fears, phobias, and panic. Behavior concomitants of the syndrome usually show themselves through irritability, withdrawal, aggressiveness, obsessive–

compulsive disorder, impulsivity, sexual dysfunction, and suicidal ideation and intent. Intellectual difficulties are most often seen through poor concentration, confusion, disorientation, memory loss, and difficulty in attending. Lunde *et al.* (1980) describe a similar cluster of symptoms in more than 200 torture survivors.

The conditions under which prisoners of war were treated during their captivity vary considerably from war to war and theatre to theatre. Nelson (1989) provides the following descriptions of the various wartime POW experiences. During World War II, the European theatre, and more specifically the conditions under which prisoners were kept in German stalags were viewed by the outside world as relatively humane based on accounts of international Red Cross inspections. While the Geneva convention established rules for wartime treatment of prisoners sick and wounded, most POWs following the war indicated minimal standards for sane treatment in German stalags. Physical deprivation, while severe, was not as severe as in the Pacific theatre where POWs experienced sparse, unfamiliar diets with tropical diseases and primitive medical care. The mortality rate in the Pacific theatre was much higher than that in the European theatre. Whereas less than 1% of all POWs died during their captivity in Europe, more than 37% died during captivity in the Pacific. In the European theatre, diets low in proteins, calories and nutrients, together with strenuous labor activities and limited health care, provided the most serious environmental hazards. Malnutrition and pneumonia were most noted in the European theatre. Prisoners of war held captive in the Philippines, Japan, and Manchuria were found to be victims of severe maltreatment and malnourishment. The 100-mile, two-week experience known as the infamous baton death march realized 17 000 men falling victim to death through starvation and exhaustion (Jacobs, 1978). Physical torture was also more prevalent, with at least 90% of Pacific theatre prisoners of war identifying that they had received some form of direct physical punishment from their captors. Beheadings were most prominent during captivity in this theatre.

The Korean conflict provided somewhat different conditions of capture. In addition to extremely poor dietary conditions, the North Koreans frequently tied prisoners' hands behind their backs and bound their arms with wire. Medical care was primitive and inadequate. Prisoners of war who died while in captivity in North Korea showed severe signs of malnutrition, exposure and continued harassment, with noted respiratory infections and diarrhea. Environmental conditions imposed upon prisoners of war included extreme hunger and cold which were viewed as motivators to break down physical resistance. Prisoners of war were also separated by rank and authenticity and also received compulsory group indoctrination programs. Air crew members received more physical torture during captivity than did foot soldiers. Interrogation often accompanied solitary confinement for prisoners of war who showed signs of resistance.

Prisoners of war of the Vietnam era were more often better educated, older, and higher in rank than were prisoners of war of earlier conflicts and wars. North Vietnam POW experiences were marked by inadequate food, housing, and medical care, and by severe physical and mental torture for intelligence and propaganda purposes. Berg and Richlin (1979) indicate approximately 5% of the POWs died in captivity in the North, while in the South of Vietnam, physical deprivation but less emphasis on torture is noted, with a death rate of approximately 25% during captivity. What seems most apparent is that both physical deprivation and psychological stress are core ingredients of captivity. In addition, it is clear that both physical and mental torture are utilized within the framework of POW captivity.

Ursano et al. (1987) analyzed the debriefings of 324 repatriated prisoners of war shortly after their repatriation to obtain measures of stress related to captivity. Identified were the number and duration of all exploitation events and whether they involved maltreatment. These were subsequently coded into the following categories: (1) active (beatings, torture), (2) passive (forced standing or kneeling), (3) deprivation (denial of food, water or medical care), (4) psychological (threats of death, observing or hearing others being tortured) and (5) isolation. In the group studied, which represented US Air Force POWs released after April, 1973, it was noted that the use of solitary confinement after 1969 was less frequent than prior to that period of time. The duration of solitary confinement reported to medical personnel ranged from none to 7.5 years with a mean of more than five months. Percent of weight loss for these POWs ranged from 43% to 2%. A factor analysis with a principal axis solution and an equimax rotation was performed on the standardized debriefing measure. It resulted in seven identified stress factors experienced during captivity. These include: psychological maltreatment, number of maltreatments, time in solitary confinement, characteristics of interrogation, threats and denial of privileges, being singled out for punishment, solitary confinement.

The recognition of the long-term impact of captivity and prisoners of war status has been realized as well in international classification systems for psychiatric disorders. A torture syndrome has been recognized in the tenth revision of the Manual of the International Classification of Diseases (ICD–10) of the World Health Organization and in both the 1968 and 1980 revisions of the *Diagnostic and Statistical Manual* of the American Psychiatric Association. In the latter case, criteria appropriate to the torture syndrome are included in the category of transient situational disturbance and post-traumatic stress disorder, acute, chronic or delayed (DSM–III code numbers 308 and 309).

Within the context of the diagnostic criteria, the duration of the disturbance for each of the categories must be at least 1 month, and for delayed onset at least 6 months after the trauma.

CAPTOR–CAPTIVE RELATIONSHIP

Considerable attention has been given to the dynamics of the captor–captive relationship as it relates to torture in prisoners of war (Sherwood, 1986). Farber, Harlow and West (1957) suggest that the captor influence tactics induce in prisoners of war a state of debility resulting from pain, disease, fatigue and starvation. The anticipatory anxiety induced by unrelenting uncertainty and the threat of death, pain, and non-release become most prominent. Because captors control resources for alleviating this dreaded state, captives develop a dependency on their captors for relief. The result is clearly a negative impact on self-esteem and lessened conscious efforts to retain pre-captivity identity, group support and initiate covert action against the captor.

Hinckle and Wolfe (1956) have highlighted the power relationships developed by both Russian and Chinese captors. They include isolation, deprivation, abuse, and interrogation as the four key components. Isolation and denial of access to avenues of communication and the uncertainty in the access to information usually involve two types of tactics. Physical separation from fellow prisoners via solitary confinement is a tactic of considerable well-known recognition. It is noted that captives in solitary confinement usually remain active and involve themselves in physical activity, mental activity, fantasizing, counting, memorizing, and setting target dates for release. A second type of isolating tactic is more broadly conceptualized as psychological removal from previous sources of identification. Examples of this usually include segregating officers from non-officers, censoring mail thereby separating ties with family and friends, reporting of false captor military victories, and captive defeats and atrocities.

Sherwood (1986) indicates that isolated captives consciously strive to retain their pre-captivity identities. It should also be noted that officers seize opportunities to smuggle out messages, reestablishing command, lines of authority and routines. It is likely that captives cope with prohibitions and restrictions on exchange of information by developing codes, idiomatic languages, and utilizing humor in the course of coping with the various dimensions of isolation.

A second major component is deprivation. This usually involves deprivation of senses including food, adequate life-sustaining environmental factors, and sleep. Life-sustaining environmental factors often include adequate clothing and shelter, hygiene facilities, as well as food and water. In addition, medical care and access to avenues of constructive physical and mental activity are also a part of a deprivation routine. It is not uncommon for captors to make resources available but to withhold those resources in the presence of the captives.

Coping strategies to address deprivation often involve the sharing of deprived resources with others and resolving interpersonal conflicts early which are often the result of overcrowded environments which often cause stressful situations. Medical treatment, when not available, is often provided by fellow captives with resources, meager though they may be, from fellow captives.

Physical and psychological abuse is a critical element in Russian and Chinese captivity routines. Physical abuse involves beatings, punishment, and various forms of torture that have been summarized elsewhere. Psychological abuse often takes the forms of threats and 'contingency abuse'. With contingency abuse, captives are forced to witness the torture and punishment of other captives and realize their torture and punishment is contingent upon and determined by the compliance or lack thereof offered in the captive–captor relationship.

Coping with physical and psychological abuse is perhaps the most psychologically relevant dimension of captivity. The pain of abuse is often dealt with through conscious suppression of thoughts and feelings and can show itself through conversion hysteria and emotional anesthesia. Less complex coping strategies can include fantasy, sensate focus and self-imposed deprivation.

The fourth tactic utilized includes interrogation with structured and standardized format. Immediate post-capture interrogation tend to be most forceful, while ongoing interrogations tend to be geared more towards indoctrination and re-education. Most prominently felt emotions during interrogation are anger and frustration, together with shame, guilt, doubt, and mistrust. It is not uncommon for captives to cope with the shame, doubt and guilt involving public confessions by incorporating the same into expressions designed to communicate lack of sincerity and duress in subtle ways.

LEARNED HELPLESSNESS AND LOSS OF CONTROL

Within the context of understanding the impact of captivity as a stressful life experience, one must recognize important ingredients of a theoretical nature. Seligman and Elder (1986) suggested that perceived control becomes the most important feature for an individual in a stressful life experience. It is natural for human beings to seek indicators that reliably predict safety. In the absence of a safety signal, human beings remain in a state of anxiety and in a chronic state of fear and apprehension. Human beings are safety signal seekers. They search predictors of unavoidable danger because such knowledge also gives them knowledge of safety. The safety signal hypothesis argues that human beings who are victims of captivity and torture will be afraid all of the time except in the presence of a stimulus that reliably predicts their safety. The longer they experience unpredictability and therefore stress, the more likely they will develop depressive features which show themselves through learned helplessness. The theory of learned helplessness suggests that regardless of what efforts are attempted, the person will have no control over the outcome. It results in the individual losing hope and in most cases is recognized by the fact that the individual succumbs to the adverse experience such as captivity. Learned helplessness does the following: it may reduce the motivation to attempt control of the outcome, it may interfere with learning a response by which the person may develop some control over the outcome, and if the outcome is traumatic, it produces fear for as long as the subject is uncertain about the controllability of the outcome, thus producing a depressed state. The persistent avoidance of stimuli associated with the trauma, also known as a numbing of general responsiveness, is most characteristic of individuals who experience post-traumatic stress disorder and is consistent with the findings of the torture syndrome previously discussed.

The reformulated learned helplessness model (Abramson, Seligman and Teasdale, 1978) suggests that individuals confronted with negative events such as captivity try to explain those events. According to the model, causal explanations can be analyzed along three dimensions. Individuals who characteristically make internal, stable, and global explanations for negative events will be at greater risk for depressive deficits in the face of those events. That is to say, people who blame themselves and who believe that bad events will endure in time and will affect many areas of their lives, are more likely to become depressed.

Eberly *et al.* (1985) found that both physical and psychological torture and hardship variables defined a cluster of former prisoners of war at much higher risk for the development of psychopathology in severe post-traumatic stress disorder symptoms. The prisoners of war trauma is primarily defined by malnutrition and torture, but additional features of experiencing mental suffering, injury or delirium, being forced to relocate, and witnessing torture add to the significance of understanding these characteristics within the context of delayed stress syndrome for former prisoners of war.

METHODOLOGY

Assessed is the presence of depressive symptoms in post-traumatic stress disorder in veterans who were former prisoners of war of the Japanese and Germans during World War II. Addressed are several demographic criteria, specific aspects of capture, and prisoner of war conditions. Post-military adjustment and current psychological variables were measured through standardized psychological assessment. It is the intent of this research to assist mental health professionals in identifying the critical factors helpful in evaluating former prisoners of war and their subsequent adjustment in civilian life.

The measures employed include the National Institute of Mental Health's Center for Epidemiological Studies 20-item Depression Scale (NIMH/CES-D) and the Lie and Hysteria scales of the MMPI, history of hospitalization and medical conditions under treatment and medical conditions not being treated. The choice of the CES-D and MMPI are of special significance for this population. The CES-D was chosen as the instrument for measuring depressive symptoms because of its extensive use in community studies. Although these studies are primarily epidemiological in nature, the CES-D has been used and validated in several clinical settings. The MMPI is a well-known clinical instrument. The Hysteria scale, which includes both over-reporting (admit) and under-reporting (deny) subscales, was included to check whether the former prisoner of war might very well under-report his psychological symptoms, while the Lie scale was included to screen out for prevaricators. The use of the CES-D instrument is especially appropriate when the focus of the study is epidemiological in nature, that is, focusing on populations rather than individuals. A further advantage of the CES-D is its suitability for studies of a general population rather than of patients in a clinical setting. It should further be recognized that the CES-D was designed for use in groups in which most of the individuals are thought to be well rather than ill. Finally, the CES-D has been shown to be highly correlated with clinical diagnoses and

Table 6.1. *Demographic characteristics of former prisoners of war who were captives of Germany and Japan*

Factors	POWs who were German-held	POWs who were Japanese-held	Significance of group differential
Average age at capture	24.1	23.1	NS
Average age at repatriation	24.9	26.8	NS
Average age at discharge	25.2	29.3	NS
Rank capture			
Enlisted	92.8	85.8	NS
Officer	7.2	14.2	NS
Months in captivity	8.8	35.9	*
Marital status induction			
% Single	85.7	85.7	NS
% Married	14.3	14.3	NS
Marital status capture			
% Single	85.7	85.7	NS
% Married	14.3	14.3	NS
Marital status repatriation			
% Single	85.7	14.3	***
% Married	14.3	14.3	NS

also quite sensitive and specific when compared to clinical measures of depression.

Subjects included in this initial study involved 86 former prisoners of war who participated through voluntary screening, psychological testing along with chart review and screening measures relevant to the specific aspects of the lives of these patients, which were recorded in an attempt to identify a life-style profile, a pattern particular to prisoners of war and their susceptibility to traumatic stress disorder. Critical factors addressed include age, educational background, family background, military rank, conditions during capture and post-capture, type of discharge, years in service, and psychiatric history.

RESULTS

More than 130 000 military personnel were captured during World War II, with a ratio of 3:1 experiencing POW status in the European theatre. Of those captured, 89% survived. Survival rates among those prisoners of war in the Pacific theatre was much lower than that of the European theatre. In examining the demographic criteria of the two comparison groups, German-held POWs compared closely with Japanese-held POWs on the average age of capture (approximately 24 years of age) and average age of repatriation (approximately 25 years of age) but differ significantly on the average age of discharge (German-held 25 years of age; Japanese-held 29 years of age). Most notable on rank of capture was that those individuals captured by the Japanese were higher rank than those captured by the Germans. Fifty-seven and one-tenth percent (57.1%) of the German-held POWs held a rank of E–1 at capture, with 14.3% holding a rank of E–2. In contrast, Japanese-held POWs held ranks of E–2, E–3, and E–4, representing close to 70% of all those captured. Similar rates are realized in repatriation. Marital status through induction, capture, repatriation, and discharge compares favorably with current level of marital status suggesting a continuity when compared to more recently held prisoners of war.

The conditions of capture are of significance in this comparability study noting that German-held prisoners of war were more often captured with group intact, whereas Japanese-held prisoners of war were more often captured individually. Also consistent with this is that a higher proportion of Japanese-held prisoners of war were held in isolation. A higher percentage of German-held POWs (42.9%) were injured during capture, while only 28.6% of the Japanese-held prisoners of war were injured during their experience. During their

Table 6.2. *Captivity factor for former prisoners of war who were prisoners of Germany and Japan during World War II*

Factors	POWs who were German-held	POWs who were Japanese-held	Significance of group differential
Capture circumstances			
% Battle	64.3	14.3	***
% Shot down	14.3	0.0	NS
% Retreat	7.1	14.3	NS
Injured during capture	42.9	28.6	***
Work during capture			
% Farm	28.6	28.6	NS
% None	42.9	28.6	***
% Factory	7.1	0.0	NS
% Construction	21.4	14.3	NS
% Mines	7.1	28.8	**
Conditions during capture			
% Had escape plan	21.4	100.0	***
% Escape attempted	7.1	28.6	**
% Escape successful	0.0	0.0	NS
% Experienced intimidation	57.1	85.7	**
% Experienced beating	21.4	57.1	***
% Witnessed beating	50.0	85.7	**
% Physical torture	28.6	71.4	***
% Witnessed torture	28.6	85.7	***

% Psychological torture	28.6	71.4	***
% Isolation on ships	0.0	42.9	***
% Ship was attacked	0.0	28.6	**
% Isolation on railroad car	71.4	57.1	NS
% Railroad car attacked	42.9	14.3	**
% Solitary confinement	42.9	71.4	**
% Propaganda attacks	21.4	100.0	***
Wounded while captured			
% None	50.0	42.9	NS
During captivity, presence of:			
Anger and fear	85.7	83.3	NS
Prolonged depression	64.3	100.0	***
Prolonged helplessness	85.7	100.0	**
Isolation and loneliness	35.7	71.4	***
Nightmarish delirium	50.0	85.7	**
Forced to march	92.9	100.0	NS
March attacked	85.7	57.1	*
Thought of suicide	7.1	57.1	*
Attempted suicide	7.1	0.0	NS
Received news	64.3	83.3	*
News rare	83.3	100.0	*

Table 6.3. *Post-military adjustment*

Factors	POWs who were German-held	POWs who were Japanese-held	Significance of group differential
Served years after release in military	21.4	57.1	***
Additional years served (average in years)	1.0	5.5	NS
Attended school after release	21.4	33.4	NS
Highest education level (average in years)	11.0	11.8	NS
Years worked after release	35.1	32.6	NS
Number of jobs	3.7	5.7	NS
Longest employment (in years)	21.4	19.1	NS
% reported symptoms:			
Positive aspects	35.7	42.9	NS
Chest pain	28.6	57.1	**
Rapid heartbeat	42.9	71.4	**
Heartbeats skip and miss	50.0	57.1	NS
Numbness in extremities	57.1	100.0	***
Numbing weakness	85.7	100.0	*
Psychological, emotional distress	50.0	71.4	**

capture, both German-held and Japanese-held POWs (28.6%) were involved in farm work and there was a slightly higher figure with respect to German-held POWs participating in construction work than Japanese-held POWs. Of the Japanese-held POWs, 28.6% participated in work in mines, whereas none of the sample of German-held POWs had similar experiences.

Escape plans were of interest in reviewing the data within these two samples. Of the Japanese-held POWs assessed in the screening process, 100% indicated that an escape plan had been identified. Only 21.4% of the German-held POWs revealed a similar plan. While 28% of the Japanese-held POWs indicated a desire and an attempt to escape, only 7.1% of the German-held POWs did likewise. This may be due in part to the fact that Japanese-held POWs spent a much longer time in captivity (35.9 months) than German-held POWs (8.8 months).

The conditions experienced during capture show higher percentages of intimidations, beatings, physical torture, psychological torture and isolation on ships realized by Japanese-held POWs. While both subsamples indicated wounding during capture, a slightly higher percentage of the Japanese-held POWs were wounded during this period of time.

Psychological factors during captivity also became a critical focus, with Japanese-held POWs realizing a higher percentage of psychological depression due to loneliness, nightmares, thoughts of suicide and prolonged helplessness. Of interest is that 57.1% of the Japanese-held prisoners of war served up to 5.5 years after their capture, whereas only 21.4% of the German-held POWs served up to 1.1 years after their capture.

Physical symptomatology currently reported by former prisoners of war indicate Japanese-held POWs have a significantly higher percentage of chest pain, rapid heartbeat, numbness in the extremities, numbing weaknesses, weakness and emotional distress than German-held POWs.

With respect to work adjustment during post-discharge from the military, both Japanese and German-held POWs had a work history of approximately 35 years. However, Japanese-held POWs showed a higher number of job changes (5.7) as opposed to German-held POWs (3.7).

CORRELATES OF TRAUMATIC STRESS

Focusing on the psychological factors during captivity, it was noted that Japanese-held POWs realized higher percentages of psychological depression, with specific emphasis on loneliness, nightmares, thoughts

Table 6.4. Millon clinical multiaxial inventory for profile study groups four decades post-captivity for POWs of Germany and Japan during World War II

MCMI scale	POWs who were German-held	POWs who were Japanese-held	Significance of group differential
Schizoid (asocial)	61	56	*
Avoidant	57	73	**
Dependent (submissive)	73	58	NS
Histrionic (gregarious)	38	42	NS
Narcissistic	49	45	NS
Antisocial (aggressive)	46	62	NS
Compulsive (conforming)	66	51	NS
Passive-aggressive	49	73	**
Schizotypal (schizoid)	61	54	NS
Borderline (cycloid)	65	63	NS
Paranoid	59	60	NS
Anxiety	93	76	*
Somatoform	81	68	*
Hypomanic	19	48	**
Dysthymic	82	71	NS
Alcohol abuse	61	69	NS
Drug abuse	50	55	NS
Psychotic thinking	53	60	NS
Psychotic depression	56	64	NS
Psychotic delusions	61	60	NS

* p .05
** p .01

of suicide and prolonged helplessness. The treatment of POWs during military captivity at least measured by self-report of medical symptoms and weight loss, appears to be statistically linked to subsequent depressive symptoms. Furthermore, differences in depressive symptoms may well be attributed to differences in self-reported captivity-related factors. Tennant, Goulston and Dent (1986b), in studying 170 Australian POWs and comparable controls, found that former prisoners of war were significantly more depressed than non-POW controls some 40 years after repatriation. In explaining the persistence of depressive symptoms 40 years after release from captivity, the investigator suggests that over the long follow-up period, anxiety might diminish but depression might increase as a reaction to chronic impairment. This Australian data appear to provide an independent confirmation of the fact that depressive symptoms may persist long term as much as 40 years or more following release from captivity. Furthermore, depressive symptoms may appear not only as a manifestation of depressive illness *per se*, but also as a part of a larger constellation of symptomatology which constitutes a delayed stress syndrome. Researchers such as Egendorf *et al.* (1981) have provided clinical evidence that veterans of military combat and captivity are at greater risk for long-term psychological symptomatology. The DSM–III–R criteria for the diagnosis of post-traumatic stress disorder draws on these earlier concepts of war neurosis, shell shock, combat fatigue, and combat exhaustion. This suggests the possibility of both acute and chronic effects of stressful life events.

Of specific importance here is the recognition that depression symptomatology is clearly associated with post-traumatic stress disorder, particularly in the re-experiencing of the traumatic event, the emotional numbness experienced as a result of the traumatizing experience, and the cognitive and autonomic symptoms such as physiological reactivity, exaggerated startle response, hypervigilance, difficulty concentrating, irritability and sleep disturbance noted in the post-traumatic stress disorder criteria. Of even greater significance is the persistent avoidance of stimuli associated with the trauma or the numbing of general responsiveness to the trauma which is not present prior to the trauma and therefore including depressive symptoms. Clinical observations such as these suggest that post-traumatic stress disorder is a clear candidate for a diagnosis which might underlie the depressive symptomatology often observed in the former prisoners of war.

In realizing statistically significant differences noted in our prisoner of war sample, factors such as the number of months in captivity, isolation during capture and imprisonment, the development or lack thereof of an escape plan, attempt or lack thereof of escape, experience of intimidation, experience of beating, witnessing beating, witnessing physical torture, experiencing physical torture, experiencing psychological torture, isolation on ships, solitary confinement, experiencing of propaganda attacks, feelings of prolonged helplessness, isolation and loneliness, nightmares and delirium, thoughts of suicide, and experiencing of chest pain, rapid heartbeat, numbness in extremities, psychological stress and emotional distress 40 years post-captivity all point to a likely impact of better understanding the long-term effects of captivity for former prisoners of war.

PERSONALITY DISTURBANCE IN PTSD

Considerable discussion has occurred in the clinical literature regarding the possibility of personality disturbance or character pathology being associated with post-traumatic stress disorder. Greene, Linde and Grace (1985) discuss this in detail, identifying several possibilities for explaining the possible relationship between post-traumatic stress disorder and character pathology. Hypothesized by these clinical researchers are the possibilities that: (1) character pathology and post-traumatic stress disorder are relatively independent phenomena, (2) character pathology may predispose individuals to develop post-traumatic stress disorder, (3) character pathology may function as a selector for those who find themselves in high risk potentially traumatic situations and survive as a result of the trauma, and (4) character pathology may develop as a result of the trauma itself. There is no question but that personality development, viewed as a relatively enduring pattern of behavior that develops over the lifetime of the individual, provides both the competencies and coping that may be both necessary and beneficial from a cognitive as well as a physiological perspective and determines the manner in which an individual who experiences trauma processes the trauma and adapts to it. What is clear from the data on the long-term effects of torture in former prisoners of war, is that these individuals maintained both cognitive and physiological components of the trauma post-captivity and that such components affected both their adaptation and adjustment during the decades following their prisoner of war experience.

CLINICAL AND TREATMENT STRATEGIES

Former prisoners of war and victims of post-traumatic stress disorder often show moderate to severe anxiety and sleep disturbance. Those symptoms often disrupt the individual's ability to deal effectively with the activities of daily living. Tricyclic antidepressants may make a substantial contribution to the treatment of such patients on short term. Those medications are relatively well tolerated and have a demonstrated efficiency in controlling anxiety and a variety of sleep and dream disturbances. Since other aspects of the post-traumatic stress disorder remain virtually unchanged when medication only is prescribed, psychotherapy and cognitive behavioral models of therapy can provide key ingredients in addressing anxiety and the cognitive and behavioral manifestations associated with it in the post-traumatic stress disorder patient. Long-term implications may find post-traumatic stress disorder patients susceptible to exacerbations of symptoms and response to inter-current stress from other sources. Marks and O'Sullivan (1988), and others (Marks *et al.*, 1989) present considerable clinical data supporting the value of exposure therapies as the approach of choice in anxiety disorders, specifically where they are manifested by avoidance. These together with cognitive behavioral models (Miller & Feibelman, 1987; Rapee & Barlow, 1989) provide clinical methodologies which can be beneficial in treating components of post-traumatic stress disorder in former POWs.

The psychiatric consequences of trauma and torture best realized in prisoners of war and other captives have been summarized by Ursano *et al.* (1987). They identify seven distinct stress factors likely experienced by former prisoners of war during their captivity. The first factor emphasizes psychological maltreatment intended to make the captive feel guilty and turn against his comrades as well as his country. Factor two deals with the frequency and intensity of maltreatment experiences during captivity. Factor three indicates a time perspective on solitary confinement and associated maltreatment. Factor four addresses characteristics of interrogation that deal with both psychological and physical pain and stress. Factor five addresses denial and deprivation of privileges, while factor six deals with specific stressors associated with being singled out for punishment. Factor seven, as identified by Ursano *et al.*, deals with the duration of captivity and maltreatment. This research team has noted that while most repatriated prisoners of war cope successfully with the extraordinary stresses of captivity, both illness and resiliency post-captivity remain important considerations in understanding the long-term adaptivity of the individual and physical as well as psychological effects of captivity and torture. They further note that captivity and prisoner of war experiences may serve as useful purpose in promoting an organizational quality to adult mental life. More specifically, they note that an organizer produces a particular cluster of affects, cognitions, and behaviors which can be released under appropriate stimulus symbolic, environmental, or even biological in nature, which allows them to conclude that while the captivity and prisoner of war experience is clearly recognized as a stressful life event, it may well have positive qualities and characteristics that are realized with maturity and adaptation.

In considering the treatment approaches specifically addressing the former prisoner of war, it becomes imperative that the therapist realize that the individual to receive treatment was forced at a time in his life to live for weeks, months, or years with no safety signal and the most oppressive of outlooks. While doing so, the prisoner of war likely experienced physical and emotional deprivation, witnessed comrades die from a myriad of diseases, starvation, exposure, lack of medical care, and was committed to solitary confinement, forced marches, extreme changes in temperature, and experienced torture, mutilation, beatings, and forced heavy labor under inhumane conditions. For protracted periods of time, the prisoner of war lived under severe psychological stress, harboring thoughts of suicide, expecting to be killed, and anticipating the next trauma, whether that be physical torture, intense interrogation, or political indoctrination.

It is likely that the former prisoner of war will seek treatment for medical and psychological conditions not clearly identifiable as the result of captivity at the time of initial screening. It is likely that the individual will seek help because of symptoms related to sleep disturbance, nightmares, insomnia, depression, and anxiety. There may have been indications of suicidal ideation or intent; medical concerns which include fatigue, headache, nausea, muscle soreness, low back pain, or chest pains (Horowitz & Wilner, 1980) often show themself on initial screening. Coping styles that include alcohol or substance abuse will likely be a part of the identifiable symptoms years after the captivity experience. Kluznik *et al.* (1986) identified cases similar to our own at the VA Medical Center, Lexington, Kentucky, where former POWs had kept their history of captivity and torture secret from family, community and friends for decades.

Psychotherapy should address several issues including the resistance of the former POW to express thoughts and feelings which have been harbored for many years. Most clearly, the focus will be on atrocities and abuse, and the tendency to repress these thoughts and avoid hurt associated with the anger and guilt of the experience must be processed.

Several psychotherapists have identified the important role of 'survivor guilt' as being a critically important element of the treatment of the former prisoners of war (Swartz, 1984). The prisoner of war who has survived the multiplicity or physical and psychological experiences associated with captivity will likely at some time or another feel guilt about the fact that he survived when others did not. Associated with this will be the coping strategies that he used to maintain his survival and what he did or didn't do to help those who did not survive. The vulnerability for survival guilt appears to grow especially in the aging veteran, likely because this is a time for him to review with much greater wisdom what he could or should have done in those situations which bear serious conflict and create guilt for him at this stage in his life. The prisoner of war population is clearly one that may cope with the traumas and atrocities of their captivity during much of their life but revisit and redefine for themselves the appropriateness of their actions during their captivity and torture.

The therapeutic alliance providing trust and confidentiality is essential to the therapeutic processing of the trauma for the veteran who has been a victim of torture during prisoners of war experiences. Haley (1974) and others have argued the importance of establishing a therapeutic relationship for patients reporting atrocities and that this in fact is the treatment rather than the facilitator of treatment. The former prisoner of war who is seeking understanding and resolution of the difficulties and confusion tied to that POW experience, must find in the therapist trust and acceptance for being both victim and perpetrator.

Nelson (1989) and others have argued the importance of core facilitative conditions being present including empathy, genuineness, positive regard, concreteness, and unconditionality of regard. It must permit the patient to identify with the therapist as a benign authority (Horner, 1979) and permit a catharsis free of prejudice and rationalization. Specific symptoms often seen in the former POW include phobic responses and obsessive–compulsive features. Specific cognitive–behavioral therapeutic interventions can be of benefit in reducing symptoms that have served to protect the individual from dealing with the core guilt and trauma tied to capture and torture experiences of former prisoners of war.

ISSUES FOR FUTURE CLINICAL RESEARCH

The former prisoners of war and the victims of captivity experience similar aspects to other major catastrophies but differ significantly in the way in which this information can be processed. For the victim of captivity, key issues include the following:

1 Captivity experience. Treatment by captors becomes a crucial issue in understanding and assessing adaptation. Medical, health-related activities and diet are critically important in understanding the physical implications of captivity.
2 Duration is a critical element. The length of captivity appears directly related to the degree of experienced stress as a result of the captivity experience.
3 The level of group support and the ability of individuals who are prisoners of war or victims of captivity have in relating to other captures or whether they experience isolation.
4 The level and extent to which contact with families and significant others is maintained is critically important to the adaptation of the victim of captivity.
5 The preparedness for reintegration once captivity is terminated becomes a critically important ingredient in the adaptation process. Issues related to separation, guilt feelings, and the subsequent impact on family members and significant others is a crucial factor which needs to be addressed.

Functional adaptation involves a series of stages which become critically important to successful adaptation. It needs to involve appropriate preparation, adequate communication, and effective support services to both the victim and captivity and his significant others. It needs to address a multiplicity of issues including the following:

1 Acknowledging and accepting the changes that have occurred and the subsequent impact they have on the life of the victim as well as significant other.
2 Commitment by family members and support systems toward providing a safe and individualized process or readaptation.
3 Pursuing active and full support and involvement of government agencies.
4 Maintaining a life-centered focus on the adaptation process necessary for successful adjustment.

The trauma of captivity and subsequent adaptation provide for many an opportunity for personal growth and stronger resolve in the face of adversity. To provide a growing fund of information and education, the following suggestions and recommendations are made:

1 World governments, governmental agencies and governmental planners must work toward eradicating dehumanizing experiences, torture and captivity because of its negative impact on human beings.
2 For former POWs and victims of torture and captivity, support systems need to be adequately developed and in place at the time they are needed.
3 Prompt attention and specific treatment methodologies for victims and their significant others needs to be a critical element in preparedness.
4 A research-based theory of processing trauma needs further development to help us understand conceptualization and those factors necessary in the resolution.
5 Programs aimed at educating the public on understanding the captivity experience and readaptation dilemmas faced by victims of torture and significant others need further development.
6 Graduate and undergraduate curriculum addressing these specific issues should be offered through departments such as psychology, sociology, and psychiatry in our major medical and health science university programs.

The long-term effects of torture in former prisoners of war leave an indelible mark on the lives of the victims as well as their significant others. The extent that we have grown in our understanding of these long-term effects is the extent to which we should implement measures that will be more effective in the processing, treatment and resolution of the symptoms that victims of torture experience at the hands of fellow human beings.

ACKNOWLEDGEMENT

Appreciation is extended to Dr Charles A. Stenger, American Ex-Prisoners of War Association, Bethesda, Maryland; Deborah Kessler, Elizabeth Lang, and Katrina Scott, Library Service, VAMC, Lexington, Kentucky; Rodonna Johnson, Department of Counseling Psychology, University of Kentucky; Tagalie Heister, Virginia Lynn Gift, and Debbie Howard, Department of Psychiatry, University of Kentucky; and Dr Perry Passaro, University of Kentucky, for their assistance in the preparation of this manuscript. Appreciation is also extended to

Dr Isaac Marks and Dr Metin Başoğlu, the Institute of Psychiatry, University of London, England.

REFERENCES

Abramson, L. Y., Seligman, M. E. P. & Teasdale, J. (1978). Learned helplessness in humans: Critique and reformation. *Journal of Abnormal Psychology*, **887**, 32–48.

Allodi, F. & Cowgill, G. (1982). Ethical and psychiatric aspects of torture: A Canadian study. *Canadian Journal of Psychiatry*, **27**, 98–102.

American Psychiatric Association. (1980). *Diagnostic and Statistical Manual of Mental Disorders* (3rd edn). Washington, DC: American Psychiatric Association.

American Psychiatric Association. (1987). *Diagnostic and Statistical Manual* (III–R). Washington, DC: American Psychiatric Association.

Amnesty International. (1984). *Torture in the 80's*. London, England: Amnesty International Publications, Inc.

Arthur, R. J. (1982). Psychiatric syndromes in prisoner of war and concentration camp survivors. In C. T. Friedman and R. A. Faguet, eds., *Extraordinary Disorders of Human Behavior*, pp. 47–68, New York: Plenum.

Başoğlu, M. & Marks, I. (1988). Torture. *British Medical Journal*, **297**, 1423–4.

Beebe, G. W. (1975). Follow-up studies of World War II and Korean War prisoners; II. Morbidity, disability, and maladjustments. *American Journal of Epidemiology*, **101**, 400–22.

Berg, W. & Richlin, M. (1979). Injuries and illnesses of Vietnam war POWs. IV. Comparisons of captivity effects in North and South Vietnam. *Military Medicine*, **142**, 678–80.

Cohen, B. M. & Cooper, M. Z. (1955). A follow-up study of World War II prisoners of war. *Veterans Administration Medical Monograph*. Washington, DC: US Government Printing Press.

Dent, O. F., Tennant, C. C. & Goulston, K. J. (1987). Precursors of depression in World War II veterans 40 years after the war. *Journal of Nervous and Mental Disorders*, **175**, 486–90.

Dickman, H. R. & Seiss, R. A. (1986, August). Post-traumatic stress disorder in a statewide sample of former POWs. Paper presented at the 94th annual convention of the American Psychological Association, Washington, DC.

Eberly, R. E., Engdahl, B. E., Rinehart, S. J. et al. (1985). Psychological adjustment and health among former prisoners of war. Paper presented at American Psychological Association 94th annual convention. Washington, DC.

Egendorf, A., Kadushin, C., Laufer, R. S., Rothbart, G. & Sloan, L. (1981). *Legacies of Vietnam: comparative adjustment of veterans and their peers*. New York: Center for Policy Research.

Eitinger, L. (1971). Acute and chronic psychiatric reactions in concentration camp survivors. In L. Levin, ed., *Society, Stress and Disease*, pp. 219–230, New York: Oxford University Press.

Engdahl, B. E. (1987). Psychological consequences of the World War II prisoner of war experience: Implications for treatment. American Psychological Association 95th annual convention, New York. Available from ERIC Document Services; accession number CG020530.

Farber, I., Harlow, H. & West, L. (1957). Brainwashing, conditioning, and DDD (debility, dependency, and dread). *Sociometry*, **20**, 271–85.

Goulston, K. J., Dent, O. F., Chapuis, P. H. *et al.* (1985). Gastrointestinal morbidity among World War II prisoners of war: 40 years after. *Medical Journal of Australia*, **143**, 6–10.

Green, B. L., Linde, J. D. & Grace, M. C. (1985). Post-Traumatic Stress Disorder. Toward DSM–IV. *Journal of Nervous and Mental Disorders*, **173(7)**, 406–11.

Haley, S. A. (1974). When the patient reports atrocities. *Archives of General Psychiatry*, **30**, 192–6.

Hinkle, L. & Wolff, H. (1956). Communist interrogation and indoctrination of 'enemies of the state'. *Archives of Neurology and Psychiatry*, **76**, 115–74.

Horner, A. (1979). *Object Relations and the Developing Ego in Therapy*. New York: Jason Aronson.

Horowitz, M. & Wilner, N. (1980). Life events, stress and coping. In L. W. Poon, ed., *Aging in the 1980's: Psychological Issues*, pp. 363–374, Washington, DC: American Psychological Association.

Jacobs, E. (1978). Residuals of Japanese prisoners of war: Thirty years later. *The Quan*, **32**, 4–6.

Keane, T. M. & Kaloupek, D. G. (1980). Behavioral analysis and treatment of Vietnam stress syndrome. Paper presentation at the annual meeting of the American Psychological Association, Montreal, Canada, September 12–16, 1980.

Keane, T. M., Wolfe, J. & Taylor, K. L. (1987). Post-traumatic stress disorder: Evidence for diagnostic validity and methods of psychological assessment. *Journal of Clinical Psychology*, **43**, 32–43.

Keehn, R. J. (1980). Follow-up studies of World War II and Korean conflict prisoners: Mortality to January 1, 1976. *American Journal of Epidemiology*, **111**, 194–211.

Kluznik, J. C., Speed, N., Van Valkenburg, C. *et al.* (1986). Forty-year follow-up of United States prisoners of war. *American Journal of Psychiatry*, **143**, 1443–6.

Kolb, L. C. (1987). A neuropsychological hypothesis explaining post-traumatic stress disorders. *American Journal of Psychiatry*, **144**, 989–95.

Lunde, I., Rasmussen, O. V., Lindholm, J. & Wagner, G. (1980). Gonadal and sexual functions in tortured Greek men. *Danish Medical Bulletin*, **27**, 243–5.

Marks, I. M. & O'Sullivan, G. (1988). Drugs and psychological treatments for agoraphobia/panic and obsessive–compulsive disorders: a review. *British Journal of Psychiatry*, **153**, 650–8.

Marks, I. M., Lelliott, P., Başoğlu, M., Noshirvani, H. & Monteiro, W. (1988). Clomipramine, self-exposure and therapist-aided exposure for obsessive–compulsive rituals. *British Journal of Psychiatry*, **152**, 522–34.

Miller, T. W. (1989). *Stressful Life Events*. Madison, CT: International Universities Press, Inc.

Miller, T. W. & Feibelman, N. D. (1987). Obsessional thought disturbance in gainfully employed traumatic stress disorder patients. *Journal of Occupational Health and Nursing,* **35,** 69–73.

Miller, T. W., Martin, W. & Spiro, K. (1989). Post-traumatic stress disorder in former prisoners of war. *Comprehensive Psychiatry,* **30(2),** 139–48.

Nefzger, M. D. (1970). Follow-up studies of World War II and Korean War prisoners: Study plans and mortality findings. *American Journal of Epidemiology,* **91,** 123–38.

Nelson, H. (1985). *Prisoners of War: Australians Under Nippon.* Sydney: Australian Broadcasting Corporation.

Nelson, L. F. (1989). When the war doesn't end. *Journal of Psychosocial Nursing,* **27(7),** 26–30.

Polner, M. (1986). Vietnam War stories. *Transaction,* **6,** 8–20.

Rapee, R. M. & Barlow, D. H. (1989). Psychological treatment of panic attacks in agoraphobic responses. In J. R. Walker, G. R. Norton and C. Ross eds., *Panic Disorder and Agoraphobia.* Chicago: Dorsey Press.

Seligman, M. E. P. & Elder, G. (1986). Learned helplessness and life span development. In A. Sorenson, F. Weinert and L. Sherrod, eds., *Human Development and the Life Course: Multidisciplinary Perspectives,* pp. 377–427, Hillsdale, NJ: Erlbaum.

Sherwood, E. (1986). The power relationship between captor and captive. *Psychiatric Annals,* **16(11),** 653–5.

Speed, N., Engdahl, B. E., Schwartz, J. *et al.* (1989). Post-traumatic stress disorder as a consequence of the prisoners of war experience. *Journal of Nervous and Mental Disorders,* **177,** 147–53.

Stenger, C. A. (1988). American prisoners of war in WWI, WWII, Korea, and Vietnam: Statistical data concerning numbers captured, repatriated, and still alive as of January, 1988. Unpublished manuscript.

Strange, R. E., Brown, D. E., Jr. (1976). Home from the wars. *American Journal of Psychiatry,* **127,** 488–92.

Swartz, H. J. (1984). *Psychotherapy of the Combat Veteran.* New York: S. P. Medical and Scientific Books.

Tennant, C. C., Goulston, K. J. & Dent, O. F. (1986a). The psychological effect of being a prisoner of war: Forty years after release. *American Journal of Psychiatry,* **143,** 618–21.

Tennant, C. C., Goulston, K. J. & Dent, O. F. (1986b). Clinical psychiatric illness of prisoners of war of the Japanese: Forty years after release. *Psychological Medicine,* **16,** 833–9.

Thygesen, P., Hermann, K. & Willanger, R. (1970). Concentration camp survivors in Denmark: Persecution, disease, disability, compensation. *Danish Medical Bulletin,* **17,** 65–108.

Ursano, R. J. (1985). Viet Nam era prisoners of war: Studies of U.S. air force prisoners of war. In A. S. Blank and J. A. Talbott, eds., *The Trauma of War: Stress and Recovery of Viet Nam Veterans,* pp. 341–357, Washington, DC: American Psychiatric Press.

Ursano, R. J. (1987). Commentary. Post-traumatic stress disorder: The stressor criterion. *Journal of Nervous and Mental Disorders*, **175**, 273–5.
Ursano, R. J., Wheatley, R. D., Carlson, E. H. & Rahe, A. J. (1987). The Prisoners of War. *Psychiatric Annals*, **17(8)**, 532–5.
Watson, I. P. B., Hoffman, L. & Wilson, G. V. (1988). The neuropsychiatry of post-traumatic stress disorder. *British Journal of Psychiatry*, **152**, 164–73.
Wolf, S. & Ripley, H. (1947). Reactions among allied prisoners of war subjected to three years of imprisonment and torture by the Japanese. *American Journal of Psychiatry*, **104**, 180–93.
Zeiss, R. A., Dickman, H. R. & Nicholas, B. L. (1985, August). Posttraumatic stress disorder in former prisoners of war: incidence and correlates. Paper presented at the 93rd annual convention of the American Psychological Association, Los Angeles.
Zeiss, R. A. & Dickman, H. R. (1989). PTSD 40 years later. *Journal of Clinical Psychology*, **45(1)**, 80–7.

7
THE HOLOCAUST: SURVIVORS AND THEIR CHILDREN
Norman Solkoff

INTRODUCTION

Although 55 countries have approved the United Nations Convention Against Torture, many countries continue to condone and practise brutal treatment of prisoners and political dissidents. With the steady rise in neo-fascist, religious fundamentalistic, antisemitic, and jingoistic nationalist movements, it behoves us to look again at the genocidal actions of the Nazi system.

In this chapter, the author will discuss the acts of cruelty perpetrated against men, women and children incarcerated in the concentration and extermination camps of Nazi-occupied Europe and the effects these brutalities may have had on those who survived and their children. Although systematic acts of barbarism were committed against Gypsies, Jehovah Witnesses, homosexuals, and political opponents of Nazism, especially communists, this chapter will focus upon Jewish victims and survivors, mainly because most of the English language literature on Holocaust survivors has focused upon Jews. Also addressed will be the methodological problems encountered by investigators pursuing research on survivors and their children. It is hoped that this review of past experiences with Holocaust survivors will help inform our understanding of how to deal with current problems of torture.

THE NATURE OF THE TRAUMA

Torture, as practised in the Nazi concentration and extermination camps was not primarily carried out for purposes of extortion or to extract information from inmates. Instead, physical pain and psychological degradation were inflicted as acts of gratuitous punishment, which would become a prelude to death for many, or as an extreme expression of loathing of Jews. By 1945, two out of every three Jews living in Europe in 1939 were dead. The remaining one-third survived through various combinations of luck, professional skills, physical strength, psychological coping strategies, and time and place of incarceration. It was clearly Hitler's intent to murder all of the Jews of Europe, not because they posed a political threat to the Nazi state, but simply because they were Jews.

Soon after Hitler's accession to power in 1933 there was a steady increase in the intensity and frequency of antisemitic acts, which were ultimately validated by passage of the Nuremberg Laws in 1935 (Proctor, 1988). The concentration camps, initially established to terrorize the German population and to detain political and religious opponents of National Socialism also provided a source of slave labor. These camps became the settings for 'the final solution' or the destruction of European Jewry and for carrying out life-threatening experiments, most of dubious or no scientific value, on non-informed, non-consenting individuals. For example, identical and fraternal Jewish and Gypsy twins would be injected with the same quantity of typhoid bacteria and the natural course of the disease would be followed. Or, freezing experiments were conducted on Jewish and non-Jewish Poles in an effort to determine how long exposed skin would take to freeze when submerged in freezing water and to discover the most effective thawing techniques.

The persecution experiences for the camp inmates were sustained and intense. Without forewarning, or any apparent reason, individuals, most of whom were ordinary citizens without a criminal past or a particular political agenda to implement, were forcibly uprooted from their communities and job sites leading to the dissolution of all previous family and social ties. Jews were herded into the ghettos established throughout Eastern Europe prior to being 'transported' to a camp. In these sealed off, densely populated areas, with inadequate food supplies and under unsanitary, crowded living conditions, the death rate from debilitating diseases was high.

After being removed from the ghetto and surviving the gruelling 'transportation' process to destinations which, up until the very last moment, were usually not known or only surmised, prisoners arrived at their camps. As one of many Nazi deception tactics designed to reduce resistance among the victims and make them more compliant, greeting prisoners upon their arrival would be the words, usually inscribed above the entrance gate: 'Arbeit Macht Frei' (work will make you free). What was to happen to these inmates was in direct contradiction to this message (Kogon, 1950).

So as to ensure a strong labor force, death would be instantaneous for those who appeared too young, too old, or who had obvious

F

physical disabilities. For all those who survived this initial 'selection' the tortuous ordeals were to begin. Heads were shaved under the pretext of removing lice, Jewish prisoners' identities were replaced with tattooed numbers engraved on their arms and a yellow Star of David was sewn on each Jewish prisoner's uniform. Colors differed depending upon prisoner category. With the exception of the few prisoners who had skills useful for the Nazi war effort, most other inmates were forced to perform labor designed more to test the limits of physical endurance than to achieve some productive goal. Compounding the arduousness and senselessness of the work were nutritional inadequacies – caloric intake averaging 800 – leading to states of semi-starvation. Infectious diseases, feared by the inmates because discovery would result in immediate death to those infected, were rampant due to crowded and unsanitary living conditions. Treatment facilities, if available at all, were at best primitive and often had to be housed in secret hideaways. Prisoner vulnerability was increased by the unpredictability and gratuitousness of physical assaults, especially blows to the head and buttocks. Personal hygiene could not be maintained. Water was contaminated with fecal matter and excremental relief could be neither private nor carried out when the urge presented itself. Self-soiling was therefore common and during some of the more sadistically designed orgies by the SS, inmates were forced to defecate and urinate on each other (DesPres, 1976).

Although there were differences in the intensity and duration of the cruelties perpetrated against inmates, depending upon type of camp and time during the war when incarceration took place, the goal of captivity was clear and consistent throughout: to break the psychological, physical, and spiritual resistance of Jewish prisoners, and then to stigmatize and depersonalize them in such grotesque and unsavory ways as to facilitate their extermination.

COPING STRATEGIES

What sorts of coping strategies do people employ in a world where previous moral/ethical values are shattered, often forcing people to act in ways that would have previously been repugnant to them; where neither principles of casualty nor logic determines events; and, where death is a commonplace event determined by the caprice of others? Unpredictability of one's fate was reinforced by the SS tactical use of such euphemistic words and phrases, as transportation (deporting Jews to the camps), and final solution (murdering the Jews of Europe), to disguise their true intent: genocide.

Many survivors, especially those who were able to put their thoughts and experiences into writing or artistic creations, and now, those who are offering oral testimonies of their ordeals, have described the strategies they employed while imprisoned.

Although many attribute their survival to luck or to being in the right place at the right time, most also cite specific behaviors and defenses that they believe enhanced their chances of survival. Above all, inmates had to avoid reaching a 'musulman' stage, characterized by extreme apathy, bordering on stuporousness, which would mean instant death. Based upon interviews with survivors in the United States and Jerusalem, Dimsdale (Dimsdale, 1974), described nine ways in which inmates coped with camp life:

1 seeking out small pleasures, e.g. gazing at a sunset or smelling a rose;

2 investing survival with a purpose, e.g. to bear witness to the atrocities. This is probably one reasons why many elderly survivors now wish to provide oral histories of their Holocaust experiences;

3 distancing oneself from the horrors through such defensive behaviors as intellectualization (focusing on the theological and philosophical aspects of mortality and immortality), isolation (controlling all emotional expressions), and gallows humor (trying to tell jokes and laughing at one's plight);

4 mastering the environment in even such minor ways as finding a blanket or extra piece of food for a co-inmate or carrying out a forbidden act, such as praying on the Sabbath;

5 hoping, sometimes fuelled by denial, e.g. this cannot go on forever; once the world knows about our ordeal, help will be forthcoming;

6 forming two-person friendships, even though they would be forcibly dissolved when discovered by the SS so as to discourage resistance movements;

7 trying to gain the sympathy of SS guards and other inmates, e.g. special pleading might work on those rare occasions when done in the presence of a sympathetic guard;

8 relying on fate or becoming dependent upon others, so that stress was experienced passively;

9 identifying with the SS persecutors, with the apparent acceptance of the stigmata imposed upon them.

Clearly no one strategy or combination of strategies was used by all inmates under these extreme conditions. Although previously learned defenses against anxiety may have provided some bases for current coping behaviors, even those were rendered ineffective by the unprecedented intensity and duration of stress experienced by the inmates. New coping strategies had to be learned if survival was to become even a remote possibility. Nonetheless, the available data from reconstructed case histories and extensive interviews suggest that those who employed some sort of emotional distancing or psychic numbing could maintain a semblance of equilibrium in life-in-death situations, thereby enhancing the probability for survival.

THE SURVIVORS

How did those who survived fare after repatriation? What were the effects of their Holocaust ordeal on their future psychological and physical functioning?

Based upon descriptions provided by the World Health Organization and the Red Cross, and from observations of survivors seeking monetary compensation for property losses, and/or physical, and/or psychological damage from indemnification courts in the Federal German Republic, the 'survivor syndrome' was identified (Chodoff, 1969).

The reader should bear in mind that even among investigators and clinicians convinced of the validity of the 'survivor syndrome', it was clear that there was considerable diversity among survivors in the number and intensity of the following symptoms, many of which are listed in the current DSM-III-R diagnostic category: Post-traumatic Stress Disorder:

1 chronic depression, apathy, social withdrawal and a loss of interest in one's previous activities;
2 'vigilant' insomnia or nightmares in which parts of one's persecutory experiences recur;
3 chronic anxiety accompanied by psychophysiological distress, e.g. headaches, gastrointestinal symptoms;
4 lowering of one's threshold for stimulation, and an increase in responsiveness to cues reminiscent of one's camp experiences, e.g. fire, smell.
5 guilt over having survived while family and friends perished;
6 memory and concentration disturbances related perhaps to brain damage that may have been sustained as a function of frequent blows to the head;
7 avoidance of psychiatric help, premature termination of psy-

chotherapy, or difficulties in verbalizing traumatic camp events.

Other less frequent sequelae of the persecution have been mentioned: suspiciousness (Tuteur, 1966), premature senility (Bychowski, 1986), preoccupations with the past (Chodoff, 197)), and greater vulnerability to subsequent stressors (Luchterhand, 1970). Among many survivors, a symptom-free interval occurred following repatriation which might last for several years, and which was assumed to be related to the distractions associated with evolving a new life and finding one's way in a new, often not especially welcoming country; to completion of the mourning process for dead relatives, or to fantasies and hopes that dead family members would reappear. After some stability was achieved, these survivors became more susceptible to reminders of their Holocaust experiences and such environmental cues as the death of a friend or a child going off to school, could set off debilitating symptoms. It was the presence of such symptom-free intervals that led German compensation boards initially to conclude that psychological symptoms were not compensable because no causal relationship could be established between camp experiences and subsequent psychological malfunctioning.

A controversial issue raised by researchers of survivors is the relationship between trauma and subsequent behavior disorders. More specifically, was the trauma experienced by camp survivors of sufficient intensity so that anyone exposed would develop serious psychological problems or would only those with disturbed premorbid early histories maladaptively succumb to stress? Although there is a dearth of supportive data, the consensus among investigators is that early experiences could be related both to the time it took for one's breaking point to be reached (endurance threshold) and to the clinical variations in the symptoms of the 'survivor syndrome'. Nevertheless, there was also agreement that an overwhelming degree of stress, such as was experienced in the Nazi death camps, will adversely affect almost anyone. As so eloquently stated by Eitinger (Eitinger, 1971) 'If one rides a bicycle over a flower bed, some of the flowers will be broken, others not; but if one drives a heavy bulldozer with caterpillar wheels over the same flower bed, there is little likelihood of any of the flowers ever recovering.'

METHODOLOGICAL ISSUES

Numerous methodological flaws characterize the research from which the 'survivor syndrome' was derived (Solkoff, 1982).

1 In most studies anecdotes and impressions replaced sound statistical analyses of the data. Frequency distributions and other descriptive statistics, without appropriate tests of significance, provided most of the support for investigators' conclusions.

2 When interviews, a common source for data, were conducted, neither interviewing methods and protocols nor reliability among interviewers was addressed. Furthermore, when personality or attitude questionnaires were employed, no standardization or normative data were provided. Finally, it was not infrequent for personality characteristics to be ascribed to survivors without any mention of how these descriptions were obtained.

3 Observations of symptoms and diagnoses were most often made by a single clinician who was also the major or one of the investigators, with no efforts made to determine the reliability of the observations or diagnoses.

4 Samples selected for study were often biased, consisting of survivors identified with non-representative groups in the Jewish community, e.g. Hasidic Jews. Under such conditions, generalizations to the entire Jewish survivor population were impossible.

5 In addition to samples that were biased, study subjects were more often than not inadequately described. For example, information was often unavailable on age of survivor, sex breakdown, time, place or duration of incarceration, intensity of maltreatment, the presence of physical injuries, or countries to which survivors emigrated. Without fairly complete sample descriptions, replications are virtually impossible.

6 Finally, pitifully few studies included control groups against which the Jewish survivors could be compared. For example, no controls were indicated for such potentially important variables as: immigrant status, e.g. Eastern European Jews who experienced the Holocaust and Eastern European Jews who emigrated to America or Canada prior to the Holocaust; religious/ethnic backgrounds of survivors, e.g. Polish Jewish compared with Polish Catholic survivors; mode of survival, e.g. concentration camp, extermination camp, in hiding, as a resistance fighter; country to which emigration took place, e.g. America, Israel, France. Even when control groups were included, subjects were not properly matched on such variables as age when studied, sex, education, year and age when

imprisoned and length of imprisonment, and the presence of absence of physical problems.

In the face of these methodological deficiencies, the validity of the 'survivor syndrome' as it is currently conceptualized, must be questioned. At this point in the history of the research on survivors of the Holocaust, it therefore has to be left to the reader's judgment whether or not to accept the diagnostic conclusions reached by poorly designed research.

A related issue concerns the usefulness of diagnostic labels, whatever their validity, when applied to survivors of extreme trauma deliberately inflicted upon them for political/racial reasons. A diagnostic label should shed light on etiology and should guide psychotherapeutic strategies. As noted earlier, the most significant etiology for whatever problems survivors may have had, was probably the intensity and chronicity of the trauma they experienced in the camps and not any psychological 'anlage'. In addition, the success of intervention strategies was unrelated to the particular diagnostic labels applied to survivors. In this writer's view therefore, the diagnostic enterprise for survivors of the Holocaust has been neither useful nor fruitful and should probably be abandoned altogether.

INTERVENTION STRATEGIES FOR SURVIVORS

Most survivors resisted psychiatric treatment and preferred to avoid talking about their past traumatic experiences. It has been suggested that either the culturally determined unacceptability of psychotherapy for many survivors (Grauer, 1969), the wish to ward off past memories or the perception of treatment as threat or stigma (Krystal, 1968) deterred many survivors from seeking help. Lifton (Lifton, 1968) mentioned several reasons for survivors' reluctance to request psychotherapy. Some may not have wanted to alter their unique experience of surviving or they may have perceived themselves as too different to be understood. Others might have been suspicious of any treatment which implied that they were inferior or inadequate. Finally, Lifton speculated that psychotherapists may have resisted treating survivors who threatened their own denial of death.

The usual approach for survivors who sought treatment was psychodynamically oriented and based upon psychoanalytic principles. For those individuals, the going was often rough and the results of treatment were unpredictable. The survivor patient's transference feelings often resulted in perceptions of the therapist as an enemy, a potential Nazi guard, or as someone who could never understand the patient's stressful experiences. An additional impediment arose when, if the therapist was not Jewish, the patient would presume that he/she was antisemitic. Any one or all of those factors would result in premature termination of treatment or in not starting treatment at all. The therapist's countertransference feelings also played a role in the process and outcome of treatment. Many therapists did not want to hear about the gruesome brutalities perpetrated against their patients and would therefore shy away from explicit recognition or discussion of those events. In addition, many Jewish therapists experienced personal guilt at not having done enough for the victims or at not having themselves undergone similar inhuman experiences. The guilt was then transformed into anger with the patient being blamed for being a victim. Such attitudes were clearly not conducive to establishing meaningful and trusting relationships with patients.

Although most of the reported treatment outcomes with survivors have been pessimistic, the methods for determining outcome have not been specified and few, if any, follow-up studies have been conducted. In addition, no studies have systematically compared different intervention strategies with survivor patients. Finally, we have no data by which to differentiate survivors who benefited from psychotherapy from those who did not, nor do we know why some survivors functioned admirably and creatively without any need for psychotherapy at all.

It is perhaps no surprise that when the now aging members of the survivor population currently seek help, they turn to group approaches which focus on immediate problems in a context with individuals who have had similar traumatic pasts, rather than to the more traditional psychotherapies. Perhaps the current interest among survivors to provide oral histories of their lives under the Nazis may have more significant cathartic and ameliorative effects than any of our standard treatment approaches.

A WORD ABOUT CHILDREN OF SURVIVORS

Will the extreme trauma experienced by survivors of the Holocaust affect their subsequent parenting techniques? Will the children of these survivors be negatively affected by their parents' experiences? Is there any evidence for the transgenerational effects of trauma?

As was the case with survivors, most of the research designed to consider these questions have been psychoanalytically oriented clinical studies with abundant anecdotal evidence. Few investigators included carefully constituted control groups and many used subjects from various non-representative clinical subpopulations (Solkoff, 1981). The conclusions reached by these clinicians paint a very pessimistic psychological picture of children of survivors who, though not believed to constitute a homogeneous group are nonetheless most frequently depicted as acting out the unexpressed rage of their parents, as pursuing unrealistic goals to prove themselves to their parents (Barocas & Barocas, 1973), as moderately phobic, depressed and mistrustful of others, and as feeling the need to become an audience for and therefore vindicate their parents' past suffering (Trossman, 1968).

Again, as with survivors, these conclusions were based upon studies with flawed experimental designs (Solkoff, 1982). While men and women were frequently included in the samples, rarely were the data for the two sexes separately analyzed. This is particularly troublesome in view of some findings suggesting that male and female children may respond differently to their parents' Holocaust experiences and that father and mother survivors may differentially affect their children.

A second problem concerns the assessment of dependent measures. The instruments used by investigators were often designed for their studies and were not evaluated for such psychometric properties as reliability of validity. Pilot data, even if collected, were never reported. A third and very important flaw of many of these studies concerns sampling. Appropriate controls were not used against which to compare Jewish children of survivors and samples were often biased through the non-random selection of participants, e.g. individuals involved in Jewish studies, or attendees at synagogues. In addition, it was too often the case that the demographic characteristics of samples were not properly described.

While clinical and anecdotal data point to the psychopathologic effects Holocaust survivors have on their children, results of the few more methodologically sophisticated studies generally concluded that children of survivors were not substantially different from other children, and that even where differences appeared, the adjustment patterns of the 'second generation' fell within normal limits. In those latter studies which included children of immigrant parents who had not directly experienced the Holocaust, immigrant status of parents was more important than their Holocaust experiences in determining the psychological functioning of their children (Rose & Garske, 1987). Furthermore, significant numbers of children of survivors were found to be psychologically healthy and creatively engaged in satisfying careers, many working in health and health-related professions.

CONCLUSION

A small but significant number of European Jews, perhaps half a million, survived the Nazi genocidal actions against them. Although survival strategies varied, luck was a critical, but unpredictable, factor for surviving. As survivors, these individuals experienced some of the most barbarous acts ever perpetrated against humankind. Physical assaults, life-threatening diseases, being forced to serve as subjects in sadistic experiments, starvation and psychological degradation were commonplace. Once liberated from the Nazi camps and after having emigrated to their new countries from DP camps, how did these men and women fare? The psychological sequelae of Nazi persecution have been incorporated into what is now called the 'survivor syndrome' with most conclusions about survivors based upon psychoanalytically oriented studies and case materials, neither of which has generally considered relevant comparison groups. Similarly, the results of poorly controlled studies with biased samples have concluded that there are deleterious transgenerational effects of parental trauma.

Because much of the research on survivors of the Holocaust and their children has been methodologically flawed, the conclusions based upon such research have to be treated with scepticism. It is this author's belief that the question about the effects of Holocaust-related trauma, or for that matter any extreme trauma, on survivors and the second generation has not yet been properly answered. Although the ideal study, from a scientific standpoint probably cannot be conducted on such a complex topic, fraught with emotion, the methodological ideal must at least by approached if we are to understand the diversity of effects of exposure to any intense trauma.

In addition to developing studies with adequate sampling procedures which compare traumatized individuals with properly constituted, clearly described, control groups, we have to be better able to articulate the intrafamilial patterns in homes where one of both parents may have been severely traumatized to determine whether any lasting negative effects may have been transmitted to their children and if so, what the results of intergenerational transmission may have been. For example, one might focus on communication patterns within traumatized families. What and how much do parents tell their children about their traumatic past? What are the modes of communication? At what age do children learn about parental traumas?

Finally, for both survivors and their children we must not only try to uncover the deleterious effects of traumas – we must also consider how, for the former group, trauma may have had strengthening, steeling effects while for the latter group, how perceptions of parental trauma may have produced a more sensitive, caring second generation.

REFERENCES

Barocas, C. & Barocas, H. (1973). Manifestations of concentration camp effects on the second generation. *American Journal of Psychiatry*, **130(7)**, 820–1.

Bychowski, G. (1986). Permanent character changes as an after-effect of persecution. In H. Krystal, (ed.), *Massive Psychic Trauma*. New York: International Universities Press.

Chodoff, P. (1969). Depression and guilt among concentration camp survivors. *Existential Psychiatry*, **7(26–7)**, 19–26.

Chodoff, P. (1970). The German concentration camp as a psychological stress. *Archives of General Psychiatry*, **22(1)**, 78–87.

DesPres, T. (1976). *The Survivor: An Anatomy of Life in the Death Camps*. New York: Oxford University Press.

Dimsdale, J. (1974). The coping behavior of Nazis concentration camp survivors. *American Journal of Psychiatry*, **131** (7), 792–7.

Eitinger, L. (1971). Acute and chronic psychiatric and psychosomatic reactions in concentration camp survivors. In L. Levin, (ed.), *Society, Stress and Disease*. New York: University Press.

Grauer, N. (1969). Psychodynamics of the survivor syndrome. *Canadian Psychiatric Association journal*, **14(6)**, 617–22.

Kogon, E. (1950). *The Theory and Practice of Hell*. New York: Farrar, Straus & Co.

Krystal, H. (1968). Studies of Concentration Camp Survivors. In H. Krystal, (ed.), *Massive Psychic Trauma*. New York: International Universities Press.

Lifton, R. (1968). The survivors of the Hiroshima disaster and the survivors of Nazi persecution. In H. Krystal, (ed.), *Massive Psychic Trauma*. New York: International Universities Press.

Luchterhand, E. (1970). Early and late effects of imprisonment in Nazi concentration camps: conflicting interpretations in survivor research. *Social Psychiatry*, **5(2)**, 102–10.

Proctor, R. (1988). *Racial Hygiene: Medicine Under the Nazis*. Cambridge, Mass.: Harvard University Press.

Rose, S. & Garske, J. (1987). Family environment, adjustment, and coping among children of Holocaust survivors: a comparative investigation. *American Journal of Orthopsychiatry*, **57**, 332–44.

Solkoff, N. (1982). Survivors of the Holocaust: a critical review of the literature. *Journal Supplement Abstract Service of the American Psychological Association*.

Solkoff, N. (1981). Children of survivors of the Nazi Holocaust: a critical review of the literature. *American Journal of Orthopsychiatry*, **51(1)**, 29–42.

Trossman, B. (1968). Adolescent children of concentration camp survivors. *Canadian Psychiatric Association Journal*, 13, 121–3.
Tuteur, W. (1966). One hundred concentration camp survivors: twenty years later. *Israel Annals of Psychiatry and Related Disciplines*, 4(1), 78–90.

Part II

THEORY

8
PSYCHOBIOLOGICAL CONSEQUENCES OF SEVERE TRAUMA
José A. Saporta, Jr. and Bessel A. van der Kolk

The purpose of this chapter is to introduce the reader to the complex interaction between biological, psychological, and social factors that converge to produce and perpetuate the long-term consequences of trauma. Whether by cruel intuition or by trial and error, the torturer has learned through the ages to exploit those factors which are most effective in producing a state of helplessness and submission in his victims. The principles by which torture produces its damaging consequences are those which underlie the effects of other, varied forms of catastrophic trauma. Thus, while the after-effects of torture are so frequent and uniform that those who work with its victims have identified a 'torture syndrome' (Kosteljanetz & Aalund, 1983; Lunde, 1982; Hougen, 1988; Goldfeld et al., 1988), similar immediate reactions and long-term consequences also occur in response to combat, rape, kidnapping, concentration camp experiences, spouse abuse, child abuse, and incest (for reviews, see Horowitz, 1986, and van der Kolk, 1987a, 1988). These events share common features which elicit a common psychobiological response, a response which is also affected by such features as the subjective meaning of the event and the social and interpersonal matrix in which the event occurs. By understanding the principles of the trauma response, one is in a better position to undo its damage. Thus, our discussion will also outline the treatment implications of this model.

THE NATURE OF TRAUMA

The essence of trauma is that it overwhelms the victim's psychological and biological coping mechanisms. This occurs when internal and external resources are inadequate to cope with the external threat. There are four primary features of traumatic events which account for the overwhelming nature of trauma and the overwhelming impact of the torture experience.

Incomprehensibility

Traumatic events lie outside the normal range of human comprehension. Cognitive schemas serve as a buffer against being overwhelmed. When there are no existing cognitive schemas which allow the meaning of an event to be processed, the individual reacts with speechless terror. The inability to make sense of the experience overwhelms the victim's psychological capacity to cope. This exacerbates the state of extreme physiologic arousal induced by the stress. Such levels of arousal disrupt and disorganize cognitive processes and this interferes further with processing the meaning of the event (van der Kolk and Ducey, 1989; Fish-Murray, Koby, and van der Kolk, 1987). As a result, the traumatic experience is left unassimilated and is alternately denied and then compulsively relived with its original horrific intensity (Horowitz, 1986; van der Kolk, 1988). This may occur visually through nightmares and flashbacks, motorically through behavioral reenactments, or by reexperiencing dissociated fragments of the trauma through any sensory modality, through somatic symptoms, rage reactions, or panic states.

The traumatic experience cannot be assimilated in part because it threatens basic asumptions about oneself and one's place in the world (Janoff-Bullman, 1985). These assumptions include: personal safety, security, integrity, worth, and invulnerability, a view of the world as orderly and meaningful, and a view of others as helpful and good. Incomprehensible traumatic events may be dissociated from awareness in the service of preserving some of these assumptions about oneself and the world. However, by contrasting their view of reality the trauma usually shatters cognitive assumptions, leaving the subject in a state of inner confusion. Rieker and Carmen (1986) state that, 'confrontations with violence challenge one's most basic assumptions about the self as invulnerable and worthy and about the world as orderly and just. After abuse, the victim's view of self and world can never be the same again: it must be reconstructed to incorporate the above experience.' This reconstructed sense of self is usually negative, experienced by the victim as helpless, ineffectual, and unworthy. Victims may blame themselves and direct their anger inward in order to preserve a sense of inner control and to avoid helplessness.

The experience of torture is inherently incomprehensible, which is compounded by the fact that the torturer structures the environment to maximize confusion. Unfamiliarity of the environment, unpredictability, blindfolding, and seclusion all undermine the victim's ability to make sense of the experience. As prior schemas of the self and the world are shattered by torture, the torturer can impose new organizing schemas of the self and others. The victim is receptive to the torturer's construction of reality because of a desperate need to decrease the overwhelming terror and arousal and reestablish a sense of order and security. The victim's new view of himself as helpless and submissive to a powerful authority would better serve the torturer's ends.

Disrupted attachment

Human beings have a biologically based need to form attachments with others (Bowlby, 1969; also for review see Eagle, 1987, Chap. 2). Children need a safe base in the form of secure attachments in order to explore their environment and develop socially (Field, 1985), and adults continue to be dependent on social supports for a sense of safety, meaning, power, and control (Bowlby, 1969, 1973; Kohut, 1977; MacLean, 1985).

The need to attach to others increases in times of stress and danger. Pain, fear, fatigue, and loss all evoke efforts to attract increased care from others (Becker, 1973; Fox, 1974; Rajecki, Lamb & Obmascher, 1978). People whose internal resources are inadequate to cope with a threat may cling to others to regain a sense of predictability and security. Stable attachments help to limit overwhelming physiologic arousal (Reite, Short & Seiler, 1978; Coe, Glass & Wiener, 1983; Field 1985). Other people also validate the individual's experience and help make meaning out of what has happened. Some authors have credited surviving the concentration camps and similar extreme circumstances to the capacity to preserve attachment bonds, even when bonds with others are internalized abstractly in the forms of values and other cultural ties (for review see Eagle, 1987, Chap. 18).

The inability to turn to others in the aftermath of trauma is a loss of the major external coping resource people have available. The degree of post-traumatic dysfunction has been shown to be related to the loss of attachments and interpersonal supports (Pynoos & Eth, 1985; Stoddard, 1985). There may be several reasons for this. First, rupture of attachment bonds itself is thought to produce neurochemical responses similar to other traumatic situations, exacerbating the extreme physiologic arousal in response to stress. Secondly, the unmodulated arousal is perpetuated if the victim is not able to rely on secure interpersonal attachments to help regulate arousal and affects. As discussed above, extremes of arousal interfere with adequate processing of the traumatic experience. Thirdly, significant others are not available to validate and help make sense of the experience, perpetuating the inner chaos and terror which is, again, represented on a biological level as a neurochemical response leading to overwhelming arousal.

Traumatic rupture of interpersonal attachments is integral to the torture experience as well. Victims are kept in isolation and their captors threaten them with the capture and death of family and friends (Gonsalves, 1990). Torture survivors are often exiled after their release and feel alien and estranged (Fischman & Ross, 1990; Gonsalves, 1990). As outcasts from their society they do not receive the validation and support from their countrymen needed to overcome traumatization. This may be just one contributing factor to why they show persistent interpersonal dysfunction and increased divorce (Gonsalves, 1990). Traumatized people often show enduring difficulties in forming subsequent relationships (Lindy, 1987) and tend to alternate between withdrawing socially or attaching impulsively and maladaptively. This undermining of interpersonal resources perpetuates the traumatic situation.

In government sanctioned torture, the betrayal of the victim by his government can be viewed as the loss of an important attachment bond, both real and symbolic. Regardless of one's conscious attitudes about one's government, there tends to be a hope, or aspiration that will embody parental qualities such as the provision of protection and security. The betrayal of these expectations, and thus loss of this form of attachment, compounds the impact of torture. Given the role of attachment in overcoming trauma, we suspect that strong inner ties to groups which share political or religious ideals that give meaning to the suffering may to some degree buffer the controlling influence of torture.

Traumatic bonding

One of the most pernicious effects of torture is that in their attempt to maintain attachment bonds, victims turn to the nearest source of hope to regain a state of psychologic and physiologic calm. Under situations of sensory and emotional deprivation they may develop strong emotional ties to their tormentors (Bowlby, 1969; Rajecki, Lamb & Obmascher, 1978; Dutton & Painter, 1981; Ochberg & Soskis, 1982; Finkelhor & Brown, 1985; Kempe & Kempe, 1978). This 'traumatic bonding' is thought to occur among hostages, abused children, and abused spouses (Bettelheim, 1943; Dutton & Painter, 1981; Kempe & Kempe, 1978). The need to stay attached contributes to the denial and dissociation of the traumatic experience; in order to preserve an image of safety and to avoid losing the hope of the existence of a protector, victims may then begin to organize their lives around maintaining a bond with and placating their captors. A good example is Orwell's depiction of torture, in which Winston Smith comes to love his torturer, and Big Brother comes to dominate Smith's emotional universe (Shengold, 1989, p. 2). In the service of this illusion, captive traumatized persons are prone to blame themselves for their torment. The resultant denial and distortion further undermines processing and integrating the experience. As further quoted by Shengold in his discussion of 'soul murder', Obrien tells Smith in 1984, 'You will be hollow. We will squeeze you empty and then we shall fill you with ourselves' (quoted in Shengold, 1989, p. 2). The degree to which survivors of political torture develop self-blame and bonds with their captors, and if not what protective factors exist requires investigation.

Inescapability

The trauma response occurs when all escape routes are cut off. When there is nothing that the victim can do to terminate the massive threat to safety, his ability to cope is overwhelmed. When confronted with uncontrollable stress, animals and people develop 'learned helplessness' (Maier & Seligman, 1976). This contributes to undermining the individual's sense of self as competent and in control of his or her fate.

Torture is systematically meted out in an unpredictable and inescapable manner (see Başoğlu & Mineka, this volume for a discussion of this feature of torture). Little the victim can do can control the infliction of the torture; even cooperation and confessions rarely bring an end to the torment. The inability to escape or control the stress contributes to the cascade of terror and physiologic arousal.

Physiologic response

Persistent autonomic arousal

The final common pathway for events which are incomprehensible and terrifying, which rupture attachments, and are inescapable, is a reaction of extreme physiologic arousal, a basic biological response of fight, flight, or freeze. Severe or prolonged stress may then lead to chronic inability to modulate basic biological safety and alarm mechanisms. Kardiner noted in 1941 (Kardiner, 1941) that victims of what we now call PTSD continue to live in the emotional environment of the trauma and show an enduring vigilance for and sensitivity to environmental threat. The traumatized person may experience an alternation of numbing of emotional responses with hyperreactive emotional and physiologic responses, or may show hyperreactive responses superimposed on a baseline of numbing and dissociation. Physiologic emergency responses may become conditioned to reminders of the trauma and also generalize to other charged stimuli. Numerous studies of veterans with PTSD have documented conditioned autonomic reactions to stimuli reminiscent of the original trauma as measured by heart-rate, blood pressure, and electromyogram (Dobbs & Wilson, 1960; Kolb & Multipassi, 1982; Blanchard *et al.*, 1986; Pitman *et al.*, 1987; McFall *et al.*, 1990; Pitman *et al.*, 1990) and event-related brain potential (Paige *et al.*, 1990). Other research suggests that habituation may follow exposure to the traumatic stimulus itself, but associated events continue to elicit hyperreactivity (Strian & Klicpera, 1978). Not surprisingly, stress hormones have been shown to be persistently elevated in PTSD patients, including increased norepinephrine and epinephrine secretion (Kosten *et al.*, 1987) and abnormal cortisol secretion (Mason *et al.*, 1986; Smith *et al.*, 1989). There are also changes in receptor activity consistent with down-regulation secondary to chronic exposure to elevated levels of circulating catecholamines (Lerer *et al.*, 1987; Perry *et al.*, 1987). It is not clear whether these finding represent base line, tonic levels of catecholamines, or whether there are phasic elevations of catecholamines in response to stress superimposed on a baseline of normal or even depleted catecholamine levels.

Persistent all-or-none responses

The seeming inability to modulate biological alarm and arousal mechanisms may play a role in the tendency of trauma victims to react to stimuli with extreme, all-or-none physiologic and emotional responses. Loss of physical control undermines the individual's sense of competence and consolidates a sense of being helpless and dependent. Hyperarousal in response to recurrent stress may disorganize cognitive processes and interfere with the person's ability to respond appropriately. This further gets in the way of finding ways to get over the traumatic event, and, instead, even minor provocations can send the torture victim back to the emotional and physiologic state in which he or she was at the time of the torture. Many traumatized persons shut down their inner fantasy and emotional life in order to avoid triggering these frightening emergency responses. Unable to process emotions by thinking about them, they are prone to discharge tensions and emotions directly into action. With less access to an inner world of fantasy and symbols, they are further handicapped in working through traumatic memories and in forming and internalizing new meaning systems and interpersonal attachments.

BIOLOGICAL MODELS

There are three animal models for PTSD which share important similarities with the torture experience and which help us understand the biological effects of trauma in greater detail. Since the biological building blocks of humans and our mammalian relatives are closely related, particularly with respect to basic responses to danger, such similarities are expected. These animal models are 1) inescapable stress, 2) forced isolation, and 3) disruption of attachments in nonhuman primates.

Inescapable shock

Behavioral effects

Animals exposed to inescapable shock (IS) or other inescapable aversive stimuli develop a syndrome of profound behavioral deficits known as 'learned helplessness'. These 'tortured' animals develop: (1) deficits in learning to escape new stressful situations, (2) decreased motivation to learn new response outcome relationships, (3) decreased motivation to behave for the sake of rewards, (4) decreased exploration, (5) evidence of chronic subjective distress, (Maier & Seligman, 1976), and (6) increased immunosuppression and tumorogenesis (Visintainer, Volpicelli, & Seligman, 1982). These deficits are a direct consequence of the animal's lack of control in terminating or escaping the aversive stress (Weiss *et al.*, 1975). Once the animal recovers from the effects of IS, it may remain hyperreactive to future stresses. The animal becomes conditioned to respond to ordinary stresses with the full blown learned helplessness syndrome (Anisman & Sklar, 1979).

Stress, catecholamines, and the Locus Coeruleus (LC)

Underlying this conditioned behavioral response is a conditioned neurochemical reaction. The initial inescapable stress seems to elicit an increase in both the production and utilization of catecholamines (Anisman, Ritch & Sklar, 1981). Anisman, Ritch and Sklar (1981) propose that, under extreme stress, the utilization of these neurochemicals exceeds their synthesis, accounting for the finding of depleted brain levels of norepinephrine, dopamine, and serotonin in animals following IS (Weiss, *et al.*, 1975). Overproduction followed by net depletion of norepinephrine becomes a conditioned response to milder stresses (Anisman & Sklar, 1979) or even contextual elements of the original stress (Desiderato & Newman, 1971; Cassens *et al.*, 1980).

Some of the effects of IS can be prevented or reversed by administering drugs which prevent catecholamine depletion or which restore catecholamine levels (Anisman, Suissa & Sklar, 1980; Plaznik, Danysz & Kostowski, 1985). Learned helplessness is exacerbated by drugs or lesions which directly deplete catecholamine stores, such as reserpine and alpha-methyl-para-tyrosine (AMPT) (Glazer *et al.*, 1975; Anisman, Irwin & Sklar, 1979; Anisman, Beauchamp & Zarchnko, 1984; Britton *et al.*, 1984) This suggests that some features of learned helplessness are caused and perpetuated by this conditioned depletion of catecholamines.

Agents which stimulate the locus coeruleus such as yohimbine or cocaine exacerbate the effects of IS (see Krystal *et al.*, 1989). Conversely, agents which inhibit the LC such as clonidine, the tricyclic antidepressants (TCAs), MAO Inhibitors (MAOIs) or benzodiazepines prevent or reverse IS-induced learned helplessness (Petty & Sherman, 1979; Anisman, Suissa & Sklar, 1980; Sherman & Petty, 1980; Anisman, Ritch & Sklar, 1981; Weiss & Simpson, 1986). Catecholamine production originates in the LC, a small midbrain structure which is the primary source of noradrenergic innervation of the limbic system, cerebral cortex, cerebellum, and to a lesser extent the hypothalamus (Grant & Redmond, 1981). It has been called the 'trauma center' because it mediates fear and alarm responses (van der Kolk *et al.*, 1985; Krystal *et al.*, 1989). Destruction of the locus coeruleus causes animals to carelessly engage in dangerous behaviors (Redmond, 1979; Krystal *et al.*, 1989). Hyperreactivity or disregulation of the locus coeruleus may thus contribute to the hyperarousal and increased reactivity seen to follow IS. Also, with repeated overutilization and subsequent depletion of catecholamines in response to stress, there may be resultant upregulation or hypersensitivity of postsynaptic catecholamine receptors which would then exacerbate the hyperreactivity to stress-induced catecholamine secretion.

There are striking parallels between the animal response to IS and the human response to overwhelming trauma. Aside from the conditioned hyperarousal, van der Kolk *et al.*, (1985) and Kolb (1987) have noted similarities between the learned helplessness syndrome and the symptoms of the avoidance phase of PTSD such as anhedonia, social withdrawal, occupational dysfunction, and global cognitive and affective constriction. The biphasic PTSD symptoms may be influenced by conditioned fluctuations in catecholamine levels. Repeated depletion of catecholamines may contribute to the avoidance or numbing phase which is often accompanied by various forms of depression. It may also play a role in the general memory impairment noted in chronically traumatized patients (Gold & Zornetzer, 1983; van der Kolk & Greenberg, 1987; Greenberg & van der Kolk, 1987).

Several findings in traumatized humans support the relevance of the IS model to PTSD. Grinker and Spiegel (1945) described symptoms suggestive of catecholamine depletion such as mask face, reduced eye blink, cogwheel rigidity, postural flexion, and coarse tremor in World War II soldiers suffering from acute combat stress. We have cited evidence above for altered arousal and catecholamine levels in veterans with PTSD. Furthermore, it is those medications which prevent or reverse IS-induced learned helplessness in animals which have also been found helpful in decreasing the symptoms of PTSD. They may work at several sites in the hypothesized model. TCAs, MAOIs, clonidine, and the benzodiazepines inhibit the locus coeruleus and thus reduce conditioned hyperarousal, flashbacks, and nightmares. By blocking catecholamine overproduction at the locus coeruleus, they may prevent the catecholamine depletion 'upstream' in the brain, and MAOIs and TCAs may directly increase catecholamine availability in central synapses. MAOIs and TCAs may eventually down-regulate post-synaptic catecholamine receptors directly (Charney, Menkes & Heninger, 1981), thereby possibly reversing the receptor hypersensitivity caused by repeated, transient catecholamine depletion.

The IS model focuses on catecholamines, in particular norepinephrine. However, serotonin is also depleted by IS, and the tricyclic desipramine seems to reverse the effects of IS by increasing serotonin in the septum (Sherman & Petty, 1980). Learned helplessness in rats can also be reversed by several pure serotonergic agonists (Giral *et al.*, 1988). Thus, serotonin appears to be involved in IS and the trauma response as well. The role of serotonin in trauma is highlighted by the animal model of forced isolation.

Forced isolation

Behavioral effects

Forced isolation of animals produces increased aggression and other behavioral deficits which overlap with the learned helplessness syndrome. Pets confined to kennels away from their masters may stop eating and exhibit self mutilating behaviors (for review see Crawley, Sutton & Pickar, 1985). Wild animals forced into captivity frequently develop a syndrome characterized by, 'severe malnutrition, self-mutilation, infection, and death' (Fox, 1968; Crawley, Sutton & Pickar, 1985). Experimental isolation of animals, usually rodents, consistently produces increased aggression, including increased fighting and killing (Valzelli, 1969; Welch & Welch, 1971; Waldbillig, 1979).

Serotonin, aggression, and arousal

Isolation-induced aggression has repeatedly been shown to be related to decreased serotonin levels (Valzelli, 1969, 1982; Welch & Welch, 1971; Hodge & Butcher, 1974). The degree of isolation-induced aggression in different genetic strains of mice is directly related to the degree of iso-lation-induced decreased serotonin turnover (Valzelli & Bernasconi, 1979). Moreover, direct chemical or structural depletion of serotonin also produces aggressive behavior (Waldbillig, 1979; McKenzie, 1980).

Traumatized people also have difficulty in modulating aggression, both directed at themselves and at others. When Kardiner (1941) first delineated a traumatic neurosis of war, he included irritability and a tendency to explosive aggressive outbursts as two of the defining features. Given that both forced isolation and IS deplete serotonin in animals, aggression in traumatized humans may be related to trauma-induced decreases in serotonin levels. Decreased serotonin in humans has repeatedly been correlated with impulsivity and aggression in the form of violent and impulsive suicide attempts (Asberg, Traskman Thoren, 1976; Brown et al., 1979; Mann, 1987), cruelty to animals, fire setting and other delinquent behavior in children (Kruesi, 1989; Virk-kunen et al., 1989; Kruesi et al., 1990), and psychometric measures of impulsivity and aggression in adults with personality disorders, depression (Brown et al., 1979; Coccara et al., 1989), and substance abuse (Fishbein, Lozovsky Jaffe, 1989). Low serotonin mediated impul-sive aggression seems to be a trait that cuts across diagnostic groups (van Kammen, 1987; Coccaro et al., 1989). The research papers discuss-ing low serotonin levels in these patients seem to assume that they are dealing with a genetic trait. However, other studies of patients with these problems consistently demonstrate histories of childhood trauma such as physical and sexual abuse and neglect (Green, 1978; Pattison & Kahan, 1983).

Low serotonin in animals is also related to an inability to modulate arousal, such as exaggerated startle response to air puffs (Gerson &

Baldessarini, 1980; Depue & Spoont, 1986), enhancement of sensitization of the acoustic startle response (Davis & Sheard, 1976), increased alert postures (Poschlova, Masek & Krsiak, 1977), and exaggerated arousal in response to novel stimuli, handling, or pain (Depue & Spoont, 1986). The effect of serotonin depletion in animals is characterized as hyperirritability, hyperexcitability, and hypersensitivity, and an '... exaggerated emotional arousal and/or aggressive display, (though not necessarily attack) to relatively mild stimuli ...' (Depue & Spoont, 1986). This description bears a striking resemblance to the phenomenology of PTSD.

It has been suggested that serotonin inhibits or modulates the arousal produced by catecholamines (Samanin & Garattini, 1976; Gerson & Baldessarini, 1980; Depue & Spoont, 1986). Increased or decreased serotonin inhibits or accentuates respectively the effects of amphetamines on locomotion (Breese, Cooper & Mueller, 1974; Depue & Spoont, 1986) and serotonin inhibits amphetamine-induced aggression and alert posturing (Poschlova, Masek & Krsiak, 1977). Thus, decreased serotonin may interact with and contribute to noradrenergic dysregulation to produce the difficulties in modulating arousal and aggression seen in traumatized people.

Finally, serotonin dysfunction is related to obsessive compulsive disorder (Winslow & Insel, 1990). This, and other forms of obsessive thinking, appear to respond to medications which increase serotonin (Jenike *et al.*, 1989; Goodman *et al.*, 1990). Our clinical experience with the serotonin agonist fluoxetine has taught us that PTSD patients experienced a reduction in their obsessive fixation on the trauma and could move beyond its hold on their lives.

Separation in non-human primates

Behavioral effects

Maternal separation of nonhuman primates provides a third biological model for the trauma response. Monkeys separated from their mothers, and to some extent later on from their peer group, exhibit a biphasic protest and despair response (Bowden & McKinney, 1972; Harlow & Suomi, 1974; Suomi *et al.*, 1975). Human infants also show a biphasic protest and despair response to separation from their care givers (Bowlby, 1969, 1973; Robertson & Robertson, 1971). This biphasic response shows some similarity with the biphasic hyperarousal alternating with emotional numbing seen in traumatized adults. The despair phase of separation is similar to learned helplessness and has been offered as a model for human 'anaclitic depression' as well (Harlow & Suomi, 1974).

Catecholamines and serotonin

The biphasic protest and despair response to separation is likely correlated with fluctuations of neurochemicals similar to that elicited by inescapable shock. The despair response is alleviated by the tricyclic antidepressant, imipramine (Suomi *et al.*, 1978). Furthermore, agents which deplete central catecholamines (norepinephrine and dopamine) directly produce the despair response (Redmond *et al.*, 1971) and accentuate the despair response in peer raised separated monkeys (Kraemer & McKinney, 1979). Monkeys separated from their mothers but housed with their peers show no behavioral changes in response to a low dose of a catecholamine depleting agent. However, if housed in isolation from both mothers and peers and given the same dose of drug, it now exacerbates the amount of huddling and decreased locomotion beyond that seen in drug-free isolated animals (Kraemer & McKinney, 1979). Alcohol ameliorates the protest and despair response at low doses and exacerbates the despair response at high doses (Kraemer *et al.*, 1981).

Monkeys reared apart from their mothers are more vulnerable to exaggerated separation responses in adulthood and are also more vulnerable to the effects of catecholamine depleting drugs (Kraemer & McKinney, 1979). These monkeys also have difficulty modulating their arousal in response to social stimuli and amphetamines (Kraemer *et al.*, 1984), and easily become behaviorally disorganized in response to novel stimuli (Menzel, Davenport & Rogers, 1963; Mason, 1968). They also show increased aggressive responses (Harlow & Harlow, 1971; Kraemer *et al.*, 1984). Maternally deprived monkeys actually have lower than normal resting levels of norepinephrine but abnormally high norepinephrine elevations in response to stress, social stimuli, separation, or amphetamines (Kraemer *et al.*, 1984). Monkeys reared without their mothers also show low serotonin levels, and platelet serotonin reduction following separation returns to normal when the animal resumes social interactions (Coleman, 1971). Here, again, the loss of serotonin's modulating effect on the noradrenergic system may contribute to the wide fluctuations of norepinephrine and the hyperarousal in response to later separations and stimuli.

The three biological models of trauma show consistent overlap. Learned helplessness and the despair response to separation are similar and both seem to involve catecholamine depletion. In all three conditions there is a persistent impairment in regulating arousal and the animal is hyperreactive to later stress. Following both IS and maternal deprivation there seems to be an exaggerated catecholamine response to stress superimposed on a baseline catecholamine depletion. These reactions are affected by similar pharmacologic agents. Maternally deprived animals and those experimentally isolated have persistent problems in modulating aggression. In all cases this may involve altered serotonin function. Decreased serotonin may also underlie the loss of modulation of norepinephrine responses. The fundamental similarity to human trauma is in the persistent alternation of decreased motivation and global constriction (learned helplessness, despair) with poorly modulated and disorganizing arousal states in responses to later stimuli, as well as in impaired modulation of aggression. Trauma-induced depletion of catecholamines, catecholamine receptor hypersensitivity, and dysregulation of the locus coeruleus probably interact with trauma induced alterations of the serotinin system to produce these effects.

Vulnerability to trauma

The animal models for trauma, particularly IS and maternal separation are also similar to each other and to human trauma in terms of vulnerability factors. The severity of the response depends on the duration, repetitiveness and severity of the trauma in all cases. Furthermore, a history of early separation and maternal deprivation increase the animal's susceptibility to IS-induced learned helplessness (Anisman, deCatanzaro & Remington, 1978; Anisman & Sklar, 1981) and to separation responses in monkeys (Kraemer & McKinney, 1979; Kraemer *et al.*, 1984). Animals who are housed alone as opposed to being housed with their peers are more susceptible to the later effects of IS (Anisman & Sklar, 1981) and separation (Suomi & Harlow, 1972; Suomi, 1973). Genetic strain also appears to mitigate vulnerability to all three stressful conditions (Maier & Seligman, 1976; Anisman, Grimmer *et al.*, 1979; Valzelli & Bernasconi, 1979; Sackett *et al.*, 1981).

The data from traumatized animals allow us to predict additional features of the human response to torture. We would predict that a history of maternal deprivation, repeated separations, or early traumas increase some people's vulnerability to the damaging effects of torture, and that torture survivors would also be at an increased risk of developing PTSD in response to later life stress. This is supported by existing evidence that prior trauma predisposes adults to developing full-blown PTSD in response to later life stress (Burgess & Holstrom,

1979; Hendin, Pollinger-Haas & Singer 1983; Helzer, Robins & McEvoy, 1987). It is also likely that torture victims who are kept in isolation are more vulnerable than those housed with others, and that the quality of attachments to which the victim returns upon release is a crucial outcome variable. These factors seem to be biologically as well as psychologically mediated.

OTHER BIOLOGICAL EFFECTS OF TRAUMA

Endogenous opioids and trauma

Endogenous opioids also play a role in the trauma response. Inescapable stress results in a stress-induced analgesia in animals, and this decreased pain sensitivity becomes a conditioned response to subsequent stress and to previously neutral events associated with the noxious stimuli (Lewis, Cannon & Liebeskind, 1980; Maier, 1986; Fanselow, 1986). Opiate receptor blockers such as naloxone prevent stress-induced analgesia, and thus this conditioned analgesic response is opiate mediated (Maier, Davies, & Grau, 1980; Kelly, 1982). Stress causes increased production of opioids in humans also (Willer, Dehen & Cambier, 1981; Janal *et al.*, 1984), and this can become a conditioned response as well. van der Kolk, Pitman, and colleagues (van der Kolk *et al.*, 1989; Pitman *et al.*, 1990) have recently demonstrated that combat veterans with PTSD, but not those without PTSD, developed a naloxone reversible stress-induced analgesia in response to viewing combat films, which was correlated with a secretion of endogenous opioids equivalent to 8 mg of morphine. Indeed, this change in the pain response was the most significant factor differentiating the PTSD from the control group's response to a traumatic stimulus.

van der Kolk, Pitman, and colleagues speculate that this endogenous opioid release may be involved in the psychic numbing and dissociation which accompany trauma. In their study self reports accompanying the analgesic response to the stimulus indicated a relative blunting of emotional responses to the traumatic stimulus. Survivors of severe trauma have repeatedly described a triad of physical analgesia, psychic numbing, and depersonalization. Opioids also seem to be involved in mediating attachment behaviors; very small doses of morphine will abolish the protest response to separation in monkeys more powerfully than any other psychotropic agent (Newman, Murphy & Harbough, 1982; Panksepp, Sivey & Normansell, 1985). Affiliative behavior is increased by opiate receptor blockers (Fabre-Nys, Meller & Keverne, 1982), and brief social isolation produces opiate mediated analgesia in animals (Panksepp, 1980). Perhaps the conditioned opioid response to stress in traumatized humans contributes to their frequent social avoidance and withdrawal.

Opiates inhibit the locus coeruleus and thereby decrease the level of hyperarousal. Kosten and Krystal (1988) argue that an attempt to decrease hyperarousal underlies the abuse of such substances by traumatized patients. They point to the similarities between the hyperarousal seen in PTSD and that seen in opioid withdrawal states. Self-mutilating behaviors have also been linked to abnormally high levels of opioid production (Coid, Allolio & Rees, 1983; Richardson & Zaleski, 1983; Herman *et al.*, 1987). Numerous reports show a relationship between childhood abuse and neglect and self mutilation in nonbrain damaged patients (Green, 1978; Pattison & Kahan, 1983). Self-mutilating behavior has been reported to follow adult trauma in three cases without a prior history of child abuse (Greenspan & Samuel, 1989; Pitman, 1990). Subjectively, patients report mounting tension, arousal, and dissociation in response to stress, most notably abandonment. They are analgesic for the self-harm which is followed by a state of calm. These behaviors may be related to an attempt to modulate arousal via opioid production in an as yet undefined manner.

The psychobiology of reliving and reenactment

As early as 1889, Pierre Janet described how traumatized people become 'attached' to the trauma: 'All [traumatized] patients seem to have had the evolution of their lives checked; they are attached to an insurmountable obstacle. The struggle to continually repeat this situation leads to fatigue and exhaustion' (van der Kolk & van der Hart, 1989). Freud was confounded by patients' compulsive tendency to re-experience and repeat traumatic and painful experiences. Traumatized persons re-experience and re-enact the trauma in a variety of ways (Horowitz & Becker, 1971; Horowitz, 1986; van der Kolk, 1989). Vivid recollections, flashbacks, and nightmares repeatedly intrude into consciousness. Behavioral reenactments can take the form of stereotypic motoric acts associated with the trauma (automatisms), which occur without the subject's awareness of their significance. Reenactment behaviors can also be more complex. For example, we treated a Vietnam veteran who had lit a cigarette at night and caused the death of a friend by a sniper's bullet in 1968. From 1969–1986, on the exact anniversary of the death, to the exact hour and minute, he committed 'armed robbery' by putting a finger in his pocket and staging a 'holdup', in order to provoke gunfire from the police. This man was completely unaware of the meaning of this action during its enactment. Behavioral re-enactments may generalize to a person's entire life style. Traumatized children repeat the traumatic event in play (Terr, 1988), combat veterans may enlist as mercenaries (Solursh, 1987), incest survivors may become prostitutes (Silbert & Pines, 1981; Finkelhor & Brown, 1985), child abuse victims may abuse their children (Burgess, Hartmann & McCormack, 1987) and are more likely to be in physically abusive marriages (Gelles, 1972; Strauss, 1977; Hiberman & Munson, 1978).

Several psychological explanations for these phenomena have been advanced. The victim may intrusively re-experience traumatic memories in attempts to make sense of what has happened and to assimilate the event into existing cognitive schemas (Horowitz, 1986). Trauma may cause individuals to revert to earlier, more primitive forms of information processing and memory encoding. Thus, traumatic memories may be encoded and retrieved as motoric enactments, sensorimotor or bodily experiences, or iconic images, rather than as the linguisticaly determined concepts characteristic of adult memories (Neisser, 1967; White & Pillemer, 1979; Greenberg & van der Kolk, 1987).

Attempts at making sense of an incomprehensible experience has also been invoked to explain more general behavioral reenactments. Victims may identify with the aggressor and victimize others in efforts to combat the helplessness and powerlessness of their position. They may repeatedly reexpose themselves to the traumatic situation in the unconscious magical hope that this time the outcome will be different (Shengold, 1979). Reexposure to danger may also appease unconscious survivor guilt (Horowitz, 1986). Finally, severe trauma seems to disrupt the individual's capacity to notice danger cues and assess their own safety, leaving the traumatized person a 'sitting duck' for subsequent victimization (Kluft, 1989).

Trauma-induced neurobiological factors contribute to reexperiencing and reenactment also. Flashbacks, nightmares, and specific behavioral reenactments are usually reactive to high arousal states (Delaney, Tussi & Gold, 1983; Rainey et al., 1987) often in response to even mild stresses, and thus may be tied to those biological mechanisms which modulate arousal. The locus coeruleus (LC) plays a role in memory retrieval facilitation by means of tracts from the LC to the hippocampus and amygdala (Foot, Bloom & Aston-Jones, 1983). Long-term activation of memory tracts is observed in animals exposed to a highly stressful stimulus (Gold & Zornetzer, 1983; Kihlstrom, 1984), which is thought to be due to the massive noradrenergic activity at the time of stress (Squire, 1987). van der Kolk *et al.*, (1985) propose that hyperpotentiation of these tracts underlies the repetitive intrusive reliving of the trauma and may explain why subsequent stress is experienced as a return of the trauma. Memories laid down under massive autonomic arousal are reactivated by subsequent stress and the attendant hyperarousal, and these reactivated memories powerfully influence the victim's actions and interpretation of events.

State-dependent learning may explain why memories and behaviors of the trauma are evoked by arousal, as opposed to other memories and behaviors. Information which is acquired in an aroused, intoxicated, or otherwise altered state of mind is retrieved more readily when the altered state of mind is reintroduced (Overton, 1966; Phillips & Lepaine, 1980; Rawlins, 1980). Traumatic memories and behavioral responses which are laid down in a hyperaroused state, as well as trauma-induced dissociated or hypnotic like states of mind (Putnam, 1985; Spiegel, Hunt & Dondershine, 1988) are more accessible when people later find themselves in similar states. These states can be inadvertently triggered by subsequent stresses and internal reminders such as particular affects, and contextual stimuli associated with the trauma can evoke stored memories and state-dependent learned phenomena as well (Eich, 1980). This 'state-dependent thinking' influences how contemporary events are interpreted and responded to, and leads to inappropriate responses which were learned during times of danger. Brain stimulation experiments suggest that memories can become restricted to the 'state' of brain stimulation in which they were acquired (Phillips & Lepaine, 1980; Rawlins, 1980; Gray, 1987, p. 112). This may explain why traumatized persons can be wholly or partially amnestic for memories or behaviors enacted in the altered state of mind when they return to more habitual states of mind.

Trauma-induced alterations in serotonin function may directly contribute to behavioral reenactments. Animals with decreased serotonin function will emit behaviors which have previously been punished. Soubrié (1986) argues that serotonin systems are particularly relevant when there is competition or conflict between acting and restraining action, as when a previously rewarded behavior is now punished, and thus a tendency to act must be suppressed. In this circumstance, serotonin promotes restraint towards action. Decreased serotonin results in a shift towards facilitation of responding in circumstances where action and restraint compete.

Gray (1987) and Depue and Spoont (1986) propose a model whereby behavior is modulated by the balanced interaction of a behavioral facilitation system (BFS) and a behavioral inhibition system (BIS). The BFS is primarily dopaminergic and activates conditioned and unconditioned behavioral response systems. It is also mediated by noradrenergic fibers from the locus coeruleus which activates those structures necessary for emergency responses. It is thus activated in the presence of an expected reward or when goal oriented aggressive attack patterns require motivated motor support. The opposing system, the BIS, primarily depends upon serotonergic input and is mediated by the septal hippocampal system. In addition to inhibiting behavior in response to cues associated with punishment and nonreward, it functions to compare actual environmental circumstances with expected outcomes of behavior. In case of a mismatch the BIF:

> ... arrests ongoing behavior via inhibiting the BFS until other response strategies are formulated. The conditions constituting 'mismatch' are nonreward, punishment, and uncertainty ... the BIS responds selectively to signals of these conditions (Depue & Spoont, 1986, p. 51).

Decreased serotonin function weakens the BIS and shifts the balance from behavioral inhibition to facilitation.

These models suggest a mechanism whereby decreased serotonin functioning secondary to trauma can contribute to reactivation of traumatic memories in words, images, or actions. Behaviors which were learned and may have been adaptive during the original trauma are maladaptive in response to most ordinary stresses and must therefore be suppressed. Arousal counteracts this inhibition of learned responses: in addition to the factors argued above by which arousal leads to trauma-induced behavioral responses, conditioned catecholamine secretion in response to stress activates the behavioral facilitation system. Thus, there is a competition between behavioral response and restraint, the outcome of which is in part determined by the inhibiting function of serotonin tracts to the septo-hippocampal system. If, as we hypothesize, trauma causes decreased serotonin function, previously learned and by now maladaptive and even punished behaviors can be more easily activated by stress: the drive to repeat overcomes the victim's hope that this time they will act differently.

The comparator function of the septo-hippocampal system, in the assessment of environmental cues for impending punishment and nonreward may be impaired due to trauma-induced altered neurotransmitter function. This could explain why traumatized persons 'ignore' danger cues, repeatedly expose themselves to dangerous situations, and seem unable to learn from their painful mistakes. Heeding danger cues and learning from mistakes entails being able to compare current exigencies with expected outcomes based on prior learning and inhibiting ongoing behavior in case of a mismatch. Psychoanalysts attribute reenactments to the victim's persistent hope and need to prove that this time the outcome of the traumatic circumstance will be different (Shengold, 1979). While aligning one's hopes and expectations to real circumstances clearly involves many complex neuropsychological functions, it appears to be strongly influenced by serotonin functioning, which in turn affects the ability of the BIS-comparator to assess whether one's expectations (hopes) are likely to be realized in the current circumstance and to modulate behavior accordingly. With relative impairments in this function, traumatized persons are left to act according to their hopes and fears without the modulating influence of external reality.

Thus, torture victims may reenact aspects of their torture on themselves and others. They may respond to later stress in ways that were originally learned to cope with the torture and are now maladaptive. When frightened, they may respond to their treaters as if the helpers were torturers. They may also show 'bad judgment' in repeatedly re-exposing themselves to danger of revictimization, and may even 'provoke' such victimization.

TREATMENT IMPLICATIONS

The goal of treatment is to reduce the effect of traumatic memories on current feelings, thoughts, and actions. We assume that trauma victims ultimately must put words to their experience, and thereby integrate the traumatic experience into existing cognitive schemas or find new meanings for themselves and their place in the world.

An essential feature for recovery from trauma is reestablishing and normalizing attachments to others. Group psychotherapy is powerfully suited to mobilize the healing power of interpersonal attachments. The shared experience of group members provides shared understanding and validation. Trauma-induced obstacles to forming relationships can be observed and more adaptive relationship schemas can be learned. A group may be more able to contain traumatic material and overwhelming affects, which empowers the members and restores a sense of competence.

Biologically based post-traumatic symptoms often interfere with the patient's ability to give voice to the experience and place it in historical perspective. Overwhelming physiologic and affective responses to any reminder of the trauma, or to any charged stimulus in general under-mines these patients' sense of personal safety which is necessary to remembering and working through painful and frightening material. When therapy induces these bodily reactions without providing alter-native ways of coping, then therapy perpetuates the loss of control and feeling of incompetence initiated by the trauma. Finally the cognitive and emotional constriction seen in these patients cuts off their access to an inner world of symbols, fantasy, and language. Symbols, fantasies and words are necessary for most psychotherapies and are needed to explore and find new meanings for oneself. The person is left to act out feelings and memories rather than explore and verbalize them.

The goal of medications, then, is to reduce hyperarousal, restore the individuals' control over their bodily reactions, establish a sense of inner safety, and allow greater access to their inner world. There are reviews of pharmacotherapy of PTSD in the literature (van der Kolk, 1987b; Friedman, 1988; Davidson *et al.*, 1990) and in this volume (Keane *et al.*, this volume). Curiously, only medications which seem to be of limited therapeutic usefulness have been the subject of adequate scientific scrutiny. Tricyclic antidepressants and MAO inhibitors have a modest effect at best on hyperarousal, intrusive experiences and nightmares, and in alleviating depression (Frank *et al.*, 1988; Reist *et al.*, 1989; Davidson *et al.*, 1990). They may require trials of up to 8 weeks before response can be assessed (Davidson *et al.*, 1990), and appear to be less successful for emotional numbing and cognitive constriction. Clonidine, propranalol, and carbamazepine have all been found helpful for arousal and intrusive symptoms in open trials (Kolb, Burris & Griffiths, 1984; Lipper *et al.*, 1986; Famularo, Kinscherff & Fenton, 1988; Wolf, Alavi & Mosnaim, 1988). Benzodiazepines help decrease overwhelming affects and help sleep, but should be used cautiously in this population at risk for substance abuse. We have found clonaze-pam particularly helpful for this and for intrusive symptoms. Lithium can be very helpful in modulating affects and decreasing impulsive, explosive reactions (van der Kolk, 1987b). We have found the serotonin agonist fluoxetine especially promising in alleviating both intrusive and numbing symptoms and in bringing about a decrease in impulsi-vity, rage, and obsessive fixation on the trauma. Much remains to be learned about the role and mechanisms of medications in the treatment of trauma. This chapter has argued that the thrust of biological treatments of torture related syndromes is to restore normal neuromodulatory functions, which can be done, in part, by normaliz-ing the interaction of noradrenergic and serotonergic systems in the central nervous system.

ACKNOWLEDGEMENTS

The authors wish to thank Anne Ling Li, MD and José Saporta, Sr, MD for editorial assistance and comments.

REFERENCES

Anisman, H. L., Beauchamp, C. & Zarchanko, R. M. (1984). Effects of inescapable shock and norepinephrine depletion induced by DSP4 on escape performance. *Psychopharmacology*, **83**, 56–61.

Anisman, H., deCatanzaro, D. & Remington, G. (1978). Escape performance following exposure to inescapable shock: deficits in motor response maintenance. *Journal of Experimental Psychology [Animal Behavior]*. **4**, 197–218.

Anisman, H. L., Grimmer, L., Irwin, J. *et al.*, (1979). Escape performance after inescapable shock in selectively bred lines of mice: response maintenance and catecholamine activity. *Journal of Comparative Physiological Psychology* **93**, 229–41.

Anisman, H. L., Irwin, J. & Sklar, L. S. (1979). Deficits of escape performance following catecholamine depletion: implications for uncontrollable stress. *Psychopharmacology*, **64**, 163–70.

Anisman, H. L., Ritch, M. & Sklar, L. S. (1981). Noradrenergic and dopaminergic interactions in escape behavior. *Psychopharmachology*, **74**, 263–8.

Anisman, H. L. & Sklar, L. S. (1979). Catecholamine depletion in mice upon re-exposure to stress: mediation of the escape deficits produced by inescapable shock. *Journal of Comparative and Physiological Psychology*, **93**, 610–25.

Anisman, H. L. & Sklar, L. S. (1981). Social housing conditions influence escape deficits produced by uncontrollable stress: assessment of the contribution of norepinephrine. *Behavioral Neural Biology*, **32**, 406–27.

Anisman, H. L., Suissa, A. & Sklar, L. S. (1980). Escape deficits induced by uncontrollable stress: antagonism by dopamine and norepinephrine agonists. *Behavioral Neural Biology*, **28**, 37–47.

Asberg, M., Traskman, L. & Thoren, R. (1976). 5–HIAA in the cerebrospinal fluid: a biochemical suicide predictor. *Archives of General Psychiatry*, **33**, 93–7.

Becker, E. (1973). *The Denial of Death*. New York: The Free Press.

Bettelheim, B. (1943). Individual and mass behavior in extreme situations. *Journal of Abnormal Social Psychology*, **38**, 417–52.

Blanchard, E. B., Kolb, L. C. & Gerardi, R. J. *et al.* (1986). Cardiac response to relevant stimuli as an adjunctive tool for diagnosing post traumatic stress disorder in Vietnam veterans. *Behavior Therapy*, **17**, 592–606.

Bowden, D. M. & McKinney, W. T. (1972). Behavioral effects of peer separation, isolation, and reunion on adolescent male rhesus monkeys. *Developmental Psychobiology*, **5**, 353–62.

Bowlby, J. (1969). *Attachment and Loss, Volume I, Attachment*. New York: Basic Books.

Bowlby, J. (1973). *Attachment and Loss, Volume II, Separation*. New York: Basic Books.

Breese, G. R., Cooper, B. R. & Mueller, R. A. (1974). Evidence for involvement of 5-hydroxytryptamine in the actions of amphetamine. *British Journal of Pharmacology*, **52**, 307–14.

Brown, G. L., Goodwin, F. K., Ballenger, J. C. et al., (1979). Aggression in humans correlates with cerebrospinal fluid metabolites. *Psychiatry Research*, **1**, 131–9.

Burgess, A. W., Hartmann, C. R. R., McCormack, A. (1987). Abused abuser: antecedents of socially deviant behavior. *American Journal of Psychiatry*, **144**, 1431–6.

Burgess, A. W. & Holstrom, E. (1979). Adaptive strategies in recovery from rape. *American Journal of Psychiatry*, **136**, 1278–82.

Cassens, G., Roffman, M., Kuruc, A. et al. (1980). Alterations in brain norepinephrine metabolism induced by environmental stimuli previously paired with inescapable shock. *Science*, **209**, 1138–40.

Charney, D. S., Menkes, D. B. & Heninger, G. R. (1981). Receptor sensitivity and the mechanism of action of antidepressant treatment: implications for the etiology and therapy of depression. *Archives of General Psychiatry*, **38**, 1160–80.

Coccaro, E. F., Siever, L. J., Klar, H. M. et al. (1989). Serotonergic studies in patients with affective and personality disorders: correlates with suicidal and impulsive aggressive behavior. *Archives of General Psychiary*, **46**, 587–99.

Coe, C. L., Glass, J. C. & Wiener, S. G. (1983). Behavioral, but not physiological adaptation to repeated separation in mother and infant primates. *Psychoneuroendocrinology*, **8**, 401–9.

Coid, J., Allolio, B. & Rees, L. H. (1983). Raised plasma metenkephalin in patients who habitually mutilate themselves. *Lancet.* **ii**, 545–6.

Coleman, M. (1971). Platelet serotonin in disturbed monkeys and children. *Clinical Proceedings of the Children's Hospital*, **7**, 187–94.

Crawley, J. N., Sutton, M. E. & Pickar, D. (1985). Animal models of self-destructive behavior and suicide. *Psychiatric Clinics of North America*, **8(2)**, 299–310.

Davidson, J., Kudler, H., Smith, R. et al. (1990). Treatment of posttraumatic stress disorder with amitriptyline and placebo. *Archives of General Psychiatry*, **47**, 259–66.

Davis, M. & Sheard, M. H. (1976) p-Chloroamphetamine (PCA): acute and chronic effects on habituation and sensitization of the acoustic startle response in rats. *European Journal of Pharmacology*, **35**, 261–73.

Delaney, R., Tussi, D. & Gold, P. E. (1983). Long-term potentiation as a neurophysiological analog of memory. *Pharmacological and Biochemical Behavior*, **18**, 137–9.

Depue, R. A. & Spoont, MR. (1986). Conceptualizing a serotonin trait: a behavioral dimension of constraint. *Annals of the New York Academy of Sciences*, **487**, 47–62.

Desiderato, O. & Newman, A. (1971). Conditioned suppression produced in rats by tones paired with escapable or inescapable shock. *Journal of Comparative and Physiological Psychology*, **77**, 427–31.

Dobbs, D. & Wilson, W. P. (1960). Observations on the persistence of traumatic war neurosis. *Journal of Mental and Nervous Disorders*, 21, 40–6.

Dutton, D. & Painter, S. L. (1981). Traumatic bonding; the development of emotional attachments in battered women and other relationships of intermittent abuse. *Victimology*, 6, 139–55.

Eagle, M. (1987). *Recent Developments in Psychoanalysis, A Critical Evaluation.* Cambridge, Mass: Harvard University Press.

Eich, J. E. (1980). The cue-dependent nature of state dependent retrieval. *Memory Cognition*, 8, 157–68.

Fabre-Nys, C., Meller, R. E. & Keverne, E. G. (1982). Opiate antagonists stimulate affiliative behavior in monkeys. *Pharmacological and Biochemical Behavior*, 6, 653–9.

Famularo, R., Kinscherff, R. & Fenton, T. (1988). Propranolol treatment for childhood posttraumatic stress disorder; acute type. *American Journal of Disorders of Childhood.* 142, 1244–47.

Fanselow, M. S. (1986). Conditioned fear-induced opiate analgesia: a competing motivational state theory of stress analgesia. *Annals of the New York Academy of Sciences*, 467, 40–54.

Field, T. (1985). Attachment as psychobiological attunement: being on the same wavelength. In M. Reite, and T. Field, (eds.), *The Psychobiology of Attachment and Separation.* Orlando: Academic Press.

Finkelhor, D. & Brown, A. (1985). The traumatic impact of child sexual abuse. *American Journal of Orthopsychiatry.* 55, 530–41.

Fischman, Y. & Ross, J. (1990). Group treatment of exiled survivors of torture. *American Journal of Orthopsychiatry*, 60, 135–42.

Fishbein, D. H., Luzovsky, D. & Jaffe, J. H. (1989). Impulsivity, aggression, and neuroendocrine responses to serotonergic stimulation in substance abusers. *Biological Psychiatry*, 25, 1049–66.

Fish-Murray, C. C., Koby, E. V., van der Kolk, B. A. (1987). Evolving ideas: the effects of abuse on children's thought. In B. A. van der Kolk, ed. *Psychological Trauma.* Washington: American Psychiatric Press.

Foot, S. L., Bloom, F. E. & Aston-Jones, G. (1983). Nucleus locus coeruleus: new evidence of anatomical and physiological specificity. *Physiology Review.* 63, 844–914.

Fox, M. W. (1968). Psychomotor disturbances. In M. W. Fox, ed. *Abnormal Behavior in Animals.* Philadelphia: W. B. Saunders Company.

Fox, R. P. (1974). Narcissistic rage and the problem of combat aggression. *Archives of General Psychiatry.* 311, 807–11.

Frank, J. B., Giller, E. L. & Koster, T. R. (1988). Randomized clinical trial of phenelzine and imipramine for posttraumatic stress disorder. *American Journal of Psychiatry*, 145: 1289–91.

Friedman, M. J. (1988). Toward rational pharmacotherapy of posttraumatic stress disorder: an interim report. *American Journal of Psychiatry*, 145, 281–5.

Gelles, R. J. (1972). *The Violet Home.* Beverly Hills: Sage Publications.

Gerson, S. C. & Baldessarini, R. J. (1980). Motor effects of serotonin in the central nervous system. *Life Sciences.* 27, 1435–51.

Giral, P., Martin, P., Soubrié, P. et al. (1988). Reversal of helpless behavior in rats by putative 5-HT1A agonists. Biological Psychiatry, 23, 237–42.

Glazer, H. I., Weiss, J. M., Poherecky, L. A. et al. (1975). Monoamines as mediators of avoidance–escape behavior. Psychosomatic Medicine, 37, 535–43.

Gold, P. E. & Zornetzer, S. F. (1983). The mnemon and its juices: neuromodulation of memory processes. Behavioral and Neural Biology, 38, 151–89.

Goldfeld, A. E., Mollica, R. F., Pesavento, B. H. et al. (1988). The physical and psychological sequelae of torture; symptomatology and diagnosis. Journal of the American Medical Association, 259, 2725–9.

Gonsalves, C. J. (1990). The psychological effects of political repression on Chilean exiles in the US. American Journal of Orthopsychiatry, 60, 143–54.

Goodman, W. K., Price, L. H., Delgado, P. L. et al. (1990). Specificity of serotonin reuptake inhibitors in the treatment of obsessive–compulsive disorder: comparison of fluvoxamine and desipramine. Archives of General Psychiatry, 47, 577–85.

Grant, S. J. & Redmond, D. E. Jr. (1981). The neuroanatomy and pharmacology of the nucleus locus coeruleus. In H. Lala and S. Fielding, eds. Pharmacology of Clonidine. New York: Alan R. Liss.

Gray, J. F. (1987). The Neuropsychology of Anxiety: An Enquiry Into the Functions of the Septo-hippocampal System. New York: Oxford University Press.

Green, A. H. (1978). Self-destructive behavior in battered children. American Journal of Psychiatry, 135, 579–82.

Greenberg, M. S. & van der Kolk, B. A. (1987). Retrieval and integration of traumatic memories with the 'painting cure'. In B. A. van der Kolk, ed. Psychological Trauma. Washington: American Psychiatric Press.

Greenspan, G. S. & Samuel, S. E. (1989). Self-cutting after rape. American Journal of Psychiatry, 146, 789–90.

Grinker, R. R. & Spiegel, J. J. (1945). Men Under Stress. New York: McGraw-Hill.

Harlow, H. F. & Harlow, M. K. (1971). Psychopathology in monkeys. In H. D. Kimel, ed. Experimental Psychopathology. New York: Academic Press.

Harlow, H. F. & Suomi, S. J. (1974). Induced depression in monkeys. Behavioral Biology, 12, 273–96.

Helzer, J. E., Robins, L. N. & McEvoy, L. (1987). Post-traumatic stress disorder in the general population. New England Journal of Medicine, 26, 1630–34.

Hendin, Pollinger-Haas, A. & Singer, P. (1983). The influence of precombat personality on post-traumatic stress disorders. Comparative Psychiatrty, 24, 530–4.

Herman, B. H., Hammock, M. K., Arthur-Smith, A. et al. (1987). Naltrexone decreases self injurious behavior. Annals of Neurology, 22, 550–2.

Hiberman, E. & Munson, M. (1978). Sixty battered women. Victimology, 2, 460–1.

Hodge, G. K. & Butcher, L. L. (1974). 5-Hydroxytryptamine correlates of isolation-induced aggression in mice. European Journal of Pharmacology, 28, 326–37.

Horowitz, M. J. (1976). Stress Response Syndromes. New York: Jason Aronson.

Horowitz, M. J. & Becker, S. S. (1971). The compulsion to repeat trauma:

experimental study of intrusive thinking after stress. *Journal of Nervous and Mental Disorders.* **153**, 32–40.

Hougen, H. P. (1988). Physical and psychological sequelae to torture. A controlled clinical study of exiled asylum applicants. *Forensic Science International*, **39**, 5–11.

Janal, M. N., Colt, E. W. D., Clark, W. C. *et al.* (1984). Pain sensitivity, mood, and plasma endocrine levels in man following long-distance running: effects of naloxone. *Pain*, **19**, 13–25.

Janoff-Bullman, R. (1985). The aftermath of victimization: rebuilding shattered assumptions. In C. R. Figley, ed. *Trauma and Its Wake: The Study and Treatment of Post-traumatic Stress Disorder.* New York: Brunner/Mazel.

Jenike, M. A., Buttol, P. H. L., Baer, L. *et al.* (1989). Fluoxetine in obsessive compulsive disorder: a positive open trial. *American Journal of Psychiatry*, **146**, 909–11.

Kardiner, A. (1941). *The Traumatic Neurosis of War.* New York: Hoeber.

Kelly, D. D. (1982). The role of endorphins in stress-induced analgesia., *Annals of the New York Academy of Sciences*, **398**, 260–1.

Kempe, R. S. & Kempe, C. H . (1978). *Child Abuse.* Cambridge: Harvard University Press.

Kihlstrom, J. F. (1984). Conscious, subconscious, unconscious: a cognitive perspective. In K. S. Bowers, and D. Meichenbaum, eds. *The Unconscious Reconsidered.* New York: John Wiley and Sons.

Kluft, R. P. (1989). Treating the patient who has been sexually exploited by a previous therapist. *Psychiatric Clinics of North America*, **12**, 483–500.

Kohut, H. (1977). *The Restoration of the Self.* New York: International Universities Press.

Kolb, L. (1987). Neuropsychological hypothesis explaining post-traumatic stress disorder. *American Journal of Psychiatry*, **144**, 989–95.

Kolb, L. C., Burris, B. & Griffiths, S. (1984). Propranolol and clonidine in treatment of the chronic posttraumatic stress of war. In B. A. van der Kolk, ed. *Posttraumatic Stress Disorder: Psychological and Biological Sequelae.* Washington: American Psychiatric Press.

Kolb, L. C. & Multipassi, L. R. (1982). The conditioned emotional response: a subclass of chronic and delayed posttraumatic stress disorder. *Psychiatric Annals*, **12**, 979–87.

Kosteljanetz, M. & Aalund, O. (1983). Torture: a challenge to medical science. *Interdisciplinary Science Reviews.* **8**, 320–7.

Kosten, T. R. & Krystal, J. (1988). Biological mechanisms in posttraumatic stress disorder; relevance to substance abuse. In M. Galanter, ed. *Recent Developments in Alcoholism.* New York: Plenum Press.

Kosten, T. R., Mason, J. W., Giller, R. B., *et al.* (1987). Sustained urinary norepinephrine and epinephrine elevation in post-traumatic stress disorder. *Psychoneuroendocrinology*, **12**, 13–20.

Kraemer, G. W., Ebert, M. H., Lake, C. R. *et al.* (1984). Hypersensitivity to D-amphetamine several years after early social deprivation in rhesus monkeys. *Psychopharmacology*, **92**, 266–71.

Kraemer, G. W., Lin, D. H., Moran, E. C. *et al.* (1981). Effects of alcohol on the despair response to peer separation in rhesus monkeys. *Psychopharmacology*, 73, 307–10.

Kraemer, G. W. & McKinney, W. T. (1979). Interactions of pharmacological agents that alter biogenic amine metabolism and depression: an analysis of contributing factors within a primate model for depression. *Journal of Affective Disorders*, 1, 33–54.

Kruesi, M. J. P. (1989). Cruelty to animals and csf 5HIAA. *Psychiatry Research*, 28, 115–16.

Kruesi, M. J. P., Rapoport, J. L., Hamburger, S. *et al.* (1990). Cerebrospinal fluid monoamine metabolites, aggression and impulsivity in disruptive behaviors disorders of children and adolescents. *Archives of General Psychiatry*, 47, 419–26.

Krystal, J. H., Kosten, T. R., Perry, B. D. *et al.* (1989). Neurobiological aspects of PTSD: review of clinical and preclinical studies. *Behavior Therapy*, 20, 177–98.

Lerer, B., Ebstein, R. P., Shestatsky, M. *et al.* (1987). Cyclic AMP signal transduction in posttraumatic stress disorder. *American Journal of Psychiatry*, 144, 1324–7.

Lewis, J. W., Cannon, J. T. & Liebeskind, J. C. (1980). Opioid and opioid mechanisms of stress analgesia. *Science*. 208 , 623–5.

Lindy, J. (1987). *Vietnam, a Case Book*. New York: Brunner/Mazel.

Lipper, S., Davidson, J. R., Gradym, T. A. *et al.* (1986). Preliminary study of carbamazepine in post-traumatic stress disorder. *Psychosomatics*, 27, 849–54.

Lunde, I. (1982). Mental sequelae to torture. *Manedsskrift for Praktisk Laegegerning*. 60, 476–88.

MacLean, P. D. (1985). Brain evolution relating to family, play and the separation call. *Archives of General Psychiatry*, 42, 505–17.

Maier, S. F. (1986). Stressor controllability and stress-induced analgesia. *Annals of the New York Academy of Sciences*, 467, 55–72.

Maier, S. F., Davies, S. & Grau, J. W. (1980). Opiate antagonists and long term analgesic reaction induced by inescapable shock in rats. *Journal of Comparative Psychology*, 105, 3–46.

Maier, S. F., Seligman, M. E. (1976). Learned helplessness: theory and evidence. *Journal of Experimental Psychology [Gen]*, 105, 3–46.

Mann, J. D. (1987). Psychobiologic predictors of suicide. *Journal of Clinical Psychiatry*, 48, 39–43.

Mason, W. A. (1968). Early social deprivation in the nonhuman primates: implications for human behavior. In D. C. Glass, *Environmental Influences*. New York: Rockefeller University Press and Russel Sage Foundation.

Mason, J. W., Giller, E. L. & Kosten, T. R. (1986). Urinary free cortisol levels in post-traumatic stress disorder. *Journal of Nervous and Mental Disorders*, 174, 145–9.

McFall, M. E., Murburg, M., Grant, N. K. *et al.* (1990). Autonomic responses to stress in Vietnam combat veterans with posttraumatic stress disorder. *Biological Psychiatry*, 27, 1165–75.

McKenzie, G. (1980). Dissociation of the antiaggression and serotonin-depleting effects of fenfluramine. *Canadian Journal of Physiology and Pharmacolaogy,* 59, 830–6.

Menzel, E. W., Davenport, R. K., Rogers, C. M. (1963). Effects of environmental restriction upon the chimpanzee's responsiveness to novel situations. *Journal of Comparative Physiological Psychology,* 56, 329–34.

Neisser, U. (1967). *Cognitive Psychology.* Englewood Cliffs, NJ: Prentice-Hall.

Newman, J. D., Murphy, M. R. & Harbough, C. R. (1982). Naloxone-reversible suppression of isolation cell production after morphine injections in squirrel monkeys. *Social Neurosciences Abstracts,* 8, 940.

Ochberg, F. M. & Soskis, D. A. (1982). *Victims of Terrorism.* Boulder: Westview.

Overton, D. A. (1966). State-dependent learning produced by depressant and atropine-like drugs. *Psychopharmacologia.* 10, 6–31.

Paige, S. R., Reid, G. M., Allen, M. G. *et al.* (1990). Psychophysiologic correlates of posttraumatic stress disorder. *Biological Psychiatry,* 27, 419–30.

Panksepp, J. (1980). Brief social isolation, pain responsivity and morphine analgesia in young rats. *Psychopharmacology,* 72, 110–12.

Panksepp, J., Sivey, S. M. & Normansell, L. A. (1985). Brain opioids and social emotions. In M. Reite, T. Fields, eds. *The Psychobiology of Attachments and Separation.* Orlando: Academic Press.

Pattison, E. M. & Kahan, J. (1983). The deliberate self-harm syndrome. *American Journal of Psychiatry,* 140, 867–72.

Perry, B. D., Giller, E. L. & Southwick, S. M. (1987). Altered plasma alpha-2 adrenergic receptor affinity states in PTSD. *American Journal of Psychiatry,* 144, 1511–12.

Petty, F. & Sherman, A. D. (1979). Reversal of learned helplessness by imipramine. *Communications in Psychopharmacology,* 3, 371–73.

Phillips, A. G. & Lepaine, F. G. (1980). Disruption of conditioned taste aversion in the rat by stimulation of amygdala: a conditioning effect, not amnesia. *Journal of Comparative Physiological Psychology,* 94, 664–74.

Pitman, R. K. (1990). Self-mutilation in combat-related PTSD (letter). *American Journal of Psychiatry,* 147, 123–34.

Pitman, R. K., Orr, S., Laforgue, D. *et al.* (1987). Psychophysiology of PTSD imagery in Vietnam combat veterans. *Archives of General Psychiatry,* 44, 970–6.

Pitman, R. K., Orr, S. P. & Forgue, D. F. (1990). Psychophysiologic responses to combat imagery of Vietnam veterans with posttraumatic stress disorder versus other anxiety disorders. *Journal of Abnormal Psychology.* 99, 49–54.

Pitman, R. K., van der Kolk, B. A., Orr, S. P. *et al.* (1990). Naloxone-reversible analgesic response to combat-related stimuli in posttraumatic stress disorder: a pilot study. *Archives of General Psychiatry,* 47, 541–7.

Plaznik, A., Danysz, W. & Kostowski, W. (1985). A stimulatory effect of intraacumbens injections of noradrenaline on the behavior of rats in the forced swim test. *Psychopharmacology,* 87, 119–23.

Poschlova, N., Masek, K. & Krsiak, M. (1977). Amphetamine-like effects of 5, 6-dihydroxytryptamine on social behavior in the mouse. *Neuropharmacology,* 16, 317–21.

Putnam, F. W. (1985). Dissociation as a response to extreme trauma. In R. P.

Kluft, ed. *The Childhood Antecedents of Multiple Personality.* Washington: American Psychiatric Press.

Pynoos, R. S. & Eth, S. (1985). Developmental perspective on psychic trauma in childhood. In C. R. Figley , ed., *Trauma and Its Wake: The Study and Treatment of Posttraumatic Stress Disorder.* New York: Brunner/Mazel.

Rainey, J. M., Aleem, A., Ortiz, A. *et al.* (1987). Laboratory procedures for the inducement of flashbacks. *American Journal of Psychiatry,* **144,** 1317–19.

Rajecki, D. W., Lamb, M. E. & Obmascher, P. (1978). Toward a general theory of infantile attachment; a comparative review of aspects of the social bond. *Behavioral Brain Sciences,* **3,** 417–64.

Rawlins, J. N. P. (1980). Associative and non-associative mechanisms in the development of tolerance for stress: the problem of state-dependent learning. In S. Levine, and H. Ursin, eds. *Coping and Health.* New York: Plenum Press.

Redmond, D. E. Jr. (1979). New and old evidence for the involvement of a brain noradrenergic system in anxiety. In W. E. Fann, I. Karacan, A. D. Pakorner, *et al.* eds. *Phenomenology and Treatment of Anxiety.* New York: Spectrum.

Redmond, D. E. Jr, Maas, J. W., Kling, A. *et al.* (1971). Social behavior of monkeys selectively depleted of monoamines. *Science,* **174;** 428–31.

Rieker, P. P. & Carmen, E. H. (1986). The victim to patient process: the disconfirmation and transformation of abuse. *American Journal of Orthopsychiatry,* **56,** 369–70.

Reist, C., Kauffman, C. D., Haier, R. J. *et al.* (1989). A controlled trial of desipramine in 18 men with posttraumatic stress disorder. *American Journal of Psychiatry,* **146,** 513–16.

Reite, M., Short, R. & Seiler, C. *et al.* (1978). Physiological correlates of separation in surrogate reared infants: a study in altered attachment bonds. *Developmental Psychobiology,* **11,** 427–35.

Richardson, J. S., Zaleski, W. A. (1983). Naloxone and self-mutilation. *Biological Psychiatry,* **18,** 99–101.

Robertson, J., Robertson, J. (1971). Young children in brief separation: a fresh look. *Psychoanalytic Study of the Child,* **26,** 264–315.

Sackett, G. P., Ruppenthaal, G. C., Fahrenbruch, C. E. *et al.* (1981). Social isolation rearing effects in monkeys varies with genotype. *Developmental Psychology.* **17,** 313–18.

Samanin, R. & Garattini, S. (1976). The serotonergic system in the brain and its possible functional connections with other aminergic systems. *Life Sciences,* **17,** 1201–10.

Shengold, L. (1979). Child abuse and deprivation: soul murder. *Journal of the American Psychoanalytic Association,* **27,** 533–59.

Shengold, L. (1989) *Soul Murder.* New Haven: Yale University Press.

Sherman, A. D. & Petty, F. (1980). Neurochemical basis of the action of antidepressants on learned helplessness. *Behavioral and Neural Biology.* **30,** 119–34.

Silbert, M. H. & Pines, A. M. (1981). Sexual child abuse as an antecedent of prostitution. *Child Abuse and Neglect,* **5,** 407–11.

Smith, M. A., Davidson, J., Ritchie, J. C. *et al.* (1989). The corticotropin releasing hormone tests in patients with posttraumatic stress disorder. *Biological Psychiatry*, 26, 349–55.

Solursh, L. (1987). Combat addiction: implications in symptom maintenance and treatment planning. Paper presented at the Third Annual Meeting of the Society of Traumatic Stress Studies. Baltimore, Maryland.

Soubrié, P. (1986). Reconciling the role of central serotonin neurons in human and animal behavior. *Behavioral and Brain Sciences*, 9, 319–64.

Spiegel, D., Hunt, T. & Dondershine, H. E. (1988). Dissociation and hypnotizability in posttraumatic stress disorder. *American Journal of Psychiatry*. 145, 301–5.

Squire, L. R. (1987). *Memory and the Brain.* New York: Oxford University Press.

Stoddard, F. (1985). Stress disorders in burned children and adolescents. Paper presented at the Annual Meeting of the American Psychiatric Association.

Strauss, M. A. (1977). Sociological perspectives on the prevention and treatment of wife-beating. In M. Roy, ed. *Battered Women: A Psychosociological Study of Domestic Violence.* New York: Van Nostrand Reinhold.

Strian, F. & Klicpera, C. (1978). Die bedeuting psycho-autonomische Reaktionen im Enstehung und Persistenz von Angstzustanden. *Nervenartzt*, 49, 576–83.

Suomi, S. J. (1973). Repetitive peer separation of young monkeys: effects of vertical chamber confinements during separations. *Journal of Abnormal Psychology*, 81, 1–10.

Suomi, S. J., Eisele, C. D., Grady, S. A. *et al.* (1975). Depressive behavior in adult monkeys following separation from family environment. *Journal of Abnormal Psychology*, 5, 576–8.

Suomi, S. J. & Harlow, H. F. (1972). Depressive behavior in young monkeys subjected to vertical chamber confinement. *Journal of Comparative Physiological Psychology*, 180, 11–18.

Suomi, S. J., Seamen, S. F., Lewis, J. K. *et al.* (1978). Effects of imipramine treatment of separation induced social disorders in rhesus monkeys. *Archives of General Psychiatry*, 35, 321–5.

Terr, L. (1988). What happens to early memories of trauma? *Journal of the American Academy of Child and Adolescent Psychiatry*, 1, 96–104.

Valzelli, L. (1969). Aggressive behavior induced by isolation. In S. Garattini, and L. Sigg, eds. *Aggressive Behavior.* Amsterdam: Excerpta Medica.

Valzelli, L. (1982). Serotonergic inhibitory control of experimental aggression. *Psychopharmacological Research Communications*, 14, 1–13.

Valzelli, L. & Bernasconi, S. (1979). Aggressiveness by isolation and brain serotonin turnover changes in different strains of mice. *Neuropsychobiology*. 5, 129–35.

van der Kolk, B. A. (1987a). *Psychological Trauma.* Washington: American Psychiatric Press.

van der Kolk, B. A. (1987b). The drug treatment of posttraumatic stress disorder. *Journal of Affective Disorders*, 13, 203–13.

van der Kolk, B. A. (1988). The trauma spectrum: the interaction of biological and social events in the genesis of the trauma response. *Journal of Traumatic Stress*, **1**, 273–90.

van der Kolk, B. A. (1989). The compulsion to repeat the trauma; re-enactment, revictimization, and masochism. *The Psychiatric Clinics of North America*, **12**, 389–411.

van der Kolk, B. A. & Ducey, C. P. (1989). The psychological processing of traumatic experience: Rorschach patterns in PTSD. *Journal of Traumatic Stress*, **22**, 259–74.

van der Kolk, B. A. & Greenberg, M. S. (1987). The psychobiology of the trauma response: hyperarousal, constriction, and addiction to traumatic reexposure. In B. A. van der Kolk, (ed) *Psychological Trauma*. Washington: American Psychiatric Press.

van der Kolk, B. A., Greenberg, M. S., Boyd, H. *et al.* (1985). Inescapable shock, neurotransmitters, and addiction to trauma: toward a psychobiology of posttraumatic stress. *Biological Psychiatry*, **20**, 314–25.

van der Kolk, B. A., Greenberg, M. S., Orr, S. P. *et al.* (1989). Endogenous opioids, stress-induced analgesia, and post-traumatic stress disorder. *Psychopharmacology Bulletin*, **25**, 417–21.

van der Kolk, B. A., van der Hart, O. (1989). Pierre Janet and the breakdown of adaptation in psychological trauma. *American Journal of Psychiatry*, **146**, 1530–40.

van Kammen, D. P. (1987). 5-HT, a neurotransmitter for all seasons? *Biological Psychiatry*, **22**, 1–3.

Virkkunen, M., De Jong, J., Bartfo, J. *et al.* (1989). Psychobiological concomitants of history of suicide attempts among violent offenders and impulsive fire setters. *Archives of General Psychiatry*, **46**, 604–6.

Visintainer, M. A., Volpicelli, J. R. & Seligman, M. E. P. (1982). Tumor rejection in rats after inescapable shock. *Science*, **216**, 437–9.

Waldbillig, R. (1979). The role of the dorsal and median raphe in the inhibition of muricide. *Brain Research*, **160**, 341–6.

Weiss, J. M., Glazer, H. I., Pohorecky, L. A. *et al.* (1975). Effects of chronic exposure to stressors on subsequent avoidance–escape behavior and on brain norepinephrine. *Psychosomatic Medicine*, **37**, 522–4.

Weiss, J. M. & Simpson, P. G. (1986). Depression in an animal model: focus on the locus coeruleus. In R. Porter, G. Bock, and S. Clark, eds. *Antidepressants and Receptor Function*. New York: John Wiley.

Welch, A. S. & Welch, B. L. (1971). Isolation, reactivity, and aggression: evidence for an involvement of brain catecholamines and serotonin. In B. E. Eleftheriou, and J. P. Scott, eds. *Physiology of Aggression and Defeat*. New York: Plenum Press.

White, S. H. & Pillemer, D. B. (1979). Childhood amnesia and the development of a socially accessible memory system. In J. F. Kihlstrom, and F. J. Evans, *Functional Disorders of Memory*. NJ: Hillsdale.

Willer, J. C., Dehen, H. & Cambier, J. (1981). Stress-induced analgesia in humans: endogenous opioids and naloxone-reversible depression of pain reflexes. *Science*, **212**, 689–91.

Winslow, J. T. & Insel, T. R. (1990). Neurobiology of obsessive compulsive disorder: a possible role for serotonin. *Journal of Clinical Psychiatry*, **51(suppl)**, 27–35.

Wolf, M. E., Alavi, A. & Mosnaim, A. D. (1988). Posttraumatic stress disorder in Vietnam veterans. Clinical and EEG findings: possible therapeutic effects of carbamazepine. *Biological Psychiatry*, **23**, 642–4.

9
THE ROLE OF UNCONTROLLABLE AND UNPREDICTABLE STRESS IN POST-TRAUMATIC STRESS RESPONSES IN TORTURE SURVIVORS
Metin Başoğlu and Susan Mineka

INTRODUCTION

In this chapter we will review experimental models of anxiety, depression and post-traumatic stress and their relevance to human experience during and after torture. We believe that the intensive study over the past 25 years of the effects of unpredictable and uncontrollable traumatic events in animals has provided very useful experimental models for understanding the experiences of humans undergoing torture. The relevance of this animal research to understanding anxiety and depression has been known for some time (e.g. Barlow, 1988; Mineka & Kihlstrom, 1978; Mineka & Kelly, 1989; Overmier, 1988; Seligman, 1975). Recently, its relevance to understanding PTSD in humans has also been recognized (Foa, Steketee & Rothbaum, 1989; van der Kolk *et al.*, 1985; van der Kolk & Greenberg, 1987). However, it is our contention that the human experience with probably the closest parallels to these experimental models in animals is the experience of humans undergoing torture. Although these parallels cannot provide a comprehensive account of human behaviour during and after torture, they can nevertheless contribute significantly to our understanding of the mechanisms involved in the development of post-trauma symptoms and help us in identifying principles of effective treatment for torture survivors.

In order to avoid the difficult definitional problems torture poses, the details of the torture methods reviewed in this chapter are mainly derived from interviews with political detainees subjected to systematic torture. These methods are by no means meant to be an exhaustive list of all forms of torture used in the world. We have instead focused on the most commonly reported forms of torture by the survivors we have interviewed. These are also the most commonly reported forms of torture in the literature (Allodi & Cowgill, 1982; Stover & Nightingale, 1985; Amnesty International, 1984; Benfeldt-Zachrisson, 1985; for a review, see also Goldfeld *et al.*, 1988, and

Mollica, this volume). Similarly, we do not mean to provide a comprehensive account of coping strategies under captivity and torture but rather to focus on those which are illuminated by research on unpredictability and uncontrollability. More detailed accounts can be found in the literature (e.g. Nardini, 1962; Wolf & Ripley, 1947; Sledge, Boydston & Rahe, 1980; Spaulding & Ford, 1972; Ford and Spaulding, 1973; Rahe & Genender-Sherwood, 1983; Hinkle & Wolff, 1956; Farber, Harlow & West, 1957; Sherwood, 1986; see also chapters by Solkoff & Miller in this volume).

To facilitate the study of potential predictors of acute and post-traumatic stress symptoms, the experience of torture survivors can be broadly divided into four phases, which vary in both the forms and the degrees of uncontrollable and unpredictable stress: 1) pre-arrest/detention phase, 2) detention/torture, 3) trial/imprisonment, and 4) post-imprisonment phase. Sometimes these phases overlap with respect to some of these parameters, and phase 4 may merge into phases 1 and 2 because of repeated arrests and torture. For some, phase 3 does not apply because they are released after detention and torture. Thus, although we recognize these distinctions are somewhat arbitrary, we nevertheless think it is useful to divide discussion of torture experiences into these four phases. Broadly speaking, the analogue of phase 1 in animal research concerns questions of what pre-treatment variables serve to attenuate or potentiate the effects of subsequent exposure to uncontrollable or unpredictable aversive events. The analogue of phases 2 and 3 in animal research concerns study of the acute and short-term reactions to unpredictable and uncontrollable stress. The analogue of phase 4 concerns study of long-term sequelae of exposure to uncontrollable and unpredictable aversive events.

SYMPTOMS FOLLOWING TORTURE

Before providing a review of the myriad psychological and physiological consequences of exposure to unpredictable and uncontrollable traumatic events, we first provide a brief overview of the psychological symptoms following torture in order to facilitate the reader's understanding of the close parallels that will be documented in more detail later in the chapter.

The psychological symptoms which follow torture have been amply documented. They include psychosomatic symptoms (pains, nervousness, insomnia, nightmares, tremors, weakness, fainting, sweating, diarrhoea), behavioural changes (withdrawal, suspiciousness, irritability, aggressiveness, impulsiveness, suicide attempts, depression, fears, phobias), and cognitive impairment (confusion, disorientation, memory defects, loss of concentration) (Allodi & Cowgill, 1982). Other studies have concurred on the nature of post-torture symptoms (e.g. Rasmussen & Lunde, 1980; Lunde, 1982; Domovitch *et al.*, 1984; see Goldfeld *et al.*, 1988; Ortmann *et al.*, 1987; Somnier & Genefke, 1986; Reid & Strong, 1988; Mollica, Wyshak & Lavelle, 1987; Mollica *et al.*, 1990). It should, however, be borne in mind that some of these symptoms (e.g. concentration and memory impairment, headaches) may be due to organic pathology in the brain secondary to head traumas because such cases have been documented (Jensen *et al.*, 1982). Further discussion of symptoms will occur below in the context of discussing the four different phases of torture.

UNPREDICTABLE AND UNCONTROLLABLE TRAUMATIC STIMULI: ANIMAL LITERATURE

Overview

Study of the psychological and physiological consequences of exposure to traumatic stimuli has seen significant advances in the past 25 years. Of major importance in the progress that has been made has been the identification of two variables that have dramatic effects on whether exposure to such stimuli produces deleterious consequences. These two variables concern the degree of predictability and controllability that the organism has over the occurrence of the traumatic stimuli. In general, exposure to aversive events that are predictable and/or controllable has less adverse consequences than does exposure to the same amount and intensity of unpredictable and/or uncontrollable aversive events. Some of the behavioural and physiological consequences of manipulating the controllability and predictability of aversive events are manifested primarily in the acute situation, but other effects persist for hours or days following the termination of the stressor, and some effects may persist for weeks, months, or even years. Furthermore, manipulations of predictability and/or controllability at one point in time may have substantial impact on the consequences of subsequent exposure to unpredictable and/or uncontrollable traumatic stimuli. In the literature review that follows, we will highlight the findings from this vast literature that we believe may of be greatest importance in understanding the symptoms experienced by torture survivors – both during torture itself, and in the days, weeks, and months following torture.

In this review of the relevant literature, we will discuss the effects of predictability and controllability separately for the sake of simplicity. However, we should note at the outset that in actuality the effects of control and prediction are very closely intertwined, both functionally and operationally (Mineka & Hendersen, 1985), and so this arbitrary separation can be somewhat misleading. In places we will allude to the functional intertwining of these variables, but full discussion of these issues is beyond the scope of this chapter (see Mineka & Hendersen, 1985; Overmier, 1985; Weiss, 1977; for more elaborate discussion of these issues).

Predictability and unpredictability

Preference for predictability

If given a choice, animals generally show a strong preference for predictable or signalled aversive events in comparison to unpredictable or unsignalled aversive events (for a review see Badia, Harsh & Abbott, 1979). One early theory accounting for this preference for signalled aversive events was that the signal allows the animal to prepare for the upcoming event and thereby potentially reduce its impact (e.g. Lykken, 1962; Perkins, 1968). However, Miller & Mangan (1983) showed that rats actually judged the intensity of signalled shock to be greater than the intensity of unsignalled shock, even though they preferred the signalled shock. Thus, it does not seem likely that the preference for predictability can derive from any simple function that a possible preparatory response might serve in reducing the impact of the shock.

Another prominent theory accounting for the preference for predictability is Seligman's safety signal theory (Seligman 1968; Seligman & Binik, 1977; Weiss, 1977). According to this theory, preference for predictability derives not so much from what the signal can do to reduce the impact of the traumatic stimulus, but from the fact that having a signal when the event is going to happen also means functionally that when the signal is not on, the organism can relax and feel safe. That is, when the organism has a reliable signal for when bad things are going to happen, the absence of the signal can be used as a safety signal. For organisms experiencing unsignalled or unpredictable aversive events, the absence of a reliable signal also means the absence of a reliable safety signal. If the organism is in a context where aversive events are occurring unpredictably, this means that they may be in a state of chronic fear (Seligman, 1968; Seligman & Binik, 1977). Although the safety signal theory has fared reasonably well, there are a number of findings in the literature for which it does not easily account (e.g. Fanselow, 1980; for a discussion see Mineka & Hendersen, 1985). Nevertheless, it is our impression that this theory captures the essence of much of what goes on in the human torture situation. Torture survivors often do not have signals regarding either when their next session of torture will occur, or when the next shock or beating will occur within a given session of torture. Thus, they can be expected to experience a chronic state of fear in their cell over the timing of their next torture session. In addition, during each torture session itself (which may last for hours), they may experience intense fear and terror regarding when the next shock or beating will occur.

A third theory accounting for the preference for predictability is that it reduces uncertainty (see Imada & Nageishi, 1982), which may in, and of, itself be rewarding. This theory also remains controversial (see Mineka & Hendersen, 1985). In humans, the kind of information that is provided about an upcoming stressful event determines whether that information will alleviate or potentiate distress. For example, if people are told about the sensory properties of a painful stimulus that they are about to experience (e.g. cold pressor test or an endoscopic examination by a physician), they show reduced distress. However, if they are also given information about the painfulness of the stimulation this effect is blocked (e.g. Leventhal et al., 1979). Thus, giving only objective information about the stimulus properties of a painful stimulus has very different effects than does also giving more emotion-laden information about the threat value of the stimulus. In addition, Leventhal et al. 1978, cited in Leventhal et al., 1979) found that simply asking subjects to monitor and pay attention to the sensations in their hand during a cold pressor task was sufficient to lead to lowered distress (more rapid habituation). Thus, sensation monitoring even in the absence of accurate information as to what sensations to expect, may be sufficient to reduce distress, presumably by 'focusing attention on the objective features and away from pain distress' (Leventhal, 1979: page 32). Given that any information the torturer gives about the nature of painful stimulation to be delivered is likely to be emotion laden, one would not expect it to alleviate distress.

In humans, there also appear to be strong individual differences in whether predictability in the form of information about the nature of upcoming stressors is preferred or not, especially in more naturalistic settings than have typically been used in laboratory experiments on this issue. For example, Miller (1980, 1989; Miller & Mangan, 1983) noted that some people prefer to cope with stressful experiences by monitoring the details of what is happening, whereas others prefer to distract themselves by attending to other things. Subjects of the former type (high monitors/low blunters) show less distress in stressful situations when given much predictive information, whereas subjects of the latter type (low monitors/high blunters) show more distress when given much predictive information. This pattern of results has been corroborated by manipulating the amounts and kinds of information given to patients about to undergo various stressful medical procedures (Miller, 1989). Thus, only high monitors (as determined by self-report) seem to profit from receiving extensive preparatory and sensory information about the stressful medical procedures they are about to undergo.

Predictability and stress

Common to each of these three theories attempting to explain the preference for predictability is the assumption that exposure to predictable traumatic stimuli will, on average, be less stressful than exposure to the same frequency and intensity of unpredictable traumatic stimuli. Unfortunately, the literature on this topic is mixed. In many experiments, animals exposed to predictable aversive events (usually shocks) show less evidence of chronic fear and less stress-induced ulceration than do animals exposed to the same amount of unpredictable shocks (e.g. Seligman 1968; Seligman & Binik, 1977; Weiss, 1968, 1977). But other studies find the opposite pattern of results (for reviews see Weinberg & Levine, 1980; Weiss, 1977). Although there has never been a completely satisfactory resolution of these apparent inconsistencies, it does appear that at least some of the inconsistencies in the studies on stress-induced ulceration and in the studies measuring levels of stress hormones derive from complex ways in which the effect of predictability may interact with the effects of controllability. For example, if signals for shock lead an animal to make unsuccessful coping attempts, the signalled shocks may cause more stress-induced ulceration than do unsignalled shocks (Weiss, 1977; for a more complete discussion see Mineka & Hendersen, 1985).

In addition, even in situations where predictable shocks do not result in reduced stress in the short-term, they may have a beneficial proactive effect, manifested by reduced reactivity to future test shocks. For example, Dess *et al.* (1983) found that dogs exposed to predictable versus unpredictable shocks did not show a significant difference in cortisol response when blood was drawn immediately after the series of shocks. However, when subsequently tested with test shocks, the dogs previously exposed to the predictable shocks showed a smaller cortisol response than did the dogs previously exposed to the unpredictable shocks. Thus, even when predictability appeared to have no immediate effects in reducing stress, it none the less had proactive ameliorative effects.

Furthermore, there are now a fairly large number of studies consistently showing that, when shocks are signalled, modifications in pain reactivity are triggered (for reviews, see Bolles & Fanselow, 1982; Fanselow, 1991). This analgesia that occurs to aversive Pavlovian CSs appears to be opiate mediated because it is generally reversed by opiate antagonists such as naloxone. These reductions in pain reactivity to fear signals have been demonstrated in laboratory experiments with rats using a variety of indices of analgesia (for a review, see Fanselow, 1991). In addition, they have also been demonstrated in a Vietnam veteran with PTSD when he was presented with a naturalistic CS consisting of an ambush scene from the movie Platoon which was about the Vietnam war. This analgesia was also reversible by naloxone (Pitman *et al.*, 1990).

In the research discussed so far, predictability has been operationalized by giving the organism information about when a traumatic event is going to happen, or about what the nature of the traumatic stimulus is going to be. Relatively speaking, very little is known about what the effects are of giving the organism information about where on the body an aversive stimulus is going to be applied. Yet it would seem that this kind of predictability might be quite important in moderating the effects of the stressor. Consistent with this hypothesis were the findings of Erofeeva (1912, cited in Pavlov, 1927) in Pavlov's laboratory. In this experiment, three dogs first received a number of pairings of a mild electric shock to the skin as a conditioned stimulus (CS), preceding the occurrence of meat powder as an unconditioned stimulus (US). After a stable conditioned salivary response to the CS occurred, the intensity of the shock was gradually increased and the salivary conditioned response (CR) to the intense shocks remained stable. However, when the experimenter next attempted to generalize the CR by applying the strong shock CS to other places on the skin, the dogs showed a 'violent defense reaction' and lost all traces of the original conditioning. Thus, a traumatic stimulus (being used as a CS rather than a US here) was well tolerated as long as it occurred in the same place on the skin, but when this predictability was lost the animals showed intense behavioural disturbance. Indeed, Pavlov cited this as one of his classic examples of 'experimental neurosis' (Pavlov, 1927; for further discussion see Mineka & Kihlstrom, 1978).

Summary

In summary, there is ample evidence that on average animals and humans prefer signalled to unsignalled traumatic stimuli, and often find exposure to the signalled traumatic stimuli to be less stressful, as evidenced by behavioural and physiological measures (for reviews, see Fanselow, 1991; Mineka & Hendersen, 1985; Weinberg & Levine, 1980). When no differences in the immediate impact of predictable versus unpredictable stressors are found, differences may still be found in the impact of future stressors (Dess *et al.*, 1983). In humans, when predictability is provided by giving information about the nature of the traumatic stimuli to be encountered, sensory-based information appears to reduce stress, but emotion-laden information may block such effects. Furthermore, there are individual differences in coping style which may moderate this preference for information, with some individuals (low monitors/high blunters), doing better by distracting themselves than by attending to the stimulus information (e.g. Miller, 1980, 1989).

Controllability and uncontrollability

Uncontrollable stress produces associative and motivational deficits

Even more consistent and dramatic than the effects of predictability are the effects of controllability over traumatic events. It has long been thought that humans strive for a sense of what has variously been called control, competence, effectance, or mastery over their environments (e.g. Rotter, 1966; White, 1959), and research indeed shows that a majority of animals and humans, when given a choice, prefer to exert control (for reviews, see Mineka & Hendersen, 1985; Overmier, 1988). However, extensive experimental study of the differential effects of exposure to controllable versus uncontrollable stimulation only began in the late 1960s. The seminal investigations in this area were those of Overmier, Seligman, and Maier (Overmier & Seligman, 1967; Seligman & Maier, 1967). These investigators first coined the term 'learned helplessness' to describe a syndrome appearing in a majority of animals exposed to a long series of inescapable (or uncontrollable) shocks, but not in animals exposed to the same amount of escapable (or controllable) shocks. As first described, the most prominent aspect of this syndrome was the striking failure of animals initially exposed to uncontrollable shocks to later learn to escape or avoid shocks that were potentially controllable in a different situation. These investigators hypothesized that when an organism is exposed to uncontrollable traumatic events, it may learn to expect that it has no control over outcomes. Such learning was thought to produce both associative and motivational deficits. The motivational deficit was presumed to involve a reduced incentive to attempt to gain control in future situations resulting from a belief that responses would be ineffective in producing relief. The associative deficit was presumed to involve an impaired ability to detect response–outcome contingencies in future situations where responses to exert control over outcomes (e.g. Seligman, Maier & Solomon, 1971). A third emotional deficit was also hypothesized based on observations of increased passivity and apparent reductions in emotional reactivity to the shock.

From the outset, this learned helplessness theory, which postulates associative, motivational and emotional deficits as mediating the effects that occur following exposure to uncontrollable traumatic events, was quite controversial. Over the years, a variety of alternative theories were put forth to explain the same class of effects (often known as proactive interference or learned helplessness effects). Although space constraints preclude a review of all the various theoretical accounts that have emerged (e.g. for reviews, see Anisman, Kokinidis & Sklar, 1981; Maier & Seligman, 1976; Maier & Jackson, 1979; Mineka & Hendersen, 1985; Weiss, Glazer & Poherecky, 1976), it is important to detail at least some of the vast array of additional consequences of exposure to uncontrollable stressors that has emerged in the past two decades. Many of these effects were discovered, at least in part, through efforts to test competing theoretical accounts of the basic learned helplessness effects first reported in 1967. The primary focus of this brief review will be on results found in the animal literature because the intense physical stressors that have been used in animal experiments (e.g. electric shocks, near drowning from cold water swims, defeats in fighting) closely resemble in strength and modality those used in the human torture situation. Human experimental research on the learned helplessness phenomenon has typically used somewhat less intense stressors (at least in the physical sense) such as insoluble discrimination problems and uncontrollable loud noise. Furthermore, the human experiments on this phenomenon have generally not used as wide a range of dependent variables as have been used in the animal literature.

Emotional deficits?

Although early research on this topic had difficulty teasing apart the motivational and associative deficits postulated by learned helplessness theory, later research has tended to support the existence of both. Uncontrollable shock results in passivity and major activity deficits in the face of later controllable shocks (and other stressors). However, even in situations where these activity deficits are not manifested, uncontrollably shocked animals have difficulty learning new response–outcome contingencies (e.g. Jackson, Alexander & Maier, 1980; Maier, Jackson & Tomie, 1987; Minor, Jackson, & Maier, 1984). Recent evidence strongly suggests that this associative deficit may stem from reduced attention to internal response-related cues (Lee & Maier, 1988). In addition, animals exposed to uncontrollable shocks, but not to controllable shocks, show decreased aggressiveness and decreased competitiveness in a variety of situations (e.g. Rapaport & Maier, 1978; Williams, 1982), which may also result in a loss of rank in a dominance hierarchy. Loss of appetite and/or weight is also common (e.g. Weiss, 1968; Desan, Silbert & Maier, 1988), although more transient than long-term reductions in general activity in the home environment (Desan *et al.*, 1988). Additional evidence that inescapable shock produces other signs of anhedonia derives from an experiment showing that it reduces rates of self-stimulation from reward centres in the brain such as the substantia nigra (Bowers, Zacharko & Anisman, 1987; cited in Overmier & Hellhammer, 1988).

Although evidence supportive of the originally postulated motivational and associative deficits seems strong, the original idea of an emotional deficit seems to have been overly simplistic. Indeed, inescapable shock relative to escapable shock produces much higher levels of conditioned fear (e.g. Desiderato & Newman, 1971; Mineka, Cook & Miller, 1984; for a recent review, see Warren, Rosellini, & Maier, 1989). In addition, stress-induced ulceration is also dramatically potentiated by uncontrollable shock, relative to controllable shock (e.g. Weiss, 1971*a*, *b*, and *c*, 1977). Thus, the early observations of dogs exposed to inescapable shocks showing an emotional deficit because they were passive and appeared no longer to react to the shocks did not give a complete picture of the emotional state of the animals (Overmier, 1985).

Physiological effects

Given these disruptions in a wide variety of motivational and emotional systems, it is probably not surprising that uncontrollable shocks, relative to controllable shocks, have also been shown to produce alterations in levels of cortisol and a number of important neurotransmitters (e.g. Anisman & Sklar, 1979, Anisman *et al.*, 1981,

Dess et al., 1983; Weiss et al., 1976, 1981), as well as alternations in in vivo generation of specific antibodies to a novel antigen (Laudenslager et al., 1988). Importantly, increased susceptibility to the growth of certain kinds of cancer following exposure to inescapable shocks has also been observed in a number of laboratories (e.g. Sklar & Anisman, 1981; Visintainer, Volpicelli & Seligman, 1982). Finally, prolonged exposure to uncontrollable shocks is known to produce an opiate-mediated analgesia which dissipates fairly rapidly, but is reinstatable 24 hours later by exposure to several shocks (e.g. Maier, Drugan & Grau, 1982, Maier et al., 1983a, b). This opiate-mediated analgesia is, of course, accompanied by an increased pain threshold and seems to depend on the organism learning that the shock is inescapable (Maier, 1989).

Important extensions of this work using physical stressors such as shock have also been made in recent studies using social defeat as the stressor. In these studies subjects are intruder male rats that are placed in an established colony with a high ranking adult male rat known to react in a territorially defensive manner. The intruder rat subjects are almost invariably defeated. In a summary of recent studies on this topic, Fleshner et al. (1989) noted that the defeated intruder animals typically show the same range of physiological indices of stress as are seen following exposure to physical stressors such as inescapable shock. These include (but are not limited to) a rise in central endogenous opioids accompanied by decreased pain sensitivity (Miczek, Thompson & Shuster, 1982) and alterations in immune function (Fleshner et al., 1989). In both cases, the opioid analgesia and the altered immune function were more highly correlated with the time the subject had spent in submissive postures (indicative that the subject had given up) than with the actual number of times the subject had been bitten. Thus, exhibiting a defeat reaction to the aggressive encounter was more important than the mere physical attack in producing the opioid analgesia (Miczek et al., 1982) and the altered immune function (Fleshner et al., 1989). As will be discussed below, such findings have important parallels in the experiences of humans undergoing torture.

That the opportunity to engage in aggressive encounters during exposure to uncontrollable traumatic stimuli such as shock can dramatically attenuate the stress produced by the shock was shown by Weiss et al. (1976). In this experiment, rats exposed to uncontrollable shock but allowed to engage in aggressive encounters with conspecifics during the shock showed much lower levels of shock-induced ulceration than did yoked rats not allowed to fight. Thus, even though the animals allowed to fight not only received the 'uncontrollable' shock but also the biting and wounding attacks of a partner, they showed less ulceration – indicating that the potent stress-reducing effects of aggression may be comparable to those of exerting control *per se*. Interestingly, it was the opportunity to show species-typical aggressive postures rather than physical contact with the conspecific *per se* that was critical in producing this stress–attenuation effect. That is, rats allowed to show aggressive postures toward a conspecific but prevented from actual fighting by the presence of a clear barrier showed the same reduced levels of ulceration (see also Weiss, 1977). Such studies would seem to have important implications for understanding when torture survivors may be most likely to show a maximal stress response, i.e. amount of physical torture *per se* may be less predictive than is the victim's psychological state of resistance and fighting back versus giving up and conceding defeat.

The role of uncontrollability in depression and anxiety

In human research on the learned helplessness phenomenon, exposure to uncontrollable events (of a much milder nature) results in impaired problem-solving and increased passivity just as it does in animals (for a review see Seligman, 1975). A variety of emotional changes have also been observed following exposure to uncontrollable events, including increased anxiety, hostility and/or depression (e.g. Gatchel, Paulus & Maples, 1975; Miller & Seligman, 1975; for a review see Mineka & Kelly, 1989). Until recently the most influential theorizing about effects of exposure to uncontrollable traumatic events held that these effects provided a good model of human reactive depression (e.g. Seligman, 1974, 1975). Indeed, many important similarities between the symptoms, aetiology, treatment and prevention of helplessness (in animals and humans) and reactive depression were documented (for a recent review, see Overmier & Hellhammer, 1988). However, the early version of the once influential learned helplessness model of depression began to wane in importance as the theory was modified to incorporate attributional variables (Abramson, Seligman & Teasdale, 1978). According to the reformulated helplessness model, it is not only the occurrence of uncontrollable events that is important in precipitating depressive episodes, but also the attributions that people make about why those events have occurred. In particular, people who tend to make internal, stable, and global attributions for bad events may be most prone to depression. In an even more recent revision of this theory, Abramson, Metalsky and Alloy (1989), have further argued that depression is caused and characterized not only by helplessness (perceived lack of control over important events) but also by hopelessness (certainty of negative outcomes).

As the learned helplessness theory of depression has evolved to include emphasis on attributional variables and on the importance of hopelessness as well as helplessness, there has also been increasing recognition of the important role that uncontrollability plays in the aetiology and maintenance of fear and anxiety (cf. Barlow, 1988; Mineka & Kelly, 1989). Several theorists had long argued for the importance of lack or loss of control in fear and anxiety, even before its role was strongly implicated in depression (e.g. Mowrer & Viek, 1948; Mandler & Watson, 1966; Mandler, 1972; Masserman, 1971), but these arguments seemed to have been overshadowed for well over a decade by the influential learned helplessness model of depression. Given recent evidence for the high level of comorbidity between anxiety and depressive disorders (for reviews, cf. Kendall & Watson, 1989; Maser & Cloninger, 1990), it is perhaps not too surprising that uncontrollability may play an important role in each. Indeed, Alloy, Kelly, Mineka, and Clements (1990) have recently presented an integrated helplessness/ hopelessness model of anxiety and depression that appears to be able to account for many of the important features of comorbidity between depression and anxiety disorders that have been noted in recent years (see also Garber, Miller & Abramson, 1980). In this model, perceptions of lack of control may play a shared role in anxiety, depression, and mixed anxiety/depression. What differentiates anxiety from depression in this model is that certain forms of depression are also thought to be characterized by hopelessness (certainty of negative outcomes) (see Abramson *et al.*, 1989).

Mineka and Kelly (1989) recently reviewed animal and human research implicating lack of control in the origins and maintenance of fear and anxiety. Many of these studies have demonstrated the importance of control during aversive or stressful situations in reducing fear and anxiety. For example, as noted earlier, it has been shown in animals that less fear is conditioned to neutral stimuli paired with escapable as opposed to inescapable shocks (e.g. Desiderato & Newman, 1971; Mineka *et al.*, 1984; Mowrer & Viek, 1948). In addition, human research has shown that control reduces the stressfulness of aversive stimuli such as shock and loud noise, as evidence by physiological, behavioural and cognitive (self-report) measures (for a review of this literature, see Mineka & Kelly, 1989). Indeed, in many cases, perceived or potential control over aversive stimulation may be sufficient to reduce stress even when actual control is not exerted. In one of the most dramatic demonstrations of such effects, Sanderson, Rapee and Barlow (1989) used a variation of the perceived control paradigm in panic disorder patients about to undergo a panic provocation procedure involving inhalation for 15 minutes of 5.5% carbon dioxide-enriched air (a known panic-provocation agent). Half of the patients were told that, whenever a signal light was lit, they could use a dial to reduce the concentration of carbon dioxide that they received, although they were encouraged not to use it unless absolutely necessary (in actuality the dial was inoperative). For this group, the signal light remained on for the entire 15-minute period of inhalation. The other half of the patients was given the same instructions, but for this group the signal light never came on during the 15-minute inhalation period. Thus an illusion of control was induced in the first group but not in the second group. Subjective anxiety ratings and panic symptoms were monitored throughout the inhalation period. The illusion-of-control group, reported experiencing greater control over the symptoms produced by the CO_2 inhalation, and reported fewer and less severe symptoms than did the no-illusion-of-control group. They also had fewer catastrophic thoughts and reported less subjective distress than did the no-illusion-of-control group. Furthermore, eight of ten subjects in the latter group met criteria for a panic attack, whereas only two of ten in the illusion-of-control group met these criteria. Thus, perceived control can attenuate the effects of exposure to anxiety-provoking stimuli even among clinically anxious individuals. These findings are very relevant to understanding the important sense of reduced distress that tortured individuals experience when they perceive some control over their torturer's behaviour (see below).

The importance of control or perceived control is evident not only in laboratory situations involving experimental stressors such as shock, loud noise, or panic provocation agents, but also in clinical observations of patients with anxiety disorders. As reviewed by Mineka and Kelly (1989), anxiety-disordered patients often report that they feel helpless and unable to cope when confronted with the sources of their fears or anxiety; these include phobic stimuli, panic attacks, and obsessive thoughts (e.g. Barlow, 1988; Bandura, 1977; Beck & Emery, 1985). Such anxiety-disordered patients also often report worry and concern over future helplessness, which appears to exacerbate anticipatory or generalized anxiety in patients with disorders ranging from panic disorder, to generalized anxiety disorder and obsessive-compulsive disorder.

The role of perceived controllability in reducing fear, anxiety and depression

In addition to uncontrollability playing a role in the origins and maintenance of fear and anxiety, it also appears that, once fear or anxiety has been acquired, gaining experience with control over the source of the fear or anxiety can be helpful in its reduction. These effects have been clearly demonstrated in fears induced in laboratory settings, but there are also strong indications that similar effects apply in patients with clinical anxiety disorders (for a review, see Mineka & Kelly, 1989). Especially important in the latter regard are studies implicating the role of increased control and predictability in mediating the effects of cognitive–behavioural therapies for anxiety disorders. If perceptions of lack of control are implicated in the origins and maintenance of various anxiety disorders, then perhaps it is not too surprising that therapeutic interventions targeted at increasing perceptions of control should be beneficial in reducing anxiety. Although research on this topic is still in a very preliminary stage, Barlow noted in an important comprehensive review of the cognitive–behavioural therapy literature that 'changing perceptions of helplessness is central to any therapeutic endeavor ... [Indeed] these therapeutic attempts will not be completely successful unless the patient begins to feel in control of potential upcoming events, whether environmental or somatic' (1988, pp. 313–14). Seligman (1975) and Overmier (e.g. Overmier & Hellhammer, 1988), among others, had reached a similar conclusion about the importance of regaining a sense of control over one's environment in mediating the effectiveness of various forms of therapy for depression.

Thus far, this review has focused primarily on the immediate and long-term physiological, behavioural and emotional sequelae of exposure to controllable versus uncontrollable aversive events, and briefly on the beneficial effects of experience with increased perceptions of control in overcoming fear, anxiety, and depression. The primary theme has been that exposure to uncontrollable aversive events is far more stressful than is exposure to the same amount and intensity of controllable aversive events, and that the effects of helplessness, including anxiety and depression, can be alleviated best by therapeutic techniques that restore a sense of control.

Immunization against the effects of uncontrollable stress

One important topic not yet covered is whether such deleterious consequences following exposure to uncontrollable aversive events can be prevented. Fortunately, the answer appears to be yes, at least under some circumstances. For example, in several of the first experiments on this topic, it was found that animals (dogs and rats) who were first exposed to a short series of escapable (controllable) shocks prior to receiving a long series of inescapable shocks did not show the usual learned helplessness deficits described earlier (e.g. Seligman & Maier, 1967; Williams & Maier, 1977). Thus, it appears that first learning that one has control over aversive stimulation can immunize the organism against the later effects of exposure to uncontrollable aversive stimulation. In the Williams and Maier experiment these immunization effects occurred even when different kinds of aversive stimuli were used in the immunization and helplessness induction phases (e.g. experience escaping from cold water immunized rats against the effects of exposure to uncontrollable foot shocks). More recently, it has also been shown that immunization procedures not only prevent the traditional learned helplessness deficits first studied by Maier and Seligman, but also may prevent many of the physiological changes that occur following exposure to uncontrollable shocks. For example, immunization procedures can prevent the opiate-mediated analgesia usually seen following prolonged exposure to inescapable shocks (Moye et al., 1981, 1983), as well as the activity deficits that typically develop over the course of exposure to a series of inescapable shocks (Volpicelli et al., 1983).

In the immunization experiments discussed so far, initial short-term experiences with controllable aversive stimulation effectively prevent a variety of the deficits that are typically seen following exposure to uncontrollable stimulation. In most, if not all, of these experiments immunization, helplessness induction, and test phases typically all occur within a matter of several days. Two important questions are not answered by these kinds of experiments. First, can immunization effects be demonstrated over a longer time frame? Second, can immunization effects be demonstrated if the initial experience is with controllable appetitive stimulation rather than with controllable aversive stimulation? Again, the answer to both questions appears to be yes. With regard to the first question, Hannum, Rosellini & Seligman (1976) showed that immunization experiences given to young weanling rats had a protective effect when the rats were later exposed as adults to inescapable shocks. Regarding the second question, Joffe, Rawson & Mulick (1973) reported that rats raised in environments in which they had control over access to water, food and visual stimulation later showed less emotionality and more exploratory behaviour in a novel situation than did rats reared in yoked-uncontrollable environments. And in an experiment that addressed both questions, Mineka, Gunnar and Champoux (1986) showed similar effects in monkeys reared in controllable versus uncontrollable environments from 1 ½–11 months of age. Two groups of infant monkeys (master groups) were reared in environments where they had access to operant manipulanda that controlled access to food, water and treats. Two other groups of infant monkeys (yoked groups) were reared in identical environments except that their manipulanda were inoperative; they received reinforcers when a member of the Master group successfully operated a manipulandum. Between 7 and 10 months of age, a variety of tests were performed assessing the monkeys' abilities to cope with novel and frightening situations. The master groups were bolder and habituated more quickly than did the yoked groups when tested with a fear-provoking toy monster presented in front of their home cage. In addition, the master groups showed more eagerness to enter a novel and somewhat frightening playroom situation, and also explored more once in the playroom. There was some suggestive evidence that they also adapted better to stressful separations from peers. Thus, early experience with mastery over one's environment, even when that experience is with appetitive stimulation, may promote an enhanced ability to cope with novel and stressful situations even over a relatively long time-span.

Interactions of unpredictability and uncontrollability and assorted variables that potentiate the effects of each

As noted at the outset of this discussion, we have arbitrarily separated our discussion of the effects of unpredictability from those of uncontrollability for the sake of simplicity. However, as we also briefly noted, the two constructs are in actuality intimately interrelated and many theorists have tried to reduce the effects of one to the effects of the other (for a review, see Mineka & Hendersen, 1985). For example, the onset of either a controllable or an uncontrollable traumatic event may be either predictable or unpredictable, leading to four obvious possible combinations of unpredictability and uncontrollability. However, the situation is actually more complicated than this because an organism that has control over the offset of a traumatic event also automatically has predictability over when the offset of the event will occur. Some theorists have argued that it is this predictability over when the aversive event will terminate that mediates all of the beneficial consequences that accrue from having control (e.g. Averill, 1973), and indeed much recent research supports the notion that some of the effects of control may well be mediated this way (Mineka *et al.*, 1984; Minor *et al.*, 1990).

Nevertheless, without getting into these complexities, it is still possible to review briefly what is known about the interactive effects of unpredictability over onset with uncontrollability over offset of traumatic events. In general, it appears that the most deleterious consequences stem from uncontrollable aversive events that are also unpredictable, and that the least deleterious consequences stem from predictable and controllable aversive events. Of the remaining two combinations, unpredictable but controllable aversive events generally seem to be somewhat less stressful than predictable but uncontrollable aversive events (e.g. Weiss, 1971*a*, *c*, 1977; Dess *et al.*, 1983; Overmier, 1985), although relatively few studies have made careful comparisons of all four combinations of predictability and controllability (e.g. Overmier, 1988), many of which have never been carefully studied.

If unpredictability potentiates many of the effects of uncontrollability as suggested above, what other variables are also known to potentiate the effects of uncontrollability or to attenuate the effects of controllability? There is at least suggestive evidence from the experimental neurosis literature that restraint potentiates the effects of uncontrollable shocks (cf. Liddell, 1944; for a discussion of this issue, see Mineka & Kihlstrom, 1978). That restraint could have such effects is not surprising given that restraint, by itself, appears to induce a sense of lack of control as indexed, for example, by restraint-induced ulceration (e.g. Glavin, 1980). Thus the potentiation of the effects of uncontrollable shock by restraint may simply be an additive effect produced by exposure to two uncontrollable stressors.

In addition, there is good evidence that the beneficial effects of control can be dramatically attenuated by introducing an element of conflict into the situation. For example, Weiss (1971*b*) showed that the usual beneficial effects of control over shocks on shock-induced ulceration could be reversed by adding a mild punishing shock following the escape/avoidance response. That is, rats that were initially trained to escape and avoid intense shocks subsequently had a conflict introduced by having each controlling response followed by another mild shock; in other words, the cost of exerting control over intense shocks was mild punishment. In this case the rats with control showed more shock-induced ulceration than did the yoked rats without control that received the same series of intense and mild shocks. Both of these variables which appear to potentiate the effects of uncontrollability (i.e. restraint and conflict) have clear parallels in the experiences of torture survivors.

FEATURES OF UNCONTROLLABILITY AND UNPREDICTABILITY IN THE FOUR PHASES OF TORTURE SURVIVORS' EXPERIENCE

In the section that follows we will attempt to delineate what we think are the important parallels between these effects of exposure to uncontrollable and/or unpredictable aversive events and the experiences of humans undergoing torture. As noted at the outset, the experiences of torture survivors will be divided into four phases which vary in terms of degree of unpredictable and uncontrollable stress. These four phases roughly parallel questions that have been addressed about pretreatment and acute, short-term and long-term effects of unpredictable and/or uncontrollable aversive events.

Phase 1 – Pre-arrest/detention

A potential predictor of how a detainee will react to arrest and detention is the unexpectedness of the detention and torture experience. Politically more active individuals usually estimate a greater risk of being exposed to torture than those who are only peripherally or not at all involved in political activity. The politically more active individuals are also more likely to have been exposed to other forms of repression and harsh treatment before, including persecution and harassment by the authorities, and some may even have been driven underground or into hiding. Such individuals are thus possibly more habituated than others to the sort of stress that various forms of political repression entail. They may also have developed expectations of control through their prior experiences, which may serve at least partially to immunize them against the torture experience. In fact, certain political groups are known to train their members in stoicism with a view to increasing their resistance to torture in case they get caught. Similar training programmes are also employed by the military in some countries. These experiences have an obvious analogue in animal experiments on immunization against learned helplessness where it has been shown that prior exposure to controllable or escapable aversive events may immunize the animals against the deleterious effects of subsequent exposure to uncontrollable aversive events (e.g. Seligman & Maier, 1967; Williams & Maier, 1977). By contrast, for individuals without a high degree of political involvement, arrest and detention may be highly unpredictable. This unpredictability and lack of immunization experiences would be expected to lead to higher levels of anxiety and distress than seen in the politically active individuals previously described. Unfortunately, there is little in the way of systematic data on these predictions; however, we believe they are important question for future research.

Phase 2 – Detention/interrogation

Overview and contextual factors

Systematic torture usually takes place during the detention and interrogation phase, but it may also be used for indoctrination purposes during long-term imprisonment or captivity. On one level, it is used to extract a signed confession, to get a testimony incriminating others, to obtain information, or simply as part of a routine treatment or an act of vengeance (Stover & Nightingale, 1985, p. 7). However, on another level, it also serves as an instrument of political repression designed to deter the individual and the society from political activity against the current regime.

Torture is practised in a wide variety of ways. Whatever methods are used, the common denominator appears to be the achievement of certain objectives by the torturers through induction of loss of control in the victim. The severity of trauma stems not only from what method is used but also from its frequency, duration and chronic administration over long periods of time. Methods of torture involving unpredictable presentation of traumatic stimulation and methods which block the survivors' coping efforts all seem to potentiate the effect of various forms of torture. Subjecting prisoners to unpredictable situations to maximize stress is a practice well known to people working with torture survivors (e.g. Stover & Nightingale, 1985, p. 17; Melamed *et al.* 1990, p. 16; Reid & Strong, 1988). Although one could make a case that the global aim of torture is to remove control from the victim and to maximize unpredictability, some of its applications seem to be very specifically geared towards furthering these aims. In this section, we will review some of the applications of torture with prominent features of uncontrollability and unpredictability.

After arrest, the detainee is often kept in complete isolation from other prisoners and the outside world, including relatives and even lawyers (Amnesty International, 1984). Isolation during the period of detention constitutes a major source of stress for the detainee. After arrest and transfer to an interrogation centre notorious for its treatment of detainees, the chances of avoiding severe torture can be improved if the detainee can maintain contact with the outside world. Indeed, many political groups have devised elaborate ways of

H

monitoring their members daily so that their absence is easily noticed should they be taken by the authorities overnight. Knowledge and confidence that help is available serve as safety signals to the detainee. That is, if the detainee feels confident that this is so, distress is attenuated relative to what is seen when the detainee believes his/her disappearance has not been noticed or attended to. Isolation thus deprives the detainee of such safety signals and may intensify feelings of helplessness.

Complete isolation also serves to widen the gap between powerful authorities and helpless individuals and prevents the perception of any similarity of humanly qualities between the two sides (Suedfeld, 1990). This seems to intensify the torturers' hatred and contempt for the captive and facilitate aggressive behaviour; it also enhances the captive's perception of being completely at the mercy of an unrestrained source of aggression. Indeed, these effects can be so powerful that they have even been observed in a mock prison situation where normal college student volunteers were randomly assigned to be prisoners or guards for a two-week period (cf. Haney & Zimbardo, 1977; Zimbardo, 1975).

The effect of isolation is compounded by verbal induction of helplessness and hopelessness, a common practice both before and during the infliction of torture. The torturers attempt to undermine any sense of hope or self-reassurance in the detainees by suggestions, threats, and bluffs during interrogation (e.g. s/he is completely alone; no one can come to his/her rescue; they have captured his/her comrades, too, who have already talked; s/he shouldn't count on walking out of here alive because they will torture him/her to death if necessary and make it look like a suicide). These threats usually have a significant impact because many people are known to have died in detention. Suicides during this period are not uncommon, which may not be too surprising given that hopelessness is a common precursor of suicide (Abramson *et al.*, 1989; Beck, Kovacs, & Weissman, 1975).

Forms of torture

During the detention phase, many different forms of torture are used – some physical, some psychological, but usually a combination of both. Features of unpredictability and uncontrollability are very prominent. Sessions are often conducted daily, sometimes for as long as several months or even longer. The methods are often varied from one day to another in order to find the most effective form of torture for any one individual. However, this also maximizes unpredictability and may prevent the detainee from developing psychological defences against or extensive physiological habituation to any one form of torture. Such manipulations are also reported by others (e.g. Benfeld-Zachrisson, 1985). It is, for example, known in animals that extensive exposure to identical (15 daily) sessions of uncontrollable shock may lead to some attenuation of the physiological consequences (e.g. Weiss *et al.*, 1976).

Among the physical forms of torture, brutal beatings are routine, but more refined methods include prolonged application of electricity by mouth, ears, nipples, and genitals. Experienced torturers often vary the intensity of the current. At other times they intermittently turn the shock off, pretending the session is over, but then start it up again with no warning. This can be seen to maximize the unpredictability of the already uncontrollable shock torture experience, and indeed survivors' testimonies confirm the added effect of this element. This is consistent with animal research reviewed earlier showing that unpredictability potentiates at least some of the deleterious consequences of uncontrollable shock (e.g. Overmier, 1985; Weiss, 1977).

Falanga is another common form of physical torture which involves the beating of the soles of the feet with a baton. Conventionally, the detainee is laid on his/her back on the floor while the feet are lifted up and the exposed soles beaten up with a baton. The upper half of the body is left free to move. A recent variation on this method said to maximize the pain involves seating the detainee in the middle of few automobile tyres placed on top of each other such that s/he is completely immobilized while the beating takes place. As discussed earlier, restraint in animals is thought to potentiate the effects of exposure to uncontrollable stressors (Liddell, 1944; Mineka & Kihlstrom, 1978), although research on this topic is scant. Another version of the technique thought to increase the perceived pain is serving the blows at irregular intervals rather than in a rhythmic fashion; this, of course, can be seen to maximize unpredictability of the uncontrollable stressor.

There are also many more psychological manipulations which are used as forms of torture, either by themselves or in combination with physical torture. For example, blindfolding during torture is a common practice which not only helps the torturers remain unidentified, but also appears to increase the impact of torture. Blindfolding is highly aversive even when not combined with other forms of torture. Loss of visual monitoring of the environment distinctly intensifies feelings of helplessness and introduces a significant element of unpredictability regarding imminent aversive events. When blindfolding is combined with other forms of torture, it appears to potentiate their effects.

Certain combinations are reported to be particularly distressing. For instance, the torturers sometimes form a ring around the blindfolded detainee during interrogation, and randomly take turns serving blows to the detainee's face, often varying the intervals between blows. The detainee is thus unable to know when and from which direction the blows will come. As noted earlier, there is some evidence in animals that unpredictability about where on the body an aversive stimulus is to be applied can be highly stressful (Pavlov, 1927; Mineka & Kihlstrom 1978). Another combination involves making the blindfolded detainee walk and give him the false impression that s/he is about to hit his/her head against a hard object. S/he is repeatedly subjected to false alarms by shouting 'mind your head', the effect of which is intensified by occasionally not warning the detainee when the feared collision is actually about to occur. Unpredictability and helplessness appear to be maximized by this procedure. Blindfolding is also used to intensify the terror induced by apparent threats to life. The blindfolded detainee is first made to stand on a table and then given a push after being led to believe that s/he is dangerously close to an open window that is at considerable height from the ground; s/he is then given a push out the window which is actually only a few feet from ground. Thus, for the detainee the blindfolding magnifies a realistically minor threat into an apparently life-endangering situation.

Stripping the detainee naked is another common practice during detention. Nakedness seems to induce a sense of helplessness and danger in the face of imminent danger by depriving the detainee of the sense of protection and illusory security that clothing affords. Because of the sexual connotations of nakedness, stripping also raises a possible but uncertain threat of sexual assault.

Sham executions are a well-known and frequently reported form of torture (e.g. Allodi & Cowgill, 1982; Benfeldt-Zachrisson, 1985; Goldfeld et al., 1988). Sometimes the detainee is subjected to a prolonged threat of execution. For instance, s/he is told that s/he is going to be shot the next morning. The next day s/he is taken from, his cell, blindfolded and taken to another room where the torturer(s) holds an unloaded gun at her/her head and pulls the trigger. The same procedure may be repeated for days or weeks on end. The fact that the threat has not been realized after several occasions provides no disconfirmation of the threat because the detainee is aware of the real possibility that execution may occur one day. Thus the detainee is repeatedly subjected to an unreliable signal of the ultimate uncontrollable threat – his/her own death. This chronic high level of uncertainty over an uncontrollable threat might be expected to result in greater distress and anxiety than would be seen in an uncontrollable but predictable situation, e.g. being certain of one's execution the next day. The latter might be expected to induce a sense of hopelessness and hence depression (Abramson *et al.*, 1989; Alloy *et al.*, 1990).

The impact of torture in inducing a sense of helplessness is often compounded by suggestions that the effects of torture will be irreversible. Indeed, it seems that situations of extreme stress or pain may increase suggestibility – a phenomenon perhaps associated with dissociative states observed during traumatic situations (Spiegel & Fink, 1979; Speigel, Hunt & Dondershine, 1988). There is also some evidence to suggest that detainees can show increased suggestibility during ordinary police interrogation without physical torture (Gudjonsson & Clark, 1986). One detainee, for example, was told during electrical torture to her genitals that she would never be able to get pregnant again. Although she knew this did not make any sense, she was nevertheless horrified at the thought and had obsessive thoughts of this comment for two years after her release until she actually gave birth to a healthy baby. Similarly, a male detainee was told, while a baton was being inserted into his anus, that he had now lost his 'manhood' and that he would never be able to return to normal sexual functioning again. This, again, became a theme for recurrent nightmares later. Such threats of irreversible damage to sexual organs (or any other part of the body) are not always merely bluffs as serious damage is known to have been inflicted on sexual organs through mutilation, venereal disease, and forced abortions (Goldfeld *et al.*, 1988; Lunde & Ortmann, this volume).

Another common form of torture is confronting the detainee with an impossible choice. For example, the detainee is told that if s/he refused to comply, close relatives will be arrested, raped, and tortured in front of him/her. If s/he speaks, he/she will save him/herself and loved ones but will have to reveal information about comrades leading to their arrest, torture, or even death. In animals, it is known that inducing conflict of this sort (e.g. being punished with a mild shock for choosing to exert control and avoid a strong shock) is highly stressful (Weiss, 1971*b*).

Survivors often report as one of the most distressing aspects of their past experience being forced to witness other people being tortured. Other people may include friends, close relatives, or even total strangers. A variation of this method is forced engagement of the victim in the torture of others. Some state such treatment is even more distressing than being tortured oneself. This vulnerability, obviously well known to the torturers, is sometimes exploited by also having the detainees listen to audio- or videotape recordings of torture sessions of others. Such methods have also been reported by others (e.g. Benfeldt-Zachrisson, 1985; Goldfeld *et al.*, 1988; Roth *et al.*, 1987). Survivors also report this as distressing as oneself being tortured. That this forced exposure (visual and/or auditory) to others being tortured is so distressing is not surprising given that other non-human primates also react with high levels of distress when observing fear and distress in conspecifics (Mineka, 1987; Mineka & Cook , submitted for publication). Furthermore, it is tempting to speculate that the conditioned release of endogenous opiates which may mediate habituation and the numbing experience during physical torture (see below) may not occur simply in response to the sight of torture in others. This may help to account for why witnessing torture may be more distressing than torture itself which causes release of these endogenous opiates.

Another particularly stressful experience is the anticipation of torture. This vulnerability is often exploited by the torturers who make verbal threats of torture. Many survivors report that having to wait to be taken from their cell to the torture chamber can be even more distressing than torture itself. For example, one survivor stated that he almost felt relieved once electrical torture had started. He had learned to cope with it after several occasions and every time the session started, he realized it was not as bad as he feared it would be. The anticipatory distress seems to be greater if the intervals between sessions are variable and/or if there is an uncertainty about the nature of the next torture session; both of these factors obviously maximize unpredictability. Such observations are corroborated by research in animals showing that shocks delivered at variable intervals (as opposed to fixed intervals) produce greater heart rate elevations (Bersh *et al.*, 1952) and more ulceration (Guile, 1987).

Certain forms of torture seem to have a much greater impact than others in inducing loss of control and feelings of helplessness in the detainee. Those that involve a perceived risk to death during the process appear to be more traumatic than the ones that merely involve physical pain but no real threat to life. Submersion of the head under water until near-asphyxiation or sham executions are examples of such methods. Another commonly reported method is extreme humiliation of the detainee. Humiliation is usually achieved by attacking the individual's integrity and by violating taboos, political and religious beliefs or other values upheld by the detainee. In the case of a male detainee, inserting a baton into the anus, for instance, is not only extremely painful but a powerful insult to his 'manhood'. Near-drowning is not only exposure to an uncontrollable threat to life but also profoundly humiliating when it is carried out in a bucket full of vomit and faeces, as is often the case. Threats of rape or actual rape is not only a form of uncontrollable violence but also an attack on the individual's social standing, particularly in traditional societies. Torturing the victim's loved ones is not only an extremely distressing sight to witness but also a powerful assault on his/her sense of responsibility for others. Verbal abuse and insults often damage the individual's sense of identity and self-esteem. Numerous examples of such treatment can be given which all induce feelings of helplessness in the victim through not being able to act on anger and hostility generated by such aversive treatment. There is a substantial body of evidence that animals and humans respond with anger, hostility and aggression to threats to physical and psychological well-being (Baron, 1977; Averill, 1982), but that they give up over time (e.g. Seligman, 1975).

Psychological reactions

Psychological responses during this phase seem broadly to fall into two groups: those occurring between episodes of torture and those in response to the infliction of physical pain during torture. Not surprisingly, anticipation of the next torture episode provokes intense fear and anxiety. Animal research leads one to predict that this anticipatory fear and anxiety may be particularly intense if the waiting occurs in a dangerous context relative to in a safe context (e.g. Overmier & Murison, 1989).

Hyperarousal, hypervigilance, startle responses, restlessness, increased auditory acuity, and reduced sleep are characteristic of this phase. As reviewed above, many of these symptoms have also been observed in animals that have undergone prolonged exposure to uncontrollable and unpredictable aversive events (Mineka & Kihlstrom, 1978; Mineka & Hendersen, 1985). Intense terror and panic may lead to serious suicide attempts. Near-catatonic reactions or milder forms of negativistic behaviour may also occur. Acute cognitive impairment such as disorientation may also be observed, perhaps paralleling attentional and learning deficits seen in animals following exposure to unpredictable and uncontrollable aversive events (Jackson *et al.*, 1980; Lee & Maier, 1988; Maier *et al.*, 1987; Minor *et al.*, 1984).

Psychological responses during torture itself include many reports of depersonalization ('this is not happening to me, this is not my body'), derealization ('this is not real'), and analgesia ('feeling numb all over'). For example, one survivor said the difficult part of electrical torture was the beginning; after a while he felt numb all over his body and completely dissociated from the situation. It is quite possible that such numbness is mediated by conditioned release of endogenous opiates as seen in animals exposed to uncontrollable shock who later show opiate release following the first few shocks, which have become conditioned stimuli controlling the conditioned response of opiate release (e.g. Maier, *et al.*, 1983*a*, *b*). Dissociative states have also been reported in other traumatic situations (Spiegel & Fink, 1979).

Torture may also induce extremely submissive behaviour or dependency on the torturers (Suedfeld, 1990), an effect torturers count on. This may be functionally analogous to the defeatist postures adopted by formerly dominant mice who have been exposed to uncontrollable shock prior to being placed with an unfamiliar conspecific (e.g. Fleshner *et al.*, 1989).

Phase 3 – Imprisonment

Overview and contextual factors

For most detainees who are transferred to a prison either to await trial or to serve a sentence if they have already been convicted, this phase is often a relief because it signifies survival from a life-threatening ordeal. Although some may still be taken away from time to time for further interrogation and torture, this phase, by and large, offers less uncertainty and poses less threat to life than does the detention phase. The living conditions, however, are still very harsh and oppressive. Overcrowding, poor sanitary conditions, poor nutrition, and inadequate medical care are common. Lengthy court trials and waiting for an impending sentence contribute to uncertainty about the future. Some prisoners face life imprisonment or even capital punishment.

Psychological responses

The psychological reactions observed during detention continue into the early stages of the prison phase. In addition, nightmares, night terrors, intrusive recollections of torture, and phobic and anxiety responses may occur. If there is any likelihood of further interrogation and torture, anxiety reactions may persist. Full-blown PTSD may develop and persist throughout the prison phase, particularly in those deprived of emotional support and when there is anticipation of further torture. Otherwise, acute traumatic stress reactions tend to diminish during a prolonged prison phase. Life in prison becomes more stable and predictable. Contacts with the outside world sometimes can be re-established and help from friends and relatives some-times becomes more available.

Phase 4 – Post-imprisonment

Overview and contextual factors

The events following the prison phase are highly variable. They may range from going back to normal activity to going into hiding, internal exile, or fleeing the country to seek political asylum elsewhere. Job loss, separation from the family, loss of friends or relatives, disruption of educational studies, and other social and financial difficulties are common. Harassment and persecution by the authorities may con-tinue, and there may be threats of further arrest and torture. In fact, some may have to go through the same cycle many more times.

A critical factor during this phase seems to be the availability of social support. An important ingredient of social support is approval and acceptance by comrades and being able to resume social and political functioning. Whether such support is available partly depends on the survivor's past behaviour during detention or prison and whether s/he has adhered to the moral codes and values upheld by their political group. Divulging critical information under torture or any other form of surrender may be regarded as a violation of an important code and hence a proof of untrustworthiness. Such indi-viduals may be ostracized or held at a distance from their political group.

Lack of social support may also be manifest on a different level. In countries where political resistance has largely been crushed by a totalitarian regime, many activists come out of prison to face the bitter reality of a 'lost cause.' Some of the realities that such survivors will have to cope with include: all political activity banned, political organizations disbanded, friends imprisoned, killed, or in exile, and no hope of immediate recuperation. Moreover, they may have to face the additional stress of being stigmatized as troublemakers, traitors, or criminals. Such a political vacuum deprives them of the ideological support so vital in maintaining their sense of control over their lives and the environment they had sacrificed so much to change. Under these circumstances, many find it difficult to give meaning to their traumatic experience. Lack of social support and societal disapproval of the survivor's cause is thought to be an important factor in the high incidence of PTSD among American Vietnam veterans (Keane *et al.*, this volume). Torture survivors may also have to face an unsympathetic attitude from the public who blame them for having brought their misfortune upon themselves (for a review of 'the psychology of bystanders' and 'just-world thinking', see Staub, 1985, 1989, 1990). If they have to flee the country to seek political asylum elsewhere, their plight often poses an additional sequence of traumatizing events which may reinforce feelings of helplessness.

In brief, social and emotional support is an important factor for recovery during this phase. To the best of our knowledge, there are no animal parallels for the role of social support in recovery from the effects of uncontrollable stress.

Psychological symptoms

The most common symptoms during this phase are those commonly seen in PTSD, including nightmares, intrusive recollections of past events, hypervigilance, hyperarousal, suspiciousness, mistrust of authority, loss of meaning in life, emotional numbing, irritability, aggressivity, depressed mood, generalized anxiety, exacerbation of symptoms by reminders of past experience, phobic avoidance of trauma-related cues, sleep disturbance, night terrors and/or panics, fear of sleep, memory and concentration impairment, difficulty in learning, and somatic symptoms. Somatic symptoms include dyspepsia (Hougen *et al.*, 1988; Petersen *et al.*, 1985), peptic ulcers, and other gastrointestinal symptoms such as alternating bouts of constipation and diarrhoea (Petersen *et al.*, 1985). Psychotic reactions are not uncommon and are often of the paranoid type. These symptoms are usually more severe during the first 6 months after release from detention/prison and tend to resolve thereafter. In some cases, though, symptoms are known to persist years after the torture experience (Petersen *et al.* 1985). Some of these symptoms (e.g. hypervigilance, hyperarousal, suspiciousness, irritability, generalized anxiety, phobic avoidance, sleep disturbance, fear of sleep, panics, and night terrors) are more prominent when the individual faces threats of further arrest and torture. Such threats can sometimes evoke panics and agoraphobia-like reactions with extensive avoidance of outdoor situations and even complete housebondage. In situations where the environment is relatively safe, other symptoms such as intrusive thoughts, emotional numbing, depressed mood, cognitive impairment, and somatic symptoms may be more salient. However, the former set of symptoms can still predominate in a safe environment such as a new country when the individual overestimates the likelihood of re-arrest and further torture. A refugee from an African country, for instance, presented with intense fear and anxiety evoked by an unrealistic thought of being hunted down by government teams from her home country. Another refugee in London could not go home at night because of a similar fear and spent his nights in night buses travelling in town.

COPING WITH STRESS: ATTEMPTS TO MAINTAIN AND REGAIN CONTROL AND PREDICTABILITY

Detention/torture phase

Struggle for control to avoid, or at least to minimize torture starts from the first moment of arrest. Coping attempts during this phase come under broadly two overlapping categories: 1) those that are geared towards reducing the stress generated by isolation (e.g. solitary confinement) and the uncertainty about if and when torture is likely to occur and 2) those that serve to minimize the physical and psychological pain during torture.

Uncertainty about torture is a major stressor during detention. In situations where torture is likely to be used for interrogation, the uncertainty can be reduced by assessing how informed the authorities already are on the detainees. Attempts are thus made using every possible means to contact other detained comrades (or those outside) to find out what exactly the authorities want from them, who else has been arrested, who has said what during interrogation and so on. Special codes of communication may be developed and used to smuggle out messages via other inmates or bribed wardens, or through verbal or non-verbal communication with other inmates during brief outings to the lavatory. A realistic appraisal of the risk of torture reduces the unpredictability of the situation and consequent stress even when the perceived likelihood approaches certainty. Similar attempts at re-establishing contact with important others have also been frequently observed in prisoners of war (Sherwood, 1986).

When communication is not possible, knocking on the neighbour's wall can be psychologically important in coping with isolation, even when the only message that can be conveyed by doing so is no more than 'I'm alive'. It has also long been known that an effective way of coping with prolonged isolation is to follow a structured programme of activities and engage in some mental or behavioural exercises that help retain control over some areas of life (Suedfeldt, 1990, p. 113). The effects of isolation is maximized when it is coupled with severe restriction of movement (e.g. in a small 'cage') which seems to remove such possibilities for maintaining control.

Coping with torture takes place on three overlapping levels: psychophysiological, behavioural and cognitive. Psychophysiological processes include responses to physical pain described earlier, namely depersonalization, derealization, and analgesia, the latter possibly involving the release of endogenous opioids. Behavioural and cognitive coping strategies seem to be geared towards maintaining a sense of perceived control. The availability of behavioural defences against physical pain depends largely on the form of torture used. If pain is inflicted while parts of body are left free to move such as in beating while untied or in falanga with the upper part of the body mobile, the self-defensive body movements, however ineffective they might be, seem to be useful in reducing pain and preserving a sense of control. One of the most dreaded forms of torture is hanging by the wrists tied at the back ('Palestinian hanging') which causes excruciating pain at shoulder joints that becomes unbearable after 10–15 minutes. No defensive bodily movement is possible because the slightest movement increases the strain on shoulder joints and aggravates the pain. Even then certain gestures can be helpful in reducing the frustration caused by helplessness. For example, one female survivor urinated forcefully while hanging naked from the ceiling – an act which she perceived to spoil the torturers' fun who were mocking and laughing at her.

Survivors often point to the importance of exerting some control over events even when this is most likely to incur further punishment. For instance, deliberate disobedience or refusal to display any sign of distress during torture is designed to frustrate the torturers. To do so may be a gratifying (or anger/frustration reducing) experience in the sense that one ceases to be a passive recipient of others' actions. For example, one survivor noted that, during torture when blindfolded, his senses were acutely tuned in to the torturer's responses for signs of frustration which he could 'turn on and off' at will.

Some coping processes can be better understood within the context of torturer–victim relationship and of the group processes in which systematic torture takes place (for a review of culture of torture and torturers, see Staub, 1985, 1990). Torturers are often part of an ideological system, with shared values, goals, a common jargon, and a common enemy (Staub, 1990, p. 66). They often believe that their victims are enemies of the people, the state and of their own values, morality and everything else they stand for. The victims therefore deserve the treatment they get. The torturers' duty is to obey orders and serve their country by annihilating the traitors. They get credit for executing their job successfully.

Coping behaviours of the kind described earlier may assume a special meaning for the victim when the detainees are kept in groups and when the power struggle generalizes to the larger group of torturers and detainees. The detainees may come to view any hint of surrender on their part as the personal success of the torturers. Thus, resisting torture may be an effective way of retaliation when the torturer's failure to break the 'tough nut' is likely to cause embarrassment and loss of prestige among the torturer's colleagues. Such dynamics explain why some torturers develop personal vendettas against certain prisoners and also why some 'accidental' deaths occur during torture.

Cognitive style and attributional processes play an important role in coping with both the immediate and the long-term psychological effects of torture. Individuals who have greater awareness of the socio-political context of torture and its objectives seem to be better protected against the traumatic effects of torture.

Imprisonment phase

Life in prison is often regulated by extremely oppressive measures. Indoctrination procedures, daily beatings and other forms of punishment such as solitary confinement, banning visitors, and withholding mail are common. Such treatment, however, becomes a predictable feature of daily life, and prisoners learn ways of coping and regain some sense of control.

One survivor's account illustrates the anxiety-reducing effect of predictability and perceived control. A group of 30 inmates received daily beatings for refusing to comply with instructions regarding daily inspections. Twice every day they were ordered to count from left to right when they were lined up for inspections and the last one in the row was supposed to complete the counting by saying 'everybody present, commander'. The group decided to resist this procedure by having the last person in the row remaining silent. This person would then get a beating from the infuriated wardens. The group devised a rota so that each time a different person would get what they humorously called 'the beating of the last'. In contrast to similar treatment during detention, these beatings posed little or no distress; rather, they became a joke among the prisoners and enhanced group solidarity.

Availability of emotional support from other inmates seems to be a critical factor in speeding up recovery from the effects of torture. A supportive group affords opportunity for the newcomer to be 'debriefed' and his/her traumatic experience shared. An important coping strategy under oppressive prison conditions is collective hunger strikes. Such actions often attract considerable national and international media attention, thereby putting intense pressure on the prison authorities as well as the government concerned. Resistance often serves to enhance solidarity and sense of control among the prisoners. Hunger strikes can sometimes lead to starvation and even death. Starving oneself to death in response to uncontrollable stress can be regarded as an ultimate form of control.

To summarize, the imprisonment phase may speed up recovery if the individual receives psychological support in a predictable environment over which some control can be achieved. Individuals who go through this phase seem to be better off than those who are released from detention/torture into a non-supportive environment.

Post-imprisonment phase

As noted earlier, the events following release from prison are highly variable. Those individuals who have recovered during imprisonment move into this phase without much problem. For those who have not, the outcome is determined by a variety of factors. The following discussion concerning the latter group also applies to those released after detention and torture without going through imprisonment.

An important factor in this phase which may determine outcome is the degree of further threat to one's self or to friends or relatives. As noted earlier, this phase may merge into the pre-arrest/detention phase whereby the survivor is exposed to risk of further re-arrest and torture or other forms of political repression.

Acceptance by comrades is critical during this phase. A positive attitude from peer groups not only provides vital emotional support but also enables a return to group political activity. Being part of a group also affords some protection from further threats of persecution and harassment. Such group support is vital for recovery from feelings of helplessness and loss of control experienced during torture. Political activity can be directed against the regime for its human rights violations or against particular figures known for their involvement in these violations. Suppressed anger and hostility often find expression in these activities to bring those responsible to court for punishment and to see that justice is done. Internal conflicts caused by degradation and humiliation can be resolved if the survivors enjoy esteem and respect from friends and comrades. The cognitive change necessary for re-evaluation of personal worth and recovery of self-esteem is facilitated by a supportive environment where torture is viewed as a litmus test of individual strength, integrity, commitment to the cause and reliability; those who have passed the test often enjoy considerable prestige and credibility in later political life.

The survivor will also have to cope with the long-term effects of verbally-induced helplessness. This is often achieved by cognitive change. The torturers' comments about the permanent effects of torture in the body (e.g. infertility, loss of virility, developing homosexual tendencies, etc) may lead to obsessional worries of physical health and bodily functioning, as previously noted. Such comments will have to be disconfirmed in time, as in the case of the survivor who had anxiously to wait until she got pregnant and delivered a healthy baby. Her first reaction was more of an angry sense of triumph than of a passive relief and addressed directly to the torturers: 'the victory is mine'.

In summary, the critical factor for recovery in this phase is the availability of social support in counteracting the effects of uncontrollable stress; there is evidence supporting its therapeutic role in human trauma survivors (Keane *et al.*, this volume). The mechanisms by which social support enhances recovery process are not entirely clear but several factors can be identified. It provides a relatively predictable and safe environment which possibly counteracts the effects of unpredictability and unavailability of safety signals that characterize the torture setting. Secondly, it helps positive cognitive change which leads to alterations in the survivor's negative self-perception and negative evaluations of helplessness behaviour during captivity. Such cognitive change seems to neutralize expectations of negative outcomes in future coping behaviour, thereby alleviatings feelings of helplessness and hopelessness. Third, the help provided by a supportive environment in dealing with serious life problems after imprisonment and torture reduces helplessness and allows opportunities for the survivor to exercise and regain control over the environment.

IMPLICATIONS FOR THE TREATMENT OF TORTURE SURVIVORS

If perceptions of loss of control play a role in the origins and maintenance of anxiety disorders, then treatments should be aimed at restoring a sense of control and mastery over the environment. This would be expected to reverse the effects of uncontrollable stress (helplessness and hopelessness) and reduce anxiety and depression in torture survivors. Research in this area certainly seems worthwhile.

Most rehabilitation programmes available for torture survivors today involve support for a wide range of social, political, economic, medical, legal, and family problems. As noted earlier, this can be seen to reduce feelings of helplessness in the survivor or at least prevent him/her from being overwhelmed by further uncontrollable events following the torture experience. The role of social support in therapy outcome and the mechanisms by which social support affects psychological functioning require more attention in future research. Also relevant for future studies is the question 'which kind of social support', because not all forms of social support are therapeutic in trauma survivors (see a discussion of the role of social support in trauma survivors by Keane et al., this volume).

Psychotherapy often involves cognitive interventions to help the survivor to leave the 'victim role' induced by the traumatic experience. This can be seen as helping the survivor regain a sense of control over the trauma as well as current environmental events (see Başoğlu, this volume, for a discussion of cognitive therapy in torture survivors).

The 'testimony' method used by some in treating torture survivors (Cienfuegos & Monelli, 1983; Agger & Jensen, 1990) involves the survivor documenting his/her experience in detail to be used in the future as evidence against the perpetrators. This seems to alter the survivor's cognitions of 'helplessness' resulting from the torture experience by turning the traumatic experience that hitherto meant total helplessness into an effective instrument of political struggle against torture and/or particular torturers, thereby giving a new meaning to the trauma. There is, as yet, no evidence in support of the efficacy of such interventions but research certainly seems warranted.

Helplessness and depression may be sustained by fear and anxiety responses evoked by intrusive recollections of the trauma and other environmental events and situations that resemble the torture experience (conditioned stimuli). Re-experiencing the torture may be viewed as re-experiencing helplessness induced by uncontrollable traumatic stress. Thus regaining control over fear-evoking conditioned stimuli would be expected to reduce feelings of helplessness. Exposure treatment might be useful in this connection since it is known to reduce fear and anxiety cued by conditioned stimuli (for a review of evidence, see Keane et al. and Başoğlu, this volume). Habituation to 1) anxiety-evoking recollections of the trauma and other related mental imagery through imaginal exposure (implosion) and 2) environmental cues which trigger re-experiencing phenomena through in vivo exposure can help regain perceptions of control, thereby reducing feelings of helplessness and depression. Other treatments said to be effective in torture survivors involve elements of imaginal exposure to trauma during reconstruction of the trauma story and the cathartic reactions that occur in the process (for a more detailed discussion of exposure-based treatments and the common elements between various psychotherapies, see Başoğlu, this volume).

CONCLUSION

In this chapter we have reviewed the evidence on the role of uncontrollable and unpredictable stress in anxiety and depression and drawn attention to the parallels between experimental models of anxiety/depression and human experience under torture. As noted earlier, these models may not offer a comprehensive account of human behaviour during and following torture but they are nevertheless useful in understanding psychological reactions to extreme stress. They may also have important implications for treatment of torture survivors and thus deserve closer scrutiny in future research.

ACKNOWLEDGEMENTS

The authors wish to thank J. B. Overmier for his valuable comments on the manuscript.

REFERENCES

Abramson, L., Metalsky, G. & Alloy, L. (1989). Hopelessness depression: a theory-based subtype of depression. *Psychological Review*, **96**, 358–72.

Abramson, L., Seligman, M. & Teasdale, J. (1978). Learned helplessness in humans: critique and reformulation. *Journal of Abnormal Psychology*, **87**, 49–74.

Agger, I. & Jensen, S. B. (1990). Testimony as ritual and evidence in psychotherapy for political refugees. *Journal of Traumatic Stress*, **3(1)**, 115–30.

Allodi, F. & Cowgill, G. (1982). Ethical and psychiatric aspects of torture: A Canadian study. *Canadian Journal of Psychiatry*, **27**, 98–102.

Alloy, L., Kelly, K., Mineka, S., & Clements, C. (1990). Comorbidity in anxiety and depressive disorders: a helplessness/hopelessness perspective. In J. Maser and C. R. Cloninger, (eds.) *Comorbidity in Mood and Anxiety Disorders*. American Psychiatric Press, Inc: Washington, DC.

Amnesty International (1984). *Torture in the Eighties*. London: Amnesty International Publications.

Anisman, H. & Sklar, L. (1979). Catecholamine depletion in mice upon reexposure to stress: mediation of the escape deficits produced by inescapable shock. *Journal of Comparative and Physiological Psychology*, **93**, 610–25.

Anisman, H., Kokinidis, L. & Sklar, L. (1981). Contribution of neurochemical change to stress induced behavioral deficits. In S. Cooper (ed.) *Theory in Psychopharnacology*, vol. 1. London: Academic Press.

Averill., J. (1973). Personal control over aversive stimuli and its relationship to stress. *Psychological Bulletin*, 80, 286–303.

Averill, J. R. (1982). *Anger and Aggression: An Essay on Emotion.* New York: Springer-Verlag.

Badia, P., Harsh, J. & Abbott, B. (1979). Choosing between predictable and unpredictable shock conditions: data and theory. *Psychological Bulletin*, 86, 1107–31.

Bandura, A. (1977). Self-efficacy: Toward a unifying theory of behavioral change. *Psychological Review*, 84, 191–215.

Barlow, D. (1988). *Anxiety and Its Disorders.* Hillsdale, NJ: Erlbaum.

Baron, R. A. (1977). *Human aggression.* New York: Plenum Press.

Beck, A. & Emery, G. (1985). *Anxiety Disorders and Phobias: A Cognitive Perspective.* New York: Basic Books.

Beck, A. T., Kovacs, M. & Weissman, A. (1975). Hopelessness and suicidal behaviour: An overview. *Journal of American Medical Association*, 234, 1146–1149.

Benfeldt-Zachrisson, F. (1985). State (political) torture: some general, psychological, and particular aspects. *International Journal of Health Services*, 15: 339–49.

Bersh, P., Schoenfeld, W. & Notterman, J. (1952). The effect upon heart-rate conditioning of randomly varying the interval between conditioned and unconditioned stimuli. *Proceedings of the National Academy of Sciences*, 39, 563–70.

Bolles, R. & Fanselow, M. (1982). Endorphins and behaviour. *Annual Review of Psychology*, 33, 87–101.

Bowers, W., Zacharko, R. & Anisman, H. (1987). Evaluation of stressor effects on intracranial self stimulation from the nucleus accumbens and the substantia nigra in a current intensity paradigm. *Behavioral Brain Research*, 23, 85–93.

Cienfuegos, A. J. & Monelli, C. (1983). The testimony of political repression as a therapeutic instrument. *American Journal of Orthopsychiatry*, 53(1), 43–51.

Desan, P., Silbert, L. & Maier, S. (1988). Long-term effects of inescapable stress on daily running activity and antagonism by desipramine. *Pharmacology, Biochemistry, and Behaviour*, 30, 21–29.

Desiderato, O. & Newman, A. (1971). Conditioned suppression produced in rats by tones paired with escapable or inescapable shock. *Journal of Comparative and Physiological Psychology*, 96, 427–31.

Dess, N., Linwick, D., Patterson, J., Overmier, J. & Levine, S. (1983). Immediate and proactive effects of controllability and predictability on plasma cortisol responses to shocks in dogs. *Behavioural Neuroscience*, 97, 1005–16.

Domovitch, E., Berger, P. B., Waver, M. J. *et al.* (1984) Human torture: description and sequelae of 104 cases. *Canadian Journal of Family Physician*, 30, 827–830.

Érofeeva, M. N. (1912) Electrical stimulation of the skin of the dog as a conditioned salivary stimulus. Thesis, Petrograd: Prelim. Commun. Russian Medi. Soc. in Petrograd., Vol. 79.

Fanselow, M. (1980). Signalled shock-free periods and preference for signalled shock. *Journal of Experimental Psychology: Animal Behaviour Processes*, 6, 65–80.

Fanselow, M. (1991). Analgesia as a response to aversive Pavlovian conditional stimuli: Cognitive and emotional mediators. In M. Denny (ed.), *Aversive Events and Behaviour*. Hillsdale, NJ: Erlbaum.

Farber, I., Harlow, H. & West, L. (1957). Brainwashing, conditioning, and DDD (debility, dependency, and dread). *Sociometry*, 20, 271–85.

Fleshner, M., Laudenslager, Simons, L. & Maier, S. (1989). Reduced serum antibodies associated with social defeat in rats. *Physiology and Behaviour*, 45, 1183–87.

Foa, E., Steketee, G. & Rothbaum, B. (1989). Behavioral/cognitive conceptualization of post-traumatic stress disorder. *Behavior Therapy*, 20, 155–76.

Ford, C. & Spaulding, R. (1973). The Pueblo incident: a comparison of factors related to coping with extreme stress. *Archives of General Psychiatry*, 29, 340–4.

Garber, J., Miller, S. & Abramson, L. (1980). On the distinction between anxiety states and depression: Perceived control, certainty, and probability of goal attainment. In J. Garber and M. Seligman, (eds.), *Human Helplessness: Theory and Applications*. Academic Press: New York.

Gatchel., R., Paulus, P. & Maples, C. (1975). Learned helplessness and self-reported affect. *Journal of Abnormal Psychology*, 85, 27–34.

Glavin, B. (1980). Restraint ulcer: history, current research and future implications. *Brain Research Bulletin*, 5, 51–8.

Goldfeld, A. E., Mollica, R. F., Pesavento, B. H. & Faraone, S. V. (1988). The physical and psychological sequelae of torture–symptomatology and diagnosis. *Journal of American Medical Association*, 259(18), 2725–9.

Gudjonsson, G. H. & Clark, N. K. (1986). Suggestibility in police interrogation: a social psychological model. *Social Behaviour*, 1, 83–104.

Guile, M. (1987). Differential gastric ulceration in rats receiving shocks on either fixed-time or variable-time schedules. *Behavioural Neurosciences*, 101, 139–40.

Haney, C. & Zimbardo, P. (1977). The socialization into criminality: on becoming a prisoner and a guard. In J. L. Tapp and F. L. Levine (eds.) *Law, Justice, and the Individual in Society: Psychological and Legal Issues*. pp. 198–223, New York: Holt, Rinehart and Winston.

Hannum, R., Rosellini, R. & Seligman, M. (1976). Retention of learned helplessness and immunization in the rat from weaning to adulthood. *Developmental Psychology*, 12, 449–54.

Hinkle, L. & Wolff, H. (1956). Communist interrogation and indoctrination of 'enemies of the state'. *Archives of Neurology and Psychiatry*, 76, 115–74.

Hougen, H. P., Kelstrup, J., Petersen, H. D. & Rasmussen, O. V. (1988). Sequelae to torture. A controlled study of torture victims living in exile. *Forensic Science International*, 36, 153–60.

Imada, H. & Nageishi, Y. (1982). The concept of uncertainty in animal experiments using aversive stimulation. *Psychological Bulletin*, **91**, 573–88.

Jackson, R., Alexander, J. & Maier, S. (1980). Learned helplessness, inactivity and associative deficits: effects of inescapable shock on response choice escape learning. *Journal of Experimental Psychology: Animal Behaviour Processes*, **6**, 1–20.

Jensen, T. S., Genefke, I. K., Hyldebrandt, N. *et al.* (1982). Cerebral atrophy in young torture victims. *New England Journal of Medicine*, **307**, 1341.

Joffe, J., Rawson, R. & Mulick, J. (1973). Control of their environment reduces emotionality in rats. *Science*, **180**, 1383–4.

Kendall, P. & Watson, D., eds. (1989). *Anxiety and Depression: Distinctive and Overlapping Features*. New York: Academic Press.

Laudenslager, M., Fleshner, M., Hofstadter, P., Held, P., Simons, L. & Maier, S. (1988). Suppression of specific antibody production by inescapable shock: stability under varying conditions. *Brain, Behaviour, and Immunity*, **2**, 92–101.

Lee, R. & Maier, S. (1988). Inescapable shock and attention to internal versus external cues in a water discrimination escape task. *Journal of Experimental Psychology: Animal Behaviour Processes*, **14**, 302–10.

Leventhal, H. (1979). A perceptual-motor processing model of emotion. In P. Pliner, K. Blankstein, and I. M. Spiegel eds. *Advances in the study of communication and affect: Perception of emotion in self and others*, vol. 5 New York: Plenum.

Leventhal, H., Brown, D. Shacham, S. & Engquist, G. (1979). Effects of preparatory information about sensations, threat of pain, and attention on cold pressor distress. *Journal of Personality and Social Psychology*, **37**, 688–714.

Liddell, H. (1944). Conditioned reflex method and experimental neurosis. In J. McV. Hunt ed., *Personality and the Behaviour Disorders*, vol. 1, New York: Ronald Press.

Lunde, I. (1982). Mental sequelae or torture (Psykike folger has torturofet). *Manedsskrift Praktisk Laegegerning*, **60**, 476–88.

Lykken, D. (1962). Perception in the rat: autonomic response to shock as a function of length of warning interval. *Science*, **137**, 665–6.

Maier, S. F. (1989) Determinants of the nature of environmentally induced hypoalgesia. *Behavioural Neuroscience*, **103**, 131–43.

Maier, S., Drugan, R. & Grau, J. (1982). Controllability, coping behaviour, and stress-induced analgesia in the rat. *Pain*, **12**, 47–56.

Maier, S. & Jackson, R. (1979). Learned helplessness: all of us were right (and wrong): inescapable shock has multiple effects. In G. Bower, ed., *The Psychology of Learning and Motivation, vol. 13, Advances in Theory and Research*. New York: Academic Press.

Maier, S., Jackson, R., Grau, J., Hyson, R., MacLennan, A & Moye, T. (1983a). Learned helplessness, pain inhibition, and the endogenous opiates. In *Advances in the Analysis of Behaviour*, vol. 3, New York: Wiley.

Maier, S., Jackson, R. & Tomie, A. (1987). Potentiation overshadowing, and prior exposure to inescapable shock. *Journal of Experimental Psychology: Animal Behaviour Processes*, **13**, 260–70.

Maier, S & Seligman, M. E. P. (1976). Learned helplessness: theory and evidence. *Journal of Experimental Psychology: General*, 105, 3–45.

Maier, S., Sherman, J., Lewis, J., Terman., G. & Liebeskind, J. (1983*b*). The opioid/nonopioid nature of stress-induced analgesia and learned helplessness. *Journal of Experimental Psychology: Animal Behaviour Processes*, 9, 80–90.

Mandler, G. & Watson, D. (1966). Anxiety and the interruption of behaviour. In C. Spelberger, ed., *Anxiety and Behaviour*. New York: Academic Press.

Mandler, G. (1972). Helplessness: theory and research in anxiety. In C. Spielberger, ed., *Anxiety: Current Trends in Theory and Research I*. New York: Academic Press.

Maser, J. & Cloninger, R., eds. (1990). *Comorbidity of Mood and Anxiety Disorders*. American Psychiatric Press.

Masserman, J. (1971). The principle of uncertainty in neurotogenesis. In H. Kimmel, ed., *Experimental Psychopathology: Recent Research and Theory*. New York: Academic Press.

Melamed, G., Melamed, J. L. & Bouhoutsos, J. C. (1990). Psychological Consequences of Torture: A need to formulate new strategies for research. In P. Suedfeldt, ed. *Psychology and Torture*. Hemisphere Publishing Corporation.

Miczek, K., Thompson, M. & Shuster, L. (1982). Opioid-like analgesia in defeated mice. *Science*, 215, 1520–2.

Miller, R., Greco, C., Vigorito, M. & Marlin, N. (1983). Signalled tailshock is perceived as similar to a stronger unsignalled tailshock: implications for a functional analysis of classical conditioning. *Journal of Experimental Psychology: Animal Behaviour Processes*, 9, 105–31.

Miller, S. (1980). Why having control reduces stress: if I can stop the roller coaster I don't want to get off. In M. Seligman and J. Garber eds. *Human Helplessness: Theory and Applications*. New York: Academic Press.

Miller, S. (1989). Information, coping and control in patients undergoing surgery and stressful medical procedures. In A. Steptoe and A. Appels, eds. *Stress, Personal Control and Health*. Wiley: Chichester.

Miller, S. & Mangan, C. (1983). Interacting effects of information and coping style in adapting to gynecologic stress: should the doctor tell all? *Journal of Personality and Social Psychology*, 45, 228–38.

Miller, W. & Seligman, M. (1975). Depression and learned helplessness in man. *Journal of Abnormal Psychology*, 84, 228–238.

Mineka, S. (1987). A primate model of phobic fears. In H. Eysenck & I. Martin, eds. *Theoretical Foundations of Behaviour Therapy*. Plenum Press.

Mineka, S. & Cook, M. (1992). Mechanisms involved in the observational conditioning of fear, in press.

Mineka, S., Cook, M. & Miller, S. (1984). Fear conditioned with escapable and inescapable shock: the effects of a feedback stimulus. *Journal of Experimental Psychology: Animal Behaviour Processes*, 10, 307–23.

Mineka, S., Gunnar, M. & Champoux, M. (1986). Control and early socio-emotional development: infant rhesus monkeys reared in controllable versus uncontrollable environments. *Child Development*, 57, 1241–56.

Mineka, S. & Hendersen, R. (1985). Controllability and predictability in acquired motivation. *Annual Review of Psychology*, **36**, 495–529.

Mineka, S. & Kelly, K. (1989). The relationship between anxiety, lack of control and loss of control. In A. Steptoe and A. Appels, eds., *Stress, Personal Control and Health*. Brussels: Wiley.

Mineka, S. & Kihlstrom, J. (1978). Unpredictable and uncontrollable events: a new perspective on experimental neurosis. *Journal of Abnormal Psychology*, **87**, 256–71.

Minor, T., Jackson, R. & Maier, S. (1984). Effects of task irrelevant cues and reinforcement delay on choice escape learning following inescapable shock: evidence for a deficit in selective attention. *Journal of Experimental Psychology: Animal Behaviour Processes*, **10**, 543–56.

Minor, T., Trauner, M., Lee, C-Y & Dess, N. (1990). Modelling signal features of escape response: effects of cessation conditioning in 'learned helplessness' paradigm. *Journal of Experimental Psychology: Animal Behaviour Processes*, **16**, 123–36.

Mollica, R. F., Wyshak, G. & Lavelle, J. (1987). The psychosocial impact of war trauma and torture on Southeast Asian refugees. *American Journal of Psychiatry*, **144**, 1567–72.

Mollica, R. F., Wyshak, G., Lavelle, J., Truong, T., Tor, S. & Yang, T. (1990). Assessing symptom change in Southeast Asian refugee survivors of mass violence and torture. *American Journal of Psychiatry*, **147**, 83–8.

Mowrer, H. & Viek, P. (1948). An experimental analogue of fear from a sense of helplessness. *Journal of Abnormal and Social Psychology*, **43**, 193–200.

Moye, T., Cook, Grau, J. & Maier, S. (1981). Therapy and immunization of long-term analgesia in rats. *Learning and Motivation*, **12**, 133–48.

Moye, T., Hyson, R., Grau, J. & Maier, S. (1983). Immunization of opioid analgesia: effects of prior escapable shock on subsequent shock-induced and morphine-induced antinociception. *Learning and Motivation*, **4**, 238–51.

Nardini, J. (1962). Psychiatric concepts of prisoner of war confinement. *Military Medicine*, **127**, 299–307.

Ortmann, J., Genefke, I. K., Jakobsen, L. & Lunde, I. (1987). Rehabilitation of torture victims: an interdisciplinary treatment model. *American Journal of Social Psychiatry*, **4**, 161–7.

Overmier, J. B. (1985). Toward a reanalysis of the causal structure of the learned helplessness syndrome. In F. R. Brush and J. B. Overmier, eds. *Affect, Conditioning and Cognition: Essays on the Determinants of Behaviour*, pp. 211–28. Hillsdale, NJ: Lawrence Erlbaum.

Overmier, J. B. (1988). Psychological determinants of when stressors stress. In D. Hellhammer, I. Florin and H. Weiner, eds. *Neurobiological Approaches to Human Disease*. Toronto: Hans Huber Publishers.

Overmier, J. B. & Hellhammer, I. (1988). The learned helplessness model of human depression. *Animal Models of Psychiatric Disorders*, **2**, 177–202.

Overmier, J. B. & Murison, R. (1989). Poststress effects of danger and safety signals on gastric ulceration in rats. *Behavioral Neurosciences*, **103**, 1296–301.

Overmier, J. B. & Seligman, M. E. P. (1967). Effects of inescapable shock upon subsequent escape and avoidance responding. *Journal of Comparative and Physiological Psychology*, **63**, 28–33.

Pavlov, I. P. (1927). *Conditioned reflexes: an investigation of the physiological activity of the cerebral cortex.* London: Oxford University Press.

Perkins, C. (1968). An analysis of the concept of reinforcement. *Psychological Review*, **75**, 155–72.

Petersen, H. D., Abildgaard, U., Daugaard, G. *et al.* (1985). Psychological and physical long-term effects of torture. A follow-up examination of 22 Greek persons exposed to torture 1967–1974. *Scandinavian Journal of Social Medicine*, **13**, 89–93.

Pitman, R., van der Kolk, B., Orr, S. & Greenberg, M. (1990). Naloxone reversible analgesic response to combat-related stimuli in posttraumatic stress disorder. *Archives of General Psychiatry*, **47**, 541.

Rapaport, P. & Maier, S. (1978). Inescapable shock and food-competition dominance in rats. *Animal Learning and Behaviour*, **6**, 160–5.

Rahe, R. & Genender-Sherwood, E. (1983). Adaptation to and recovery from captivity stress. *Military Medicine*, **148**, 577–85.

Rasmussen, O. V. & Lunde, I. (1980). Evaluation of investigation of 200 torture victims. *Danish Medical Bulletin*, **27**, 241–3.

Reid, J. C. & Strong, T. (1988). Rehabilitation of refugee victims of torture and trauma: principles and service provision in New South Wales. *The Medical Journal of Australia*, **148**, 340–6.

Roth, E. F., Lunde, I., Boysen, G. & Genefke, I. K. (1987). Torture and its treatment. *American Journal of Public Health*, **77**, 1404–1406.

Rotter, J. (1966). Generalized expectancies for internal versus external control of reinforcement. *Psychological Monographs*, **80** (1, Whole No. 609).

Sanderson, W., Rapee, R. & Barlow, D. (1989). The influence of an illusion of control on panic attacks induced via inhalation of 5.5% carbon dioxide-enriched air. *Archives of General Psychiatry*, **46**, 157–62.

Seligman, M. E. P. (1968). Chronic fear produced by unpredictable shock. *Journal of Comparative and Physiological Psychology*, **66**, 402–411.

Seligman, M. (1974). Depression and learned helplessness. I. M. Friedman and M. Katz eds., *The Psychology of Depression.* Washington, DC: Winston Press.

Seligman, M. (1975). *Helplessness: On Depression, Death, and Development.* San Francisco: Freeman.

Seligman, M. E. P. and Binik, Y. (1977). The safety-signal hypothesis. In H. Davies, & H. Hurwitz, eds. *Operant–Pavlovian interactions.* Hillsdale, NJ: Erlbaum.

Seligman, M. E. P. & Maier, S. F. (1967). Failure to escape traumatic shock. *Journal of Experimental Psychology*, **74**, 1–9.

Seligman, M. E. P., Maier, S. & Solomon, R. (1971). Unpredictable and uncontollable aversive events. In F. R. Brush, ed., *Aversive conditioning and learning.* Academic Press: New York.

Sherwood, E. (1986). The power relationship between captor and captive. *Psychiatric Annals*, **16(11)**, 653–5.

Sklar, L. & Anisman, H. (1981). Stress and cancer. *Psychological Bulletin*, **89**, 369–406.

Sledge, W., Boydston, J. & Rahe, A. (1980). Self-concept changes related to war captivity. *Archives of General Psychiatry*, **37**, 420–443.

Somnier, F. E. & Genefke, I. K. (1986). Psychotherapy for victims of torture. *British Journal of Psychiatry*, **149**, 323–9.

Spaulding, R. & Ford, C. (1972). The Pueblo incident: psychological reactions to the stresses of imprisonment and repatriation. *American Journal of Psychiatry*, **129**, 17–26.

Speigel, D. & Fink, R. (1979). Hysterical psychosis and hypnotizability. *American Journal of Psychiatry*, **136**, 377–81.

Speigel, D. Hunt, T. & Dondershine, H. E. (1988). Dissociation and hypnotizability in posttraumatic stress disorder. *American Journal of Psychiatry*, **145(3)**, 301–5.

Staub, E. (1985). The psychology of perpetrators and bystanders. *Political Psychology*, **6**, 61–85.

Staub, E. (1989). The evolution of bystanders, German psychoanalysts, and lessons for today. *Political Psychology*, **10**, 39–52.

Staub, E. (1990). The psychology and culture of torture and torturers. In P. Seudfeld, ed. *Torture and Psychology*. New York: Hemisphere Publishing Corporation.

Stover, E. & Nightingale, E. O. (1985). Introduction. In E. Stover & E. O. Nightingale, eds. *The Breaking of Minds and Bodies*, pp. 1–26, New York: Freeman.

Suedfeldth, P. (1990). Torture: a brief overview. In P. Suedfeldth, ed. *Psychology and Torture*, p. 3. New York: Hemisphere Publishing Corporation.

van der Kolk, B. & Greenberg, M. (1987). The psychobiology of the trauma response: Hyperarousal, constriction, and addition to traumatic reexposure. In B. van der Kolk, ed. *Psychological Trauma*. Washington, DC: American Psychiatric Press.

van der Kolk, B. Greenberg, M., Boyed, H. & Krystal, J. (1985). Inescapable shock, neurotransmitters, and addiction to trauma: Toward a psychobiology of post traumatic stress. *Biological Psychiatry*, **20**, 314–25.

Visintainer, M., Volpicelli, J. & Seligman, M. (1982). Tumor rejection in rats after inescapable or escapable shock. *Science*, **216**, 437–9.

Volpicelli, J. R., Ulm, R. R., Altenor, A., & Seligman, M. E. P. (1983). Learned mastery in the rat. *Learning and Motivation*, **14**, 204–22.

Warren, D., Rosellini, R. & Maier, S. (1989). Fear, stimulus feedback and stressor controllability. In G. Bower, ed. *The Psychology of Learning and Motivation*, vol. 24, New York: Academic Press.

Weinberg, J. & Levine, S. (1980). Psychobiology of coping in animals: The effects of predictability. In S. Levine & H. Ursin, eds., *Coping and Health*, New York: Plenum Press.

Weiss, J. (1968). Effects of coping response on stress. *Journal of Comparative and Physiological Psychology*, **65**, 251–60.

Weiss, J. (1971a). Effects of coping behaviour in different warning-signal conditions on stress pathology in rats. *Journal of Comparative and Physiological Psychology*, **77**, 1–13.

Weiss, J. (1971b). Effects of punishing the coping response (conflict) on stress pathology in rats. *Journal of Comparative and Physiological Psychology*, **77**, 14–21.

Weiss, J. (1971c). Effects of coping behaviour with and without a feedback signal on stress pathology in rats. *Journal of Comparative and Physiological Psychology*, **77**, 22–30.

Weiss, J. (1977). Psychological and behavioral influences on gastrointestinal lesions in animal models. In J. Maser & M. E. P. Seligman, eds. *Psychopathology: Experimental Models*. San Francisco: Freeman.

Weiss, J., Glazer, H. & Poherecky, L. (1976). Coping behaviour and neurochemical changes in rats: an alternative explanation for the original 'learned helplessness' experiments. In G. Serban & A. Kling, eds. *Animal Models in Human Psychobiology*. pp. 141–73, New York: Plenum Press.

Weiss, J., Goodman, P., Losito, B., Corrigan, S., Charry, J. & Bailey, W. (1981). Behavioral depression produced by an uncontrollable stressor: relationship to norephinephrine, dopamine, and serotonin levels in various regions of rat brain. *Brain Research Review*, **3**, 167–205.

White, R. (1959). Motivation reconsidered: the concept of competence. *Psychological Bulletin*, **66**, 317–30.

Williams, J. (1982). Influence of shock controllability by dominant rats on subsequent attack and defensive behaviors toward colony intruders. *Animal Learning and Behaviour*, **10**, 240–52.

Williams, J. & Maier, S. (1977). Transsituational immunization and therapy of learned helplessness in the rat. *Journal of Experimental Psychology: Animal Behaviour Processes*, **3**, 240–52.

Wolf, S. and Ripley, H. (1947). Reactions among allied prisoners of war subjected to three years of imprisonment and torture by the Japanese. *American Journal of Psychiatry*, **104**, 180–93.

Zimbardo, P. G. (1975). On transforming experimental research into advocacy for social change. In M. Deutsch and H. Dornstein eds., *Applying Social Psychology: Implications for Research, Practice, and Training*. Hillsdale, NJ: Erlbaum.

Part III

ASSESSMENT, DIAGNOSIS, AND
CLASSIFICATION

10
PSYCHOPATHOLOGY OF POST-TRAUMATIC STRESS DISORDER (PTSD): BOUNDARIES OF THE SYNDROME

Richard J. McNally

INTRODUCTION

Although the psychiatric effects of trauma have been recognized for many years, the resultant disorders have often been described in reference to the precipitating event (e.g. 'concentration camp syndrome', Chodoff, 1963; 'post-Vietnam syndrome', Shatan, 1973; 'rape trauma syndrome', Burgess & Holmstrom, 1974). The plethora of event-specific syndromes notwithstanding, diverse stressors can produce remarkably similar effects, a view acknowledged by the formal recognition of post-traumatic stress disorder (PTSD) in DSM–III (*Diagnostic and Statistical Manual of Mental Disorders* – third edition; American Psychiatric Association [APA], 1980).

The formal recognition of PTSD has prompted concerns about its syndromal validity (Goodwin & Guze, 1984, p. 82), its forensic implications (Sparr & Atkinson, 1986), and its boundaries with other well-established disorders (Sierles *et al.*, 1983). Nevertheless, ratification of the disorder has also stimulated research on traumatic stress, much of it confirming the validity of the diagnosis (March, 1990). In this chapter, I will review recent findings on the syndromal validity of PTSD.

CLINICAL DESCRIPTION OF DSM–III–R PTSD

PTSD comprises a characteristic set of symptoms that emerge following exposure to an extremely stressful event (APA, 1987). Such events provoke distress in nearly everyone, are experienced with terror and helplessness, and are exemplified by combat, horrific accidents, rape, and natural disasters. The characteristic symptoms include (1) re-experiencing the traumatic event, (2) avoidance of stimuli reminiscent of the trauma or emotional numbing, and (3) increased arousal. Symptoms must be present for at least one month for the diagnosis to be assigned. The DSM–III–R criteria are shown in Table 10.1.

Table 10.1. *DSM–III–R criteria for post-traumatic stress disorder*

Criterion A
The person has experienced an event that is outside the range of usual human experience and that would be markedly distressing to almost anyone, e.g. serious threat to one's life or physical integrity; serious threat or harm to one's children, spouse, or other close relatives and friends; sudden destruction of one's home or community; or seeing another person who has recently been, or is being, seriously injured or killed as the result of an accident or physical violence.

Criterion B
The traumatic event is persistently re-experienced in at least one of the following ways:

1 recurrent and intrusive distressing recollections of the event (in young children, repetitive play in which themes or aspects of the trauma are expressed)
2 recurrent distressing dreams of the event
3 sudden acting or feeling as if the traumatic event were recurring (includes a sense of reliving the experience, illusions, hallucinations, and dissociative [flashback] episodes, even those that occur upon awakening or when intoxicated)
4 intense psychological distress at exposure to events that symbolize or resemble an aspect of the traumatic event, including anniversaries of the trauma

Criterion C
Persistent avoidance of stimuli associated with the trauma or numbing of general responsiveness (not present before the trauma), as indicated by at least three of the following:

1 efforts to avoid thoughts or feelings associated with the trauma
2 efforts to avoid activities or situations that arouse recollections of the trauma
3 inability to recall an important aspect of the trauma (psychogenic amnesia)
4 markedly diminished interest in significant activities (in young children, loss of recently acquired developmental skills such as toilet training or language skills)
5 feeling of detachment or estrangement from others
6 restricted range of affect, e.g. unable to have loving feelings
7 sense of a foreshortened future, e.g. does not expect to have a career, marriage, or children, or a long life

Table 10.1. (*cont.*)

Criterion D
Persistent symptoms of increased arousal (not present before the trauma), as indicated by at least two of the following:

1 difficulty falling or staying asleep
2 irritability or outbursts of anger
3 difficulty concentrating
4 hypervigilance
5 exaggerated startle response
6 physiological reactivity upon exposure to events that symbol-ize or resemble an aspect of the traumatic event (e.g. a woman who was raped in an elevator breaks out in a sweat when entering any elevator)

Criterion E
Duration of the disturbance (symptoms in B, C, and D) of at least one month.
Specify delayed onset if the onset of symptoms was at least six months after the trauma.

Reprinted by permission of the American Psychiatric Association.

The trauma can be re-experienced in several ways. Patients usually have recurrent intrusive recollections of the event, and recurrent nightmares in which the event is re-experienced. Occasionally they re-experience the event during flashbacks, acting and feeling as if the event were recurring. These dissociative episodes may last from seconds to days. Finally, patients typically experience intense distress when encountering stimuli reminiscent of the trauma, including anniversaries of the event.

Avoidance symptoms include attempts to suppress thoughts or feelings about the trauma, and attempts to avoid stimuli associated with it. Psychogenic amnesia for aspects of the event may be present. Symptoms of emotional numbing include inability to feel close to others, to experience positive emotions, and to enjoy pleasurable activities.

Symptoms of increased arousal include exaggerated startle, sleep disturbance, concentration difficulties, hypervigilance, irritability, and physiological reactivity in response to reminders of the trauma.

DOES PTSD CONSTITUTE A COHERENT SYNDROME?

To reformulate the DSM–III PTSD criteria, expert clinicians relied upon phenomenological studies describing the psychiatric consequences of war, natural disasters, rape, and other traumatic events (Keane, 1989). If this description captures a valid entity, then the diagnosis should be made reliably, and the criteria should cohere as a syndrome.

PTSD can be diagnosed reliably, especially when structured interviews are used. Kappa coefficients, which express interrater reliability corrected for chance agreement, range from 0.58 for unstructured interviews (Woolfolk & Grady, 1988) to 0.78 (Davidson, Smith & Kudler, 1989a) and 0.86 (Blanchard et al., 1986a) for structured interviews.

PTSD has emerged as a coherent syndrome in studies on the internal consistency of the diagnostic criteria (Keane, 1989). Excellent values for Cronbach's alpha have been obtained for the PTSD Module of the Structured Clinical Interview for DSM–III–R (alpha = 0.93, SCID; Spitzer, Williams & Gibbon, 1987; Keane, 1989), the Structured Interview for PTSD (alpha = 0.94, SI–PTSD; Davidson *et al.*, 1989a), and the Mississippi Scale for Combat-Related Posttraumatic Stress Disorder (alpha = 0.89, M-PTSD; Keane, 1989; Keane, Caddell & Taylor, 1988).

These studies indicate that PTSD constitutes a coherent syndrome that can be diagnosed with satisfactory reliability. The validity of the diagnostic criteria will be addressed later in this chapter.

PREVALENCE OF PTSD

The prevalence of PTSD has been assessed in two ways (Davidson & Fairbank, 1989). One strategy involves estimating prevalence by interviewing representative samples of the general population. This strategy works well for disorders lacking specific precipitants (e.g. bipolar disorder), but presents complications for PTSD because population estimates are a direct function of the frequency with which interviewed samples are exposed to trauma. The other strategy involves interviewing traumatized populations 'at-risk' for the disorder.

The first strategy was employed in the Epidemiologic Catchment Area (ECA) survey in which lay interviewers used the Diagnostic Interview Schedule (DIS) to estimate the lifetime prevalence of PTSD in the general population. Prevalence rates were 1.0% and 1.3% at the St. Louis (Helzer, Robins & McEvoy, 1987) and North Carolina (Davidson et al., 1991) sites, respectively. At the St. Louis site, the rates were 3.5% among persons exposed to either civilian or military violence, and 20% among veterans wounded in Vietnam. At the North Carolina site, the rate was 3.3% among victims of sexual assault.

The second strategy was employed in two studies designed to assess psychiatric morbidity in Vietnam veterans. In the Vietnam Experience Study (VES), lay interviewers, using a slightly modified DIS, obtained lifetime and current PTSD prevalence rates of 14.7% and 2.2%, respectively, in a random sample of male veterans (Center for Disease Control, 1988). In striking contrast to these findings, the National Vietnam Veterans Readjustment Study (NVVRS) reported lifetime and current PTSD prevalence rates of 30.9% and 15.2%, respectively, for male veterans, and lifetime and current prevalence rates of 17.5% and 8.5%, respectively, for female veterans (Kulka *et al.*, 1988). For those exposed to high war zone stress, the current prevalence rates for men and women were 38.5% and 17.5%, respectively. These findings indicate that PTSD persists in approximately 478,000 of the 3.15 million veterans who served in Vietnam.

Methodological differences can explain the widely discrepant prevalence estimates obtained in the VES and NVVRS (Kulka *et al.*, 1988). In the VES, prevalence estimates were based on the lay-administered DIS, an instrument whose sensitivity for detecting PTSD is only 25% (Kulka *et al.*, 1988). In the NVVRS, prevalence estimates were based on multiple convergent measures of PTSD, including the M-PTSD (Keane *et al.*, 1988) and the clinician-administered SCID (Spitzer *et al.*, 1987). Comparisons between the VES and NVVRS methods suggests that those used in the former study greatly underestimated the true prevalence of PTSD among Vietnam veterans (Kulka *et al.*, 1988).

LONGITUDINAL COURSE OF PTSD

Following exposure to a traumatic event, most people temporarily experience at least some symptoms (APA, 1987). Of those who develop full-blown PTSD, most meet criteria immediately following exposure to trauma. The majority recover, whereas others develop chronic PTSD (Blank, 1989*a*).

The longitudinal course of the disorder in victims of rape and other violent crimes has been studied by Rothbaum and Foa (1989). They found that, among rape victims seeking clinical assistance, 95% meet PTSD criteria within two weeks of the assault. The proportion meeting criteria at one, three, and six months post-assault declined to 63.3%,

J

45.9%, and 41.7%, respectively. Among victims of nonsexual assault, 64.7% met PTSD criteria one week post-assault, whereas the proportion meeting criteria declined at one, three, six, and nine months post-assault to 36.7%, 14.6%, 11.5%, and 0%, respectively.

Degree of traumatic exposure may not only influence the occurrence of PTSD, but also influence its course. One month following a fatal sniper attack on their school playground, 77% of the children who had been on the playground had PTSD, and 67% of the children who had been inside the school had PTSD (Pynoos et al., 1987). Fourteen months later, 74% of the first group still had the disorder, whereas less than 19% of the second group did (Nader et al., 1989).

Forty-year follow-up studies of former World War II prisoners of war (POWs) indicate that severe traumatization can produce persistent PTSD (Blank, 1989a; Kluznik et al., 1986; Speed et al., 1989). Among subjects interviewed by Kluznik et al., 67% had met criteria at repatriation, and 32% still met criteria at follow-up. Among subjects interviewed by Speed et al., 50% had met criteria at repatriation, and 20% still met criteria at follow-up.

Although PTSD usually emerges immediately following the trauma, there have been reports of it emerging years later, after an intervening period of apparent mental health (e.g. van Dyke, Zilberg, & McKinnon, 1985). Some clinicians, however, question the validity of a delayed onset subtype, noting that such cases may actually constitute either delayed recognition of PTSD or the exacerbation of subclinical PTSD (e.g. Pary, Turns, & Tobias, 1986).

To investigate this controversial issue, Solomon, Kotler, Shalev and Lin (1989) assessed Israeli veterans who sought psychiatric help for war-related problems between six months and five years after the end of the 1982 Lebanon War. Solomon et al. classified them as follows: (1) delayed help-seeking for chronic PTSD (40%); (2) exacerbation of subclinical PTSD (33%); (3) reactivation of PTSD in soldiers who had recovered from PTSD stemming from the 1973 Yom Kippur War; (4) delayed onset PTSD (10%); (4) other non-PTSD psychiatric disorders (4%). Delayed help-seekers developed the disorder soon after their combat-related trauma, but did not apply for treatment until their symptoms became unbearable. Cases of exacerbated subclinical, reactivated, and delayed onset PTSD developed the full-blown disorder following exposure to subsequent (nontraumatic) stressors, such as marriage or being called up for reserve duty. Even cases of genuine delayed onset experienced at least some symptoms (e.g. nightmares) shortly after the trauma. These findings suggest that delayed onset may be confused with either delayed help-seeking or exacerbation of a subclinical condition. In any event, cases of delayed onset are clinically indistinguishable from cases of immediate onset (Watson *et al.*, 1988).

RISK FACTORS FOR DEVELOPING PTSD

Far and away the strongest predictor of PTSD is exposure to trauma (March, 1990). Most studies reveal a dose–response effect whereby the probability of developing the disorder increases as a function of stressor magnitude. This holds for combat (e.g. Center for Disease Control, 1988; Foy *et al.*, 1984; Kulka *et al.*, 1988), increasing brutality of rape (Steketee & Foa, 1987), proximity to urban violence (Pynoos *et al.*, 1987), and proximity to volcanic eruption (Shore, Tatum, & Vollmer, 1986). For example, killing noncombatants, being wounded, and witnessing or participating in atrocities enhance the magnitude of combat-related stress and increase the probability of PTSD developing (Foy *et al.*, 1987).

Davidson and Fairbank (1989) have noted that certain pre-trauma factors may increase the likelihood of PTSD, including a history of childhood conduct problems (Kulka *et al.*, 1988), parental poverty (Davidson *et al.*, 1989*b*), neuroticism, and previous psychiatric disorder (McFarlane, 1989). Low levels of post-trauma social support are associated with chronic PTSD, but one cannot easily disentangle cause from effect in studies demonstrating this relationship (e.g. Keane *et al.*, 1985; Solomon, Mikulincer & Avitzur, 1988). But as March (1990) has emphasized, variables that identify high-risk persons at low-exposure levels may lose importance at high-exposure levels. For example, Foy *et al.* (1987) investigated the family history of psychopathology in Vietnam veterans who had either low or high combat exposure, and who were either healthy or had developed PTSD. Although the PTSD group had the highest rates of family psychopathology, the role of family history was nonsignificant for veterans with high combat exposure. That is, regardless of a family history of mental illness, veterans with high combat exposure developed high rates of PTSD.

FAMILY STUDIES

Because many psychiatric disorders run in families, confidence in the validity of a syndrome is enhanced when its prevalence is increased among relatives having the greatest genetic similarity to the proband. Although one would not expect elevated rates of PTSD among non-traumatized relatives of PTSD probands, elevated rates of other anxiety disorders would imply a familial vulnerability for developing anxiety problems in general, including PTSD.

Interviewing probands with combat-related PTSD, Davidson *et al.* (1985) found that 66% reported a family history of psychopathology, with substance abuse (60%), generalized anxiety and phobic/panic states (22%), and depression (20%) the most common conditions. Davidson *et al.* compared the patterns of family psychopathology to those of patients with either generalized anxiety disorder (GAD) or depression. In the families of GAD patients, the rate of anxiety disorder was 14% and the rate of depression was 14%. In the families of depressed patients, the rate of anxiety disorder was 4% and the rate of depression was 37%. Davidson *et al.* interpreted these findings as indicating that the patterns of familial psychopathology in the PTSD group resembled that of the GAD group more than that of the depressed group.

In a subsequent investigation, Davidson, Smith and Kudler (1989*b*) compared age-corrected morbidity risks for psychopathology in families of probands with combat-related PTSD with those in families of veterans with either depression, alcoholism, or nonpsychiatric medical conditions. Davidson *et al.* found that PTSD probands were less likely than depressed probands to have a family history of depression, thus suggesting that PTSD is not a 'variant of the depression genotype, even though depression is a well-known complication of PTSD' (p. 342). PTSD was noted in the families of six PTSD probands, but in none of the families of controls. Overall, however, PTSD probands did not differ from alcoholic or nonpsychiatric probands in terms of family history of psychopathology. When Davidson *et al.* compared the families of PTSD probands with the families of the 17 nonpsychiatric controls who had been exposed to combat, they found significantly more cases of anxiety disorders in the former than in the latter. There were 15 cases of GAD, six cases of PTSD, and two cases of panic/phobic state. These findings suggest a familial vulnerability for anxiety disorders among the relatives of PTSD patients.

To investigate generational transmission of PTSD vulnerability, Solomon, Kotler and Mikulincer (1988) studied previously healthy Israeli combat stress reaction casualties from the 1982 Lebanon War, approximately half of whom were offspring of Holocaust survivors. They found significantly increased rates of PTSD among Holocaust offspring, thus implying that children of traumatized parents may be at risk for PTSD should they be exposed to trauma.

PATTERNS OF COMORBIDITY

Like many psychiatric (Boyd *et al.*, 1984) and nonpsychiatric syndromes (Feinstein, 1970), PTSD commonly presents in conjunction with other disorders (Davidson & Fairbank, 1989). For example, in the NVVRS, 98.8% of the PTSD cases had a lifetime history of at least one other psychiatric disorder, including substance abuse (Davidson & Fairbank, 1989). The most common comorbid conditions in men were alcohol abuse, depression, and GAD; the most common comorbid conditions in women were depression, GAD, alcohol abuse, and panic disorder.

Current comorbidity is nearly as high as lifetime comorbidity, at least in help-seeking Vietnam combat veterans with PTSD. Sierles and associates reported that 84% of both their inpatient and outpatient PTSD cases had an additional diagnosis, often alcoholism or antisocial personality disorder (Sierles *et al.*, 1983; Sierles *et al.*, 1986). Cultural factors may influence the pattern of comorbidity, as evinced by the absence of comorbid substance abuse and antisocial personality disorder in Israeli combat veterans with PTSD treated by Lerer *et al.* (1987). Diagnoses of panic disorder and dysthymia, however, were common in these patients.

In summary, PTSD often occurs with depression, alcohol abuse, and other anxiety disorders. This comorbidity pattern resembles that found with other anxiety syndromes (e.g. de Ruiter *et al.*, 1989), thus suggesting that PTSD is, indeed, correctly classified as an anxiety disorder (Barlow *et al.*, 1990). Future research in this area, however, needs to determine whether symptomatic overlap between PTSD and disorders such as depression produce spuriously high comorbidity rates, or whether the co-occurrence of PTSD and depression reflect genuine comorbidity of two discrete entities.

DELIMITATION FROM OTHER DISORDERS

To validate a new syndrome, one must distinguish it from other well-established disorders (Robins & Guze, 1970). Indeed, skepticism concerning the validity of PTSD has partly stemmed from its symptomatic overlap with well-established entities (e.g. Pitts, 1985). Diagnoses sharing boundaries with PTSD include depression, panic disorder, simple phobia, and factitious disorder.

Symptomatic overlap between PTSD and major depression includes social withdrawal, anhedonia, sleep disturbance, concentration

difficulties, irritability, dysphoria, and guilt (Friedman, 1988). Distinctive features of the former include exaggerated startle, re-experiencing
symptoms, and physiological reactivity to trauma-related cues.
Furthermore, the sleep disturbance of PTSD differs from that of
depression. Rapid eye movement (REM) sleep is decreased in PTSD
(Hefez, Metz & Lavie, 1987; Lavie *et al.*, 1979; Schlosberg & Benjamin,
1978), but increased in depression (Kupfer & Thase, 1983). REM latency
is lengthened in PTSD (Hefez *et al.*, 1987; Lavie *et al.*, 1978; Schlosberg
& Benjamin, 1978), but shortened in depression (Kupfer & Thase,
1983). Finally, PTSD nightmares – usually exact replicas of the traumatic event – emerge during non-REM as well as REM sleep (Friedman, 1981; van der Kolk *et al.*, 1984).

There are neuroendocrine differences between PTSD and depression (Friedman, 1988; McFall *et al.*, 1989; Pitman, 1989). In contrast to
depressed patients (Carroll *et al.*, 1981), nondepressed PTSD patients
rarely exhibit nonsuppression on the dexamethasone suppression test
(DST; Kudler *et al.*, 1987). Indeed, in one study, even depressed PTSD
patients responded normally on the DST (Halbreich *et al.*, 1988).
Urinary norepinephrine (NE) and epinephrine (EPI) levels are elevated in PTSD relative to depression (Kosten *et al.*, 1987). Mason and
associates, however, found decreased 24-hour urinary free-cortisol
(UFC) in PTSD relative to depression (Mason *et al.*, 1986). As McFall
et al. (1989) point out, this is surprising because cortisol is usually
positively correlated with levels of anxiety and depression. Indeed,
Pitman and Orr (cited in Pitman, 1989) reported increased 24-hour
UFC excretion in PTSD patients relative to healthy combat controls. In
any event, elevated NE/cortisol ratios distinguish PTSD patients from
depressives (Mason *et al.*, 1988). Finally, basal plasma levels of cortisol
are lower in PTSD patients with major depression than in patients
with major depression alone (Halbreich *et al.*, 1988). Although PTSD
can often be distinguished from depression on neuroendocrine
measures, the values obtained for PTSD patients nevertheless often fall
within normal limits (Halbreich *et al.*, 1988; Mason *et al.*, 1988; Smith *et
al.*, 1989).

There are similarities between PTSD and panic disorder (Friedman,
1988). Both are characterized by chronic anxiety, by sudden episodes
of arousal (i.e. flashbacks, panic attacks), and by fear of arousal
symptoms, as measured by the Anxiety Sensitivity Index (McNally &
Lorenz, 1987; McNally *et al.*, 1987). Lactate infusion provokes panic
attacks in panic disorder patients (Liebowitz *et al.*, 1984), and provokes
flashbacks as well as panic in PTSD patients with comorbid panic
disorder (Rainey *et al.*, 1987). The physiological symptoms of panic

occur during flashbacks as well (Mellman & Davis, 1985). Hypothalamic–pituitary–adrenal–cortical axis abnormalities in PTSD resemble those in panic disorder (e.g. abnormal corticotropin-releasing
hormone (CRH) test, normal DST, normal UFC excretion; Smith *et al.*,
1989). Finally, sleep disturbance in PTSD resembles that in panic
disorder (i.e. increased sleep latency, decreased sleep time, and
decreased sleep efficiency; Pitman, 1989).

Despite these similarities, PTSD is readily distinguishable from panic
disorder. Panic patients do not report re-experiencing phenomena or
psychic numbing. Moreover, the cognitive content of panic differs
from that of flashbacks. Panic attacks are commonly associated with
the misinterpretation of a bodily sensation (e.g. skipped heartbeat) as a
sign of impending catastrophe (e.g. heart attack; Clark, 1986; McNally,
1990), whereas flashbacks are associated with the involuntary activation of a disturbing episodic memory. In other words, panic attacks are
about impending threat, whereas flashbacks are about past threat.
Panic attacks are strongly associated with the development of agoraphobia, whereas PTSD is not. Finally, Stage 4 sleep is decreased in
PTSD, but increased in panic disorder (Friedman, 1988).

PTSD resembles simple phobia in that both are characterized by fear
and avoidance of specific stimuli. Accordingly, simple phobias that
develop following exposure to trauma may potentially be difficult to
distinguish from PTSD (McNally & Saigh, 1989). For example, automobile accidents may produce either full-blown PTSD or simple driving
phobia. Driving phobias, however, are characterized by highly circum-
scribed fears and avoidance of driving, but not by other PTSD symptoms such as emotional numbing (Kuch, 1989; Kuch, Swinson & Kirby,
1985). Post-accident psychopathology tends to be greatest in passen-
gers rather than in drivers, in persons who believe they were not
responsible for the accident, in persons with a history of automobile
accidents, and in persons with a history of another anxiety disorder
(Kuch, 1989).

Once combat-related PTSD became classified as a claim compensable
by the Department of Veterans Affairs, concerns were expressed about
veterans simulating PTSD in order to secure service-connected disability compensation (Atkinson *et al.*, 1982). Case reports of 'fictitious
PTSD' seemingly confirmed the seriousness of the problem (Sparr &
Pankratz, 1983).

In a study designed to determine whether genuine PTSD can be
distinguished from fabricated PTSD, Fairbank, McCaffrey and Keane
(1985) had Vietnam veterans with PTSD, well-adjusted Vietnam
veterans, and clinicians familiar with PTSD complete the Minnesota

Multiphasic Personality Inventory (MMPI; Hathaway & McKinley, 1967). Nonclinical subjects were instructed to respond as if they were trying to fabricate PTSD for the purposes of compensation. Results indicated that both fabricating groups scored higher than the PTSD group on the F scale and on Keane, Malloy, and Fairbank's (1984) MMPI PTSD scale. A discriminant function analysis indicated that subjects with *T* scores above 88 on the F scale correctly classified 93% of the subjects in the total sample. None of the simulators was misclassified as having PTSD.

Combat veterans without PTSD are capable, however, of simulating PTSD in a psychophysiological assessment (Gerardi, Blanchard & Kolb, 1989). When exposed to audiotaped combat sounds, simulating subjects can mimic the enhanced physiological reactivity of PTSD patients. In contrast to the responses of PTSD patients, those of simulating veterans rapidly return to baseline during the recovery period. These findings suggest that the time course of physiological reactivity to combat cues may discriminate genuine from factitious PTSD.

VALIDATION OF DIAGNOSTIC CRITERIA IN LABORATORY RESEARCH

Laboratory paradigms have provided convergent validation for certain PTSD criteria. These paradigms are not subject to the limitations associated with introspective self-report approaches to diagnostic validation.

Psychophysiological research has documented that Vietnam combat veterans with PTSD exhibit psychological distress (Criterion B4) and physiological reactivity (Criterion D6) when exposed to audiotaped battle sounds (Blanchard *et al.*, 1982, 1986*b*; Pallmeyer, Blanchard & Kolb, 1986), audiovisual combat scenes (i.e. slides and sounds; Malloy, Fairbank & Keane, 1983), and imagery scripts that describe personal combat traumas (Pitman *et al.*, 1990; Pitman *et al.*, 1987). The tendency to avoid stimuli associated with the trauma (Criterion C2) was documented by Malloy *et al.* who reported that PTSD patients were more likely than healthy combat veterans to terminate exposure to audiovisual combat stimuli (80% versus 0%). The remaining PTSD patients shut their eyes to avoid exposure to the combat scenes.

Moreover, Blanchard and his associates have demonstrated that the increases in heart rate (HR), systolic blood pressure, and electromyogram (EMG) activity exhibited by PTSD patients in response to combat sounds do not occur in healthy civilians, healthy combat veterans, combat veterans with other psychiatric disorders, and nonveteran simple phobics. Consistent with these findings, Pitman and his associates have demonstrated that the increases in skin conductance and EMG exhibited by PTSD patients when visualizing imagery scripts containing descriptions of their combat experiences do not occur in healthy combat veterans or combat veterans with other anxiety disorders.

Psychophysiological researchers have also investigated disturbed startle reflex in PTSD patients (Criterion D5). In one study, children with, and without, PTSD were exposed to non-startling acoustic prestimulation, followed, on some trials, by an acoustic startle stimulus (Ornitz & Pynoos, 1989). In contrast to normal controls, children with PTSD failed to exhibit inhibition of startle following brief prestimulation, and exhibited facilitation of startle following sustained prestimulation. Loss of inhibitory modulation of startle is consistent with chronic brainstem dysfunction.

Inconsistent with Criterion D5, Pallmeyer *et al.* (1986) reported that PTSD patients not only failed to startle when exposed to an unexpected burst of 80 dB white noise, but exhibited a HR decrease. Clearly, more research is needed to elucidate the nature of disturbed startle in this population.

Using sodium lactate infusion, Rainey *et al.* (1987) provoked flashbacks in all seven of the PTSD patients they tested (Criterion B3). These patients, six of whom had comorbid panic disorder, also panicked. Rainey *et al.* also noted phenomenological similarities between flashbacks and panic attacks. It remains to be seen whether lactate can provoke flashbacks in PTSD patients who do not also have panic disorder.

Sleep studies have documented complaints about traumatic nightmares (Criterion B2) and about difficulties falling and staying asleep (Criterion D1). PTSD patients experience nightmares that typically replicate the trauma, and that occur during non-REM as well as during REM sleep (e.g. van der Kolk *et al.*, 1984). Other abnormalities include increased sleep latency, increased REM latency, decreased REM sleep, decreased Stage 4 sleep, and diminished sleep efficiency (Hefez *et al.*, 1987; Lavie *et al.*, 1979; Ross, Ball, Sullivan & Caroff, 1989; Schlosberg & Benjamin, 1978).

To validate intrusive cognitive activity as a diagnostic criterion (Criterion B1), researchers have used the modified Stroop color-naming paradigm (McNally *et al.*, 1990). In this paradigm, subjects are shown words of varying emotional significance, and asked to name the colors in which the words are printed while ignoring the meanings of the words (Mathews & MacLeod, 1985). Delays in color-naming (i.e. Stroop interference) occur when the meaning of the word automatically attracts the subject's attention despite the subject's effort to attend to the color of the word. Because delays in color-naming reflect involuntary semantic activation, interference produced by trauma-related words may provide a quantitative index of negative intrusive activity. Consistent with this hypothesis, Vietnam combat veterans with PTSD exhibit Stroop interference for Vietnam-related words (e.g. BODYBAGS) but not for positive words (e.g. LOVE) or words related to another anxiety disorder (e.g. GERMS; McNally et al., 1990). Similar findings have been obtained in research on rape-related PTSD (Cassiday, McNally & Zeitlin, 1992; Foa et al., 1991). In all of these studies, traumatized subjects without the disorder failed to process trauma cues selectively, thus indicating that the Stroop interference effect is specific to PTSD and not simply to a history of trauma. In addition to providing experimental validation for intrusive cognitive activity, the Stroop interference effect is consistent with two additional criteria: hypervigilance for threat (Criterion D4) and concentration difficulties (Criterion D3).

CURRENT ISSUES IN THE CLASSIFICATION OF PTSD: TOWARD DSM–IV

In preparation for the publication of DSM–IV in 1994, the PTSD workgroup is considering arguments and evidence concerning proposed changes in the classification of PTSD. The workgroup is operating under a conservative mandate: no change in the diagnostic criteria or accompanying text is to be recommended without overwhelming evidence favoring the change. Several issues under deliberation are addressed below.

Should the stressor criterion be altered?

Although exposure to a catastrophic stressor is a diagnostic requirement for PTSD, some DSM–IV workgroup members favor broadening the criterion to include ordinary stressors (e.g. divorce) that may produce the disorder in persons who subjectively perceive them as traumatic. Other workgroup members advocate abolishing Criterion A in favor of a criteria set comprising only signs and symptoms.

Despite these concerns, there are good reasons for retaining the stressor criterion in more or less its current form. Overwhelming research evidence indicates a dose–response relationship whereby the severity of PTSD symptoms increases as a function of the severity of the stressor (March, 1990; McNally, 1989). More specifically, variables such as threat to life, severe injury, witnessing grotesque death, and loss of or injury to a loved one are strongly related to the development of PTSD (March, 1990). Reports of PTSD caused by divorce (Burstein, 1985), discovery of a spouse's affair, and miscarriage (Helzer *et al.*, 1987) are rare and of dubious validity. Problematically, authors of these reports failed to rule out previous *traumatic* exposure in persons whose PTSD apparently emerged in response to subtraumatic stressors. Indeed, PTSD can emerge following exposure to minor stressors in persons who had been previously exposed to traumatic stress but who failed to develop full-blown PTSD immediately (Solomon *et al.*, 1989). In any event, chronic PTSD does not always occur even in response to catastrophic stressors (March, 1990); there is little evidence that it occurs in response to subcatastrophic stressors.

Finally, as Blank (1989*b*) has cogently argued, to include subjective perception of threat *within* the stressor definition confounds an etiological agent with the patient's response to it. Indeed, specification of a traumatic event in DSM–III was never intended as a comprehensive description of etiology. Many factors contribute to etiology in addition to the trauma (e.g. subjective response to the trauma, aspects of the recovery environment).

A *tentative* revised Criterion A has been proposed by the DSM–IV workgroup (Davidson & Foa, 1990):

> The person has experienced, witnessed or learned about an event or events which involve actual or threatened death or injury, or a threat to the physical integrity of oneself or others.

This revision does not define qualifying stressors as those 'markedly distressing to almost anyone' that lie 'outside the range of usual human experience'. Indeed, many traumatic events are all too common to be considered outside the range of usual experience. For example, lifetime prevalence estimates for rape among American women range from 5% to 22% (Steketee & Foa, 1987).

Should there be a duration requirement for diagnosing PTSD?

According to DSM–III–R, PTSD is diagnosable only when symptomatic criteria have been met for at least one month. Some favor extending the duration requirement to three months because chronic PTSD only becomes likely if symptoms have not dissipated by then (Rothbaum & Foa, 1989). According to this view, 'acute PTSD' is a normal emotional response to an abnormal stressor, not a sign of mental illness (Barlow *et al.*, 1990). Thus, PTSD is pathological only if it persists for an unreasonable period of time.

On the other hand, others suggest that the duration requirement be abolished altogether. According to this view, suffering is no less severe merely because it has not yet lasted one month. Hence, immediate diagnosis and (reimbursable) treatment should be available to psychologically traumatized people just as it is for physically traumatized people. Furthermore, an acute PTSD diagnosis carries no more pejorative connotation than does the diagnosis of a broken arm. In both cases the patient has suffered a sufficient stressor that has produced pathology warranting diagnosis and immediate treatment.

In any event, the *tentative* DSM–IV criteria specify a three-month duration requirement for the diagnosis of PTSD (Davidson & Foa, 1990). A proposed V-code diagnosis, 'Uncomplicated Post-Traumatic Stress Reaction', will cover individuals with subthreshold symptoms, and those whose symptoms have not yet lasted three months.

Where should PTSD be classified in DSM–IV?

The workgroup has been considering four proposals for classifying PTSD in DSM–IV (Brett, 1989). One proposal is to form a broad, etiologically based category entitled 'Stress Response Disorders' that would include (1) acute stress disorder, (2) PTSD, (3) pathological grief, (4) uncomplicated bereavement, and possibly (5) adjustment disorders. Acute stress disorder is time-limited, caused by exposure to trauma, and phenomenologically similar to PTSD except for the absence of reexperiencing symptoms.

The second proposal is to form a narrow, etiologically based category entitled 'Disorders of Extreme Stress Not Elsewhere Classified (DESNEC)' that would include (1) acute stress disorder, (2) PTSD, and (3) disorders of extreme stress not otherwise specified (DESNOS). DESNOS was included to cover psychologically disturbed persons exposed to trauma (e.g. sexual abuse, family violence) who do not have PTSD.

The third proposal is to classify PTSD among the dissociative disorders. In reviewing evidence for this option, Brett (1989) cites unpublished studies that suggest that dissociation at time of trauma is related to subsequent PTSD. She also notes that some PTSD symptoms (e.g. flashbacks, amnesia) can be considered dissociative. Finally, multiple personality disorder, the most dramatic example of a dissociative condition, may result from chronic, extreme abuse in childhood.

The justification for the first three proposals is not strong. The database for the two etiologically based schemes is insufficiently compelling to warrant such drastic reorganization. In particular, there is little research on acute stress disorder, and most DESNOS patients (e.g. incest victims) are unlikely to be undiagnosed and untreated; most will meet criteria for other DSM–III–R disorders (e.g. depression, borderline personality disorder). Finally, as Brett points out, the evidence for reclassifying PTSD as a dissociative disorder is slim, at best.

The fourth proposal is to keep PTSD classified among the anxiety disorders. There are several reasons for doing so. First, PTSD results from exposure to traumatic events that typically produce extreme anxiety and terror. Secondly, PTSD resembles other anxiety disorders insofar as symptoms of fear, avoidance, and hyperarousal are prominent. Thirdly, patterns of comorbidity and family psychopathology resemble those of other anxiety disorders. Fourthly, the conceptualization of PTSD as the prototypical anxiety-based disorder has stimulated considerable research on psychopathology and treatment. Fifthly, retention of PTSD in the anxiety disorders category is consistent with the conservative mandate of DSM–IV.

Although this author favors retention of PTSD as an anxiety disorder, other DSM–IV workgroup members favor the establishment of a DESNEC category. Field trials are underway to evaluate the validity of the other disorders included in this category (e.g. DESNOS).

CONCLUSION

Since the formal recognition of PTSD as a discrete anxiety disorder in DSM–III, evidence has accumulated in support of its validity. However, most research has involved combat veterans, rape victims, and survivors of natural disasters. Systematic research on the psychiatric consequences of torture has scarcely begun (e.g. Goldfeld *et al.*, 1988; Mollica, Wyshak & Lavelle, 1987; Mollica *et al.*, 1990). Although some studies suggest that torture produces DSM–III–R PTSD (e.g. Weisaeth, 1989), the unique combination of physical and psychological trauma may produce a 'post-torture syndrome' (Başoğlu & Marks, 1988) distinguishable from PTSD as described in DSM–III–R. These issues are addressed in depth in the remaining chapters in this volume.

ACKNOWLEDGEMENTS

Preparation of this chapter was supported in part by National Institute of Mental Health Grant # MH 43809 awarded to Richard J. McNally.

REFERENCES

American Psychiatric Association (APA) (1980). *Diagnostic and Statistical Manual of Mental Disorders* (3rd edn). Washington, DC: American Psychiatric Association.

American Psychiatric Association (APA) (1987). *Diagnostic and Statistical Manual of Mental Disorders* (3rd edn, rev.). Washington, DC: American Psychiatric Association.

Atkinson, R. M., Henderson, R. G., Sparr, W. F. & Deale, S. D. (1982). Assessment of Viet Nam veterans for posttraumatic stress disorder in Veterans Administration disability claims. *American Journal of Psychiatry*, **139**, 1118–21.

Barlow, D. H., Brown, T. A., Jones, J. C. & Prins, A. (1990). *Commentary on Brett's proposition of PTSD as a stress response disorder.* Paper prepared for the DSM–IV workgroup on Post-Traumatic Stress Disorder.

Başoğlu, M. & Marks, I. (1988). Torture: research needed into how to help those who have been tortured. *British Medical Journal*, **297**, 1423–4.

Blanchard, E. B., Gerardi, R. J., Kolb, L. C. & Barlow, D. H. (1986a). The utility of the Anxiety Disorders Interview Schedule (ADIS) in the diagnosis of post-traumatic stress disorder (PTSD) in Vietnam veterans. *Behaviour Research and Therapy*, **24**, 577–80.

Blanchard, E. B., Kolb, L. C., Gerardi, R. J., Ryan, P. & Pallmeyer, T. P. (1986b). Cardiac response to relevant stimuli as an adjunctive tool for diagnosing post-traumatic stress disorder in Vietnam veterans. *Behavior Therapy*, **17**, 592–606.

Blanchard, E. B., Kolb, L. C., Pallmeyer, T. P. & Gerardi, R. J. (1982). Psychophysiological study of post traumatic stress disorder in Vietnam veterans. *Psychiatric Quarterly*, **54**, 220–9.

Blank, Jr., A. S. (1989a). *The longitudinal course of post-traumatic stress disorder.* Paper prepared for the DSM–IV workgroup on Post-Traumatic Stress Disorder.

Blank, Jr., A. S. (1989b). *The stressor criterion.* Paper prepared for the DSM–IV workgroup on Post-Traumatic Stress Disorder.

Boyd, J. H., Burke, Jr., J. D., Gruenberg, E., Holzer, III, C. E., Rae, D. S., George, L. K., Karno, M., Stoltzman, R., McEvoy, L. & Nestadt, G. (1984). Exclusion criteria of DSM–III: A study of co-occurrence of hierarchy-free syndromes. *Archives of General Psychiatry*, **41**, 983–9.

Brett, E. A. (1989). *Classification of PTSD in DSM–IV: as an anxiety disorder, dissociative disorder, or stress disorder.* Paper prepared for the DSM–IV workgroup on Post-Traumatic Stress Disorder.

Burgess, A. W. & Holmstrom, L. L. (1974). Rape trauma syndrome. *American Journal of Psychiatry*, **131**, 981–6.

Burstein, A. (1985). Posttraumatic stress disorder. *Journal of Clinical Psychiatry*, **46**, 300–1.

Carroll, B. J., Feinberg, M., Greden, J. F., Tarika, J., Albala, A. A., Haskett, R. F., James, N. M., Kronfol, Z., Lohr, N., Steiner, M., de Vigne, J. P. & Young, E. (1981). A specific laboratory test for the diagnosis of melancholia: Standardization, validation, and clinical utility. *Archives of General Psychiatry*, **38**, 15–22.

Cassiday, K. L., McNally, R. J. & Zeitlin, S. B. (1992). Selective processing of trauma cues in rape victims with post-traumatic stress disorder. *Cognitive Therapy and Research*, 16, 283–95.

Center for Disease Control. (1988). Health status of Vietnam veterans: I. Psychosocial characteristics. *Journal of the American Medical Association*, 259, 2701–7.

Chodoff, P. (1963). Late effects of the concentration camp syndrome. *Archives of General Psychiatry*, 8, 323–33.

Clark, D. M. (1986). A cognitive approach to panic. *Behaviour Research and Therapy*, 24, 461–70.

Davidson, J. R. T. & Fairbank, J. (1989). *Position paper on epidemiology of PTSD*. Paper prepared for the DSM–IV workgroup on Post-Traumatic Stress Disorder.

Davidson, J. & Foa, E. (1990). *Proposed DSM–IV criteria for post-traumatic stress disorder*. Paper prepared for the DSM–IV workgroup on Post-Traumatic Stress Disorder.

Davidson, J. R. T., Hughes, D., Blazer, D. & George, L. K. (1991). Post-traumatic stress disorder in the community: An epidemiological study. *Psychological Medicine*, 21, 713–21.

Davidson, J. R. T., Smith, R. D. & Kudler, H. S. (1989a). Validity and reliability of the DSM–III criteria for post-traumatic stress disorder: Experience with a structured interview. *Journal of Nervous and Mental Disease*, 177, 336–41.

Davidson, J., Smith, R. & Kudler, H. (1989b). Familial psychiatric illness in chronic posttraumatic stress disorder. *Comprehensive Psychiatry*, 30, 339–45.

Davidson, J., Swartz, M., Storck, M., Krishnan, R. R. & Hammett, E. (1985). A diagnostic and family study of posttraumatic stress disorder. *American Journal of Psychiatry*, 142, 90–3.

de Ruiter, C., Rijken, H., Garssen, B., van Schaik, A. & Kraaimaat, F. (1989). Comorbidity among the anxiety disorders. *Journal of Anxiety Disorders*, 3, 57–68.

Fairbank, J. A., McCaffrey, R. J. & Keane, T. M. (1985). Psychometric detection of fabricated symptoms of posttraumatic stress disorder. *American Journal of Psychiatry*, 14, 501–3.

Feinstein, A. R. (1970). The pre-therapeutic classification of co-morbidity in chronic diseases. *Journal of Chronic Disease*, 23, 455–68.

Foa, E. B., Feske, U., Murdock, T. B., Kozak, M. J. & McCarthy, P. R. (1991). Processing of threat-related information in rape victims. *Journal of Abnormal Psychology*, 100, 156–62.

Foy, D. W., Resnick, H. S., Sipprelle, R. C. & Carroll, E. M. (1987). Premilitary, military, and postmilitary factors in the development of combat-related posttraumatic stress disorder. *The Behavior Therapist*, 10, 3–9.

Foy, D. W., Sipprelle, R. C., Rueger, D. B. & Carroll, E. M. (1984). Etiology of posttraumatic stress disorder in Vietnam veterans: analysis of premilitary, military, and combat exposure influences. *Journal of Consulting and Clinical Psychology*, 52, 79–87.

Friedman, M. J. (1981). Post-Vietnam syndrome: recognition and management. *Psychosomatics*, 22, 931–943.

Friedman, M. J. (1988). Toward rational pharmacotherapy for posttraumatic stress disorder: An interim report. *American Journal of Psychiatry*, 145, 281–5.

Gerardi, R. J., Blanchard, E. B. & Kolb, L. C. (1989). Ability of Vietnam veterans to dissimulate a psychophysiological assessment for post-traumatic stress disorder. *Behavior Therapy*, 20, 229–43.

Goldfeld, A. E., Mollica, R. F., Pesavento, B. H. & Faraone, S. V. (1988). The physical and psychological sequelae of torture: Symptomatology and diagnosis. *Journal of the American Medical Association*, 259, 2725–9.

Goodwin, D. W. & Guze, S. B. (1984). *Psychiatric Diagnosis* (3rd ed.). New York: Oxford University Press.

Halbreich, U., Olympia, J., Glogowski, J., Carson, S., Axelrod, S. & Yeh, C. M. (1988). The importance of past psychological trauma and pathophysiological process as determinants of current biologic abnormalities. *Archives of General Psychiatry*, 45, 293–4.

Hathaway, S. R. & McKinley, J. C. (1967). *Minnesota Multiphasic Personality Inventory: Manual for Administration and Scoring.* New York: Psychological Corporation.

Hefez, A., Metz, L. & Lavie, P. (1987). Long-term effects of extreme situational stress on sleep and dreaming. *American Journal of Psychiatry*, 144, 344–7.

Helzer, J. E., Robins, L. N. & McEvoy, L. (1987). Post-traumatic stress disorder in the general population: Findings of the Epidemiologic Catchment Area Survey. *New England Journal of Medicine*, 317, 1630–4.

Keane, T. M. (1989). *Symptomatology of Vietnam veterans with post-traumatic stress disorder.* Paper prepared for the DSM–IV workgroup on Post-Traumatic Stress Disorder.

Keane, T. M., Caddell, J. M. & Taylor, K. L. (1988). Mississippi Scale for Combat-Related Posttraumatic Stress Disorder: Three studies in reliability and validity. *Journal of Consulting and Clinical Psychology*, 56, 85–90.

Keane, T. M., Malloy, P. F. & Fairbank, J. A. (1984). Empirical development of an MMPI Subscale for the assessment of combat-related posttraumatic stress disorder. *Journal of Consulting and Clinical Psychology*, 52, 888–91.

Keane, T. M., Scott, W. O., Chavoya, G. A., Lamparski, D. M. & Fairbank, J. A. (1985). Social support in Vietnam veterans with posttraumatic stress disorder: A comparative analysis. *Journal of Consulting and Clinical Psychology*, 53, 95–102.

Kluznik, J. C., Speed, N., van Valkenburg, C. & Magraw, R. (1986). Forty-year follow-up of United States prisoners of war. *American Journal of Psychiatry*, 143, 1443–6.

Kosten, T. R., Mason, J. W., Giller, E. L., Ostroff, R. B. & Harkness, L. (1987). Sustained urinary norepinephrine and epinephrine elevation in post-traumatic stress disorder. *Psychoneuroendocrinology*, 12, 13–20.

Kuch, K. (1989). Enigmatic disability after minor accidents. *Modern Medicine of Canada*, 44, 38–41.

Kuch, K., Swinson, R. P. & Kirby, M. (1985). Post-traumatic stress disorder after car accidents. *Canadian Journal of Psychiatry*, 30, 426–7.

Kudler, H., Davidson, J., Meador, K., Lipper, S. & Ely, T. (1987). The DST and posttraumatic stress disorder. *American Journal of Psychiatry*, 144, 1068–71.

Kulka, R. A., Schlenger, W. E., Fairbank, J. A., Hough, R. L., Jordan, B. K., Marmar, C. R. & Weiss, D. S. (1988). *National Vietnam Veterans Readjustment Study (NVVRS): Description, current status, and initial PTSD prevalence estimates*. Research Triangle Park, NC: Research Triangle Institute.

Kupfer, D. J. & Thase, M. E. (1983). The use of the sleep laboratory in the diagnosis of affective disorders. *Psychiatric Clinics of North America*, 6, 3–25.

Lavie, P., Hefez, A., Halperin, G. & Enoch, D. (1979). Long-term effects of traumatic war-related events on sleep. *American Journal of Psychiatry*, 136, 175–8.

Lerer, B., Bleich, A., Kotler, M., Garb, R., Hertzberg, M. & Levin, B. (1987). Posttraumatic stress disorder in Israeli combat veterans: effect of phenelzine treatment. *Archives of General Psychiatry*, 44, 976–81.

Liebowitz, M. R., Fyer, A. J., Gorman, J. M., Dillon, D., Appleby, I. L., Levy, G., Anderson, S., Levitt, M., Palij, M., Davis, S. O. & Klein, D. F. (1984). Lactate provocation of panic attacks I: Clinical and behavioral findings. *Archives of General Psychiatry*, 41, 764–70.

Malloy, P. F., Fairbank, J. A. & Keane, T. M. (1983). Validation of a multimethod assessment of posttraumatic stress disorders in Vietnam veterans. *Journal of Consulting and Clinical Psychology*, 51, 488–94.

March, J. S. (1990). The nosology of posttraumatic stress disorder. *Journal of Anxiety Disorders*, 4, 61–82.

Mason, J. W., Giller, E. L., Kosten, T. R. & Harkness, L. (1988). Elevation of urinary norepinephrine/cortisol ratio in posttraumatic stress disorder. *Journal of Nervous and Mental Disease*, 176, 498–502.

Mason, J. W., Giller, E. L., Kosten, T. R., Ostroff, R. B. & Podd, L. (1986). Urinary free-cortisol levels in posttraumatic stress disorder patients. *Journal of Nervous and Mental Disease*, 174, 145–9.

Mathews, A. & MacLeod, C. (1985). Selective processing of threat cues in anxiety states. *Behaviour Research and Therapy*, 23, 563–9.

McFall, M. E., Murburg, M. M., Roszell, D. K. & Veith, R. C. (1989). Psychophysiologic and neuroendocrine findings in posttraumatic stress disorder: a review of theory and research. *Journal of Anxiety Disorders*, 3, 243–57.

McFarlane, A. C. (1989). The aetiology of post-traumatic morbidity: Predisposing, precipitating and perpetuating factors. *British Journal of Psychiatry*, 154, 221–8.

McNally, R. J. (1990). Psychological approaches to panic disorder: a review. *Psychological Bulletin*, 108, 403–19.

McNally, R. J. (1989). *What stressors produce DSM–III–R post-traumatic stress disorder in children?* Paper prepared for the DSM–IV workgroup on Post-Traumatic Stress Disorder.

McNally, R. J., Kaspi, S. P., Riemann, B. C. & Zeitlin, S. B. (1990). Selective processing of threat cues in post-traumatic stress disorder. *Journal of Abnormal Psychology*, 99, 398–402.

McNally, R. J. & Lorenz, M. (1987). Anxiety sensitivity in agoraphobics. *Journal of Behavior Therapy and Experimental Psychiatry*, **18**, 3–11.

McNally, R. J., Luedke, D. L., Besyner, J. K., Peterson, R. A., Bohm, K. & Lips, O. J. (1987). Sensitivity to stress-relevant stimuli in posttraumatic stress disorder. *Journal of Anxiety Disorders*, **1**, 105–16.

McNally, R. J. & Saigh, P. A. (1989). *On the distinction between traumatic simple phobia and post-traumatic stress disorder*. Paper prepared for the DSM-IV workgroup on Simple Phobia.

Mellman, T. A. & Davis, G. C. (1985). Combat-related flashbacks in posttraumatic stress disorder: phenomenology and similarity to panic attacks. *Journal of Clinical Psychiatry*, **46**, 379–82.

Mollica, R. F., Wyshak, G. & Lavelle, J. (1987). The psychosocial impact of war trauma and torture on Southeast Asia refugees. *American Journal of Psychiatry*, **144**, 1567–72.

Mollica, R. F., Wyshak, G., Lavelle, J., Truong, T., Tor, S. & Yang, T. (1990). Assessing symptom change in Southeast Asia refugee survivors of mass violence and torture. *American Journal of Psychiatry*, **147**, 83–8.

Nader, K., Pynoos, R., Fairbanks, L. & Frederick, C. (1990). Children's PTSD reactions one year after a sniper attack at their school. *American Journal of Psychiatry*, **147**, 1526–30.

Ornitz, E. M. & Pynoos, R. S. (1989). Startle modulation in children with post-traumatic stress disorder. *American Journal of Psychiatry*, **146**, 866–70.

Pallmeyer, T. P., Blanchard, E. B. & Kolb, L. C. (1986). The psychophysiology of combat-induced post-traumatic stress disorder in Vietnam veterans. *Behaviour Research and Therapy*, **24**, 645–52.

Pary, R., Turns, D. M. & Tobias, C. R. (1986). A case of delayed recognition of posttraumatic stress disorder. *American Journal of Psychiatry*, **143**, 941.

Pitman, R. K. (1989). *Biological findings in PTSD: implications for DSM–IV classification*. Paper prepared for the DSM–IV workgroup on Post-Traumatic Stress Disorder.

Pitman, R. K., Orr, S. P., Forgue, D. F., Altman, B., de Jong, J. B. & Herz, L. R. (1990). Psychophysiologic responses to combat imagery of Vietnam veterans with posttraumatic stress disorder versus other anxiety disorders. *Journal of Abnormal Psychology*, **99**, 49–54.

Pitman, R. K., Orr, S. P., Forgue, D. F., de Jong, J. B. & Claiborn, J. M. (1987). Psychophysiologic assessment of posttraumatic stress disorder imagery in Vietnam combat veterans. *Archives of General Psychiatry*, **44**, 970–75.

Pitts, Jr., F. N. (1985). Editorial. *Journal of Clinical Psychiatry*, **46**, 373.

Pynoos, R. S., Frederick, C., Nader, K., Arroyo, W., Steinberg, A., Eth, S., Nunez, F. & Fairbanks, L. (1987). Life threat and posttraumatic stress in school-age children. *Archives of General Psychiatry*, **44**, 1057–63.

Rainey, Jr., J. M., Aleem, A., Ortiz, A., Yergani, V., Pohl, R. & Berchou, R. (1987). A laboratory procedure for the induction of flashbacks. *American Journal of Psychiatry*, **144**, 1317–19.

Robins, E. & Guze, S. B. (1970). Establishment of diagnostic validity in psychiatric illness: its application to schizophrenia. *American Journal of Psychiatry*, **126**, 983–7.

Ross, R. J., Ball, W. A., Sullivan, K. A. & Caroff, S. N. (1989). Sleep disturbance as the hallmark of posttraumatic stress disorder. *American Journal of Psychiatry*, **146**, 697–707.

Rothbaum, B. O. & Foa, E. B. (1989). *Subtypes of PTSD and duration of symptoms.* Paper prepared for the DSM–IV workgroup on Post-Traumatic Stress Disorder.

Schlosberg, A. & Benjamin, M. (1978). Sleep patterns in three acute combat fatigue cases. *Journal of Clinical Psychiatry*, **39**, 546–9.

Shatan, C. F. (1973). The grief of soldiers: Vietnam combat veterans' self-help movement. *American Journal of Orthopsychiatry*, **43**, 640–53.

Shore, J. H., Tatum, E. L. & Vollmer, W. M. (1986). Evaluation of mental effects of disaster, Mount St. Helens eruption. *American Journal of Public Health*, **76** (Suppl.), 76–83.

Sierles, F. S., Chen, J. J., McFarland, R. E. & Taylor, M. A. (1983). Posttraumatic stress disorder and concurrent psychiatric illness: a preliminary report. *American Journal of Psychiatry*, **140**, 1177–9.

Sierles, F. S., Chen, J. J., Messing, M. L., Besyner, J. K. & Taylor, M. A. (1986). Concurrent psychiatric illness in non-Hispanic outpatients diagnosed as having posttraumatic stress disorder. *Journal of Nervous and Mental Disease*, **174**, 171–3.

Smith, M. A., Davidson, J., Ritchie, J. C., Kudler, H., Lipper, S., Chappell, P. & Nemeroff, C. B. (1989). The corticotropin releasing hormone test in patients with posttraumatic stress disorder. *Biological Psychiatry*, **26**, 349–55.

Solomon, Z., Kotler, M. & Mikulincer, M. (1988). Combat-related posttraumatic stress disorder among second-generation Holocaust survivors: preliminary findings. *American Journal of Psychiatry*, **145**, 865–8.

Solomon, Z., Kotler, M., Shalev, A. & Lin, R. (1989). Delayed onset PTSD among Israeli veterans of the 1982 Lebanon War. *Psychiatry*, **52**, 428–36.

Solomon, Z., Mikulincer, M. & Avitzur, E. (1988). Coping, locus of control, and combat-related posttraumatic stress disorder: a prospective study. *Journal of Personality and Social Psychology*, **55**, 279–85.

Sparr, L. F. & Atkinson, R. M. (1986). Posttraumatic stress disorder as an insanity defense: medicolegal quicksand. *American Journal of Psychiatry*, **143**, 608–13.

Sparr, L. & Pankratz, L. D. (1983). Factitious posttraumatic stress disorder. *American Journal of Psychiatry*, **140**, 1016–19.

Speed, N., Engdahl, B., Schwartz, J. & Eberly, R. (1989). Posttraumatic stress disorder as a consequence of the POW experience. *Journal of Nervous and Mental Disease*, **177**, 147–153.

Spitzer, R. L., Williams, J. B. W. & Gibbon, M. (1987). *Structured Clinical Interview for DSM–III–R.* New York: New York State Psychiatric Institute.

Steketee, G. & Foa, E. B. (1987). Rape victims: Post-traumatic stress responses and their treatment: a review of the literature. *Journal of Anxiety Disorders*, **1**, 69–86.

van der Kolk, B., Blitz, R., Burr, W., Sherry, S. & Hartmann, E. (1984). Nightmares and trauma: a comparison of nightmares after combat with lifelong nightmares in veterans. *American Journal of Psychiatry*, **141**, 187–90.

van Dyke, C., Zilberg, N. J. & McKinnon, J. A. (1985). Posttraumatic stress disorder: a thirty-year delay in a World War II veteran. *American Journal of Psychiatry*, **142**, 1070–3.

Watson, C. G., Kucala, T., Manifold, V., Vassar, P. & Juba, M. (1988). Differences between posttraumatic stress disorder patients with delayed and undelayed onsets. *Journal of Nervous and Mental Disease*, **176**, 568–72.

Weisaeth, L. (1989). Torture of a Norwegian ship's crew: the torture, stress reactions and psychiatric after-effects. *Acta Psychiatrica Scandinavica*, **80** (Suppl. 335), 63–72.

Woolfolk, R. L. & Grady, D. A. (1988). Combat-related posttraumatic stress disorder: patterns of symptomatology in help-seeking Vietnam veterans. *Journal of Nervous and Mental Disease*, **176**, 107–11.

11
OVERVIEW: THE ASSESSMENT AND DIAGNOSIS OF TORTURE EVENTS AND SYMPTOMS

Richard F. Mollica and Yael Caspi-Yavin

INTRODUCTION

Few clinicians would deny the importance of knowing whether the information given by their patients is true, i.e. whether the events actually happened or the symptoms were experienced by the patient. The clinician would also like to know the degree to which this information is accurately remembered over time. Yet, few health providers challenge the historical record upon which their clinical interviews and treatments are based. Extensive clinical experience with torture survivors over the past 20 years has cast serious doubt on the effectiveness of clinical approaches which fail to recognize those many factors which interfere with the tortured patient's abilities to share their traumatic life experiences and symptoms (Mollica & Caspi-Yavin, 1991). Paradoxically, the cataclysmic impact of the torture event on an individual's personal life often makes the realities of this unique experience and its psychological sequelae difficult to obtain from torture survivors. The special problems inherent in evaluating, diagnosing and treating the torture survivor have led many clinicians to move away from traditional psychiatric assessment approaches toward structured interviewing methods similar to those used in scientific investigations (Mollica & Lavelle, 1988). Open-ended history taking has been replaced by methods which ask the torture survivor a checklist of specific questions. These newer interviewing techniques can collect necessary information as well as test the accuracy of the torture survivor's memory over time. The clinical assessment becomes a type of measurement; obtaining accurate information raises the issues of validity; monitoring the stability of memory addresses the problems of reliability.

Obtaining accurate knowledge of a torture survivor's life experience and symptoms and properly classifying this information into a diagnostic system capable of providing effective treatment and good therapeutic outcome are fundamental to this new field. The medical profession cannot simply apply the methods of traditional psychiatric approaches to torture survivors without evaluating their usefulness and efficacy (Başoğlu & Marks, 1988). Torture survivors, due to the horrific events which have damaged their lives, demand the assistance of both medical and psychiatric science and the sensitive humanistic involvement of the health provider (Mollica, 1989). Similar to those other clinical areas which deal with survivors of man-made tragedies (e.g. incest), the clinician is called upon by the survivor to abandon their clinical neutrality and acknowledge and condemn the injustice and brutality of the torture experience, as well as provide medical intervention, psychosocial support and therapeutic relief (Cienfuegos & Monelli, 1983). Integrating the human and scientific dimensions of the treatment of torture is a difficult task.

This chapter, therefore, focuses on the assessment and diagnosis of the torture survivor. It reviews many psychosocial, cultural and medical factors which are unique to the health provider's evaluation of the torture experience. The recognition and subsequent modification and adaptation of these factors will facilitate the acquisition of therapeutically valid clinical knowledge crucial to achieving successful treatment and rehabilitation.

VARIATION IN DEFINITION AND TYPES OF TORTURE

Lack of a universally accepted definition of torture prevents the clinician from assuming that their working definition of torture is similar to that used by the patient. The UN Declaration of Human Rights and the UN Convention of Torture and Other Cruel Inhuman or Degrading Treatment of Punishment (1985) is the most widely used definition of torture. It prohibits:

> Any act by which severe pain or suffering, whether physical or mental, is intentionally inflicted on a person for such purposes as obtaining from him or a third person information or a confession, punishing him for an act he or a third person has committed or is suspected of having committed, or intimidating or coercing him or a third person, or for any reason based on discrimination of any kind, when such pain or suffering is inflicted by or at the instigation of or with the consent or acquiescence of a public official or other person acting in an official capacity (p. 4).

The UN definition is an inadequate clinical reference because of its narow focus; it primarily emphasizes violence directed by governments unjustly at individuals for political purposes. For example, according to UN criteria, the incarceration and physical punishment of political opponents of a regime in power would constitute an act of torture. This definition unfortunately excludes those individuals who consider themselves victims of torture but have been affected by genocidal policies (e.g. victims of the Khmer Rouge regime in Cambodia), gender related victimizations such as rape and other forms of sexual violence, and the mass destruction associated with war and military conquest.

The physical manifestations of torture are as diverse as the oppressive societies and types of torture inflicted by them. Clinicians who care for torture survivors must learn the types of horrific human abuses that are perpetrated by different regimes in various geopolitical regions (Goldfeld *et al.*, 1988). For example, under the Khmer Rouge, Cambodian civilians were commonly subjected to starvation, brainwashing and hard labor. Physical beatings using bamboo sticks were common as well as threatened asphyxiation by tying plastic bags over the individuals' head (Mollica & Jalbert, 1989). In contrast, repressive Latin American regimes have frequently subjected their political prisoners to electric shock, solitary confinement and personal tortures such as 'submarino' (i.e. continuous dunking of the head in water which is often fouled by human waste) and 'falanga' (i.e. beatings of the soles of the feet) (Allodi, 1985).

Currently, little is known of the unique physical and psychological responses which are associated with each type of human rights abuse. The clinician cannot assume that the psychological reaction to a 'mock' execution is similar to that of having a plastic bag placed over one's head (Sluzki, 1990). While the extreme nature of the torture event has allowed clinicians and researchers to assume that the torture experience is a powerful and significant event in the life of the individual capable of producing illness regardless of the nature of the event (Miller, 1988), torture-related illness reactions must vary considerably. For example, some evidence exists that solitary confinement is potentially more psychologically damaging than physical torture. Many studies have revealed the differential impact of starvation on prisoners of war (POWs) subjected to hard labor and brainwashing (Sutker *et al.*, 1986). Considerable research is necessary to establish those patterns of pathological reactions specific to torture types. The health care worker can participate in this process by becoming familiar with the different tortures used in their patient's countries of origin and by accurately obtaining details as to the torture methods experienced by the survivor.

Torture also has many unique cultural meanings. The personal process of understanding and giving meaning to the torture experience is mediated by the survivor's language and cultural traditions. Recent investigations have demonstrated major differences in the cultural meaning of torture in Western and Asian societies (Mollica, 1988). In Western society, the word torture is derived from the Latin word *torquere*, which means 'to cause to turn, to twist' in order to extract testimony and/or evidence or to repress opposing religious or political views. Torture is associated with legal confessions and the political suppression of an individual's human rights. In contrast, in Cambodia, torture – *tieru na kam* – is derived from the Buddhist term for karma. Karma is defined as the individual's actions or thoughts (often of an evil nature) in a prior existence that affects life in the present. The torture experience is often believed by Cambodian survivors to be caused by bad actions (unrelated to the torture) and resulting karma.

The cultural attitudes and beliefs of Indochinese women associated with sexual torture illustrate the profound influence cultural norms have on their subjective reaction to the torture event (Mollica & Son, 1989). In Asian culture, emphasis is placed on a woman's sexual purity, i.e. the virginal woman is considered the essence of purity. In Cambodia, the term for virginity, *prumcaarey* is defined as purity, chastity, prosperity, holiness, piety and is associated with the Buddha. Similarly for Vietnamese women, a woman's virginity is considered her single most important asset for obtaining happiness. A traditional Vietnamese proverb states, 'If a perfumed flower has lost its stamen, the charm cannot be covered up by makeup'. Therefore, a Vietnamese woman's value is synonymous with the preservation of her virginity, which should only be given to her husband. In Indochinese societies, negative social sanctions and severe punishment fall upon women who lose their sexual purity, even under the most tragic circumstances, such as rape torture. A Vietnamese proverb regarding rape summarizes the severity of these sentiments: 'Someone ate out of my bowl and left it dirty'.

The following descriptions of torture related to the rape experience (Amnesty International, 1991) reveal the importance of determining the socio-cultural, and political background of all torture experiences (Mollica & Son, 1989).

(1) A young pregnant Vietnamese woman arrived to the Thai border refugee camp after being raped at sea. When the pirates started to take her away to their boat, she tried to hide behind her husband, and he, frightened for their lives, did nothing to rescue

his wife. She was raped by the pirates for a whole month, already pregnant with her husband's child, and then was taken to a pirate's home to be a maid. From there she eventually escaped and brought herself to safety with the local police. Although she knew that her husband was at the same refugee camp, she lied about her identity and refused to recognize him. On the baby's birth certificate the father was listed as 'unknown', and to the camp authorities she declared her husband was dead, even though the camp authorities suspected otherwise. In a confidential conversation with a local counsellor, the woman explained that she blamed her husband for not being a true husband at a time of her danger, where as partners in life, he should have risked his life to try and save her. She was also worried that if she reunited with him she would always feel guilty toward him and that the child will be a constant remainder for him of the past. She preferred that her husband would go away and that both of them set out alone on their new lives.

(2) A Cambodian woman who fled the Pol Pot regime in Cambodia to the Thai border tells of the rape torture of Cambodian women and girls. 'Many Cambodian women have suffered a great deal . . . They have been victims of rape while on their escape journey . . . Few were spared. Even preadolescent girls were raped. All ages were raped. Throughout their suffering the victims did not say anything. In our culture, those women bear the pain of shame and the guilt of blaming themselves. They have lost their self-respect and wish only to bury their feelings. The impact of rape is long lasting . . . Rape of Cambodian women resulted in loss of their honor. Some even committed suicide. Once we reached the refugee camps, the Cambodian women were still in danger. Rape occurred to young girls less than 13 years old, as well as women over 50. Many committed suicide because they didn't know what to do about the problem. Sometimes the rape was not a single incident by one man, but occurred with as many as twenty men at a time.'

(3) A South American woman sexually tortured as a political prisoner tells of her interrogations in prisons: 'I have been interrogated five times, and every single time I was completely naked . . . during each of the five interrogations I started menstruating even though it wasn't the right time for it; maybe it was due to nerves. Anyway, it resulted with me always being covered with blood. There were always at least five torturers, and they forced me to take off my clothes, . . . always making me look them

in the eyes. They then humiliated me verbally ... saying that they would rape me while they mauled me all over my body. They then lined themselves up in a row making me walk in front of them ... still making me look them in their eyes ... It felt so incredibly humiliating.'

These three vignettes reveal the impact of traditional cultural beliefs and attitudes on the reactions of three women subjected to sexual violence. The clinician caring for torture survivors must be aware of those cultural (often religious) and political factors that influence the torture survivor's subjective reactions to torture as well as the reactions of spouse and family, community social taboos, and negative social pressures which can severely limit the survivor's ability to share their experiences with health providers. For example, Southeast Asian women rarely reveal rape trauma to their therapist even after many years of treatment (Mollica & Lavelle, 1988). However, in spite of almost universal cultural prohibitions against disclosure of the torture experience, the personal desire of many survivors to share their trauma with others remains strong.

ACCURACY OF REPORTING

Tortured individuals frequently change the details of their trauma reports. Since Bartlett's classic work in 1932 ('war of the ghosts'), the influence of stress, violence and other social factors on distortions in memory have been well documented. The unique memory recall problems of the torture survivor, however, raises additional issues. Since independent prison and military records and bystander accounts of survivor reports usually do not exist, the accuracy of a torture survivor's story can never be corroborated.

The torture survivor's observed changes in remembering may be due to:

1 high emotional arousal with associated hyperbole or defensiveness;
2 The effect of trauma related illness on memory (e.g. posttraumatic stress disorder and depression);
3 impaired memory secondary to neuropsychiatric impairments caused by starvation and beatings to the head;
4 culturally prescribed sanctions that allow the trauma experience to be revealed only in highly confidential settings (e.g. rape trauma for Indochinese women);
5 coping mechanisms which utilize denial and the avoidance of memories and/or situations associated with the trauma.

Clinicians who treat torture survivors frequently describe the emotional upset associated with recalling a torture experience (Allodi, 1991; Kolb & Multipassi, 1982). Open-ended interviewing using free recall appear to generate the greatest emotional distress and limited reporting, while memory is best enhanced by using neutral retrieval cues such as reading to the torture survivor a list of possible events from a questionnaire (Tulving, 1983). Remembering is definitely enhanced by systematic methods of history taking and interviewing. Clinical experience and research findings also indicate that once an account is given both an increase in memory and an intensification of symptoms may occur (Mollica *et al.*, 1991). Thus, during the course of therapy, the clinician should be monitoring the survivor's variations in reporting historical events. These variations may signal an increase in emotional distress as the patient attempts to reveal more severely traumatizing experiences. In contrast, persistent repetition of a traumatic event may reveal severe cognitive and social damage (Mollica, 1988).

The two major psychiatric illnesses commonly associated with torture survivors, major depression and post-traumatic stress disorder (PTSD), will also affect memory recall (Eich, 1980). If the torture survivor is depressed, he or she will have difficulty remembering pleasant experiences from the past (Fogarty & Hemsley, 1983). Greater recall for unpleasant experiences will be associated with the survivor's depression and will diminish as the depression lifts.

The recurrent memory phenomena (nightmares, intrusive daytime memories and flashbacks) associated with post-traumatic stress disorder (PTSD) have been well described (Brett & Ostroff, 1985). It is not uncommon for torture survivors to have memories of their torture associated with all senses, especially smell and taste. The vivid recurrent memories of the torture associated with PTSD, however, may be misleading; it is possible that while torture survivors have easy access to past traumatic memories, their recent and past memory for other events is seriously diminished. Current investigations are in progress to determine whether PTSD is a memory disorder.

Investigations have not been able to reveal the memory disturbances associated with PTSD alone since most torture survivors have also experienced starvation and/or head injury. Recent studies have demonstrated that serious memory disturbances are associated with blunt head injury and starvation; both of these events commonly occur with torture (e.g. POWs) (Stuker *et al.*, 1986, 1991). Past research on holocaust survivors by Thygesen *et al.* (1970) and Eitinger and Strom (1973) strongly support these findings. The neurobiological mechanisms of memory disturbances associated with PTSD will only be clarified once the problem of organic co-morbidity is resolved (Petersen, 1989).

The psychological mechanisms which might affect the memory of tortured patients have been extensively described by Horowitz (1976). Denial and the avoidance of memories associated with the torture experience have been associated with attempts by highly traumatized patients to distance themselves from their painful past. Shifts in the survivor's relative state of denial or avoidance will directly influence the detail and thoroughness of reporting.

THERAPIST–PATIENT INTERACTION

Numerous clinical reports have revealed the horror confronted by clinicians when interviewing torture survivors (Kinzie *et al.*, 1990). Numerous barriers exist which prevent the clinician from obtaining a comprehensive history of the torture experience. Freud (1984) highlighted these difficulties when he warned:

> No matter how much we may shrink with horror from certain situations – of a galley-slave in antiquity, of a peasant during the Thirty Years' War, of a victim of the Holy Inquisition, of a Jew awaiting a pogrom – it is nevertheless impossible for us to feel our way into such people – to divine the changes which original obtuseness of mind, a gradual stupefying process, the cessation of expectations, and cruder or more refined methods of narcotization have produced upon their receptivity to sensations of pleasure and unpleasure. Moreover, in the case of the most extreme possibility of suffering, special mental protective devices are brought into operation (p. 89).

The emotional resistance of clinicians to hear the survivor's traumatic life history and to allow themselves to be negatively affected by their story (e.g. many will briefly develop nightmares) is only partially responsible for the reluctance of therapists to question torture survivors (Mollica, 1988).

Therapists are frequently concerned their interview will trigger off uncontrollable emotional distress, and possibly retraumatize the patient. For some clinicians, asking personal and direct questions at the onset of therapy, especially about events that are central to understanding the patient's symptoms, may represent a radical shift from their understanding of the therapeutic process. These questions may appear too intrusive, impersonal and insensitive. Obtaining the patient's trauma history is also seen by many clinicians as the central aspect of more elaborate therapeutic processes which utilize techniques such as nightmare and dream interpretation, hypnosis, psychodrama and catharsis. Many clinicians do not want to prematurely engage the emotions associated with torture events until the entire therapeutic process is ready to be initiated.

The task of accurately assessing the torture experience becomes even more complicated in bicultural settings, where the bicultural worker (who might have survived similar experiences to the client) must mediate between the torture survivor and the English speaking professional (Mollica & Lavelle, 1988). Thus the measurement of torture events and symptoms is seriously affected by both the ability of the English speaking and/or bicultural workers to objectively elicit information from the survivor.

Traditional clinical methods which ask torture survivors to tell their trauma story in their own words have frequently been found to be ineffective; it is still unknown why. Scientific investigations are necessary to elucidate those aspects of the torture response which restrict torture survivors from freely volunteering information during open-ended psychiatric interviews. Neuropsychological (e.g. improper cueing of memory), emotional (e.g. high arousal), and cultural (e.g. cultural and social taboos) factors may be all affecting the latter process.

Paradoxically, while torture survivors have difficulty recounting their experiences and symptoms to their health providers, the majority still have strong desires to give information or 'testimony' to their therapists and appreciate the health care professionals who can listen to their accounts. The Chilean psychologists (Cienfuegos & Monelli, 1983) were the first to elaborate interviewing techniques which bridged the gap between torture survivor and health professional. They were able to obtain the patient's torture history or 'testimony' by placing the clinician and torture survivor in a conversational relationship to a third entity (i.e. they successfully used a tape recorder for obtaining the trauma story). Once the torture survivor had dictated his or her history into the tape recorder, both the patient and therapist proceeded to listen to the taped history and discuss the details of meanings of particularly significant events. Similar approaches to the Chilean method have been successfully utilized by clinicians caring for Indochinese torture survivors (Mollica *et al.*, 1987). The tape recorder has been replaced by a simple checklist to elicit the Asian patient's torture experiences and symptoms. This checklist method has been well received by bicultural staff and patients. Asian torture survivors respond more readily to checklist items than to open-ended interviews; they regard the latter as a culturally appropriate medical test which 'puts words' around their feelings which they have had difficulty articulating to their therapists. The employment of a simple checklist also lessens the difficulty of communicating by mediating between the cultural and personal experiences of the survivor and of their health provider (who often cannot speak the survivor's language).

CATEGORIZING THE TORTURE RESPONSE

Assuming that accurate information can be obtained from torture survivors, clinicians are then confronted with the task of assembling clinical phenomena into a useful diagnostic system. The categorization of torture related symptoms has proceeded in two overlapping directions simultaneously. First, initial investigators studying and treating torture survivors attempted to define a torture syndrome. Goldfeld *et al.* (1988) conducted a world-wide review of the published scientific literature and found that the most common psychiatric symptoms associated with torture were anxiety, depression, memory disturbances and impairments in sleep. The medical investigations of torture survivors not only failed to demonstrate a unique torture syndrome, but demonstrated symptoms closely associated with the DSM-IIIR diagnosis of PTSD (American Psychiatric Association, 1987). Consequently, investigators have shifted their focus away from demonstrating the presence of a unique syndrome to establishing the prevalence of PTSD in torture survivors (Allodi, 1991).

Second, a unique subgroup of tortured patients have been identified; these patients have symptoms which reveal extensive neuropsychological and organic impairment. Since an early report by Bing and Vischer in 1919 on the cognitive problems of POWs, extensive research has focused on the memory and learning difficulties of POWs and holocaust survivors who have experienced torture and severe malnutrition (Sutker *et al.*, 1986, 1991). Evidence from several investigations have demonstrated that prolonged malnutrition accompanied by gruesome confinement is associated with long-term changes in cognitive functioning and problem-solving behavior. Some evidence exists (although unproven) that torture alone can produce demonstrable brain disease (Jensen *et al.*, 1982; Kellner *et al.*, 1983).

Clinical recognition of PTSD related symptoms and the neuropsychological damage associated with torture will greatly enhance all aspects of the therapeutic process from the ability to obtain useful clinical history to the ability to design successful rehabilitation strategies (Keshavan, Channabasavanna & Narayan-Reddy, 1981; Silver, Yudofsky & Hales, 1987).

POST-TRAUMATIC STRESS DISORDER (PTSD)

The diagnostic criteria for PTSD have been reviewed in a previous chapter. While the validity of PTSD as a legitimate illness has been sharply questioned in the past, recent advances in diagnostic assessment procedures and theoretical models have significantly promoted an acceptance of this disorder as a disease entity (Wolfe & Keane, 1990). Unfortunately, the usefulness of the PTSD category to the clinical care of torture survivors still remains to be demonstrated. Many issues both generic to PTSD nosology and specific to the diagnosis of the torture survivor need to be resolved.

Wolfe and Keane (1990) state that one of the most important contributions of the DSM-IIIR was a clear-cut and operationally based definition for the stressor criterion in PTSD. PTSD is a unique diagnosis since it is one of the few diseases in DSM-IIIR which relate symptoms directly to a psychosocial event. The biological and psychosocial mechanisms by which stressor (e.g. torture event) causes symptoms (e.g. psychic-numbing) is clearly implied but weakly articulated. The full range of symptom responses to individual tortures (e.g. falanga vs. mock execution) from the biological, social and psychological domains have not been elucidated. Careful phenomenological studies are necessary to establish both the range of symptom variation and the most common symptom patterns associated with different torture experiences (Sluzki, 1990). For example, it cannot be assumed that all PTSD criteria or the same PTSD criteria are associated with mock execution and sexual violence.

Recent investigations using validated standardized instruments in non-combat populations have just begun to reveal those torture symptoms (e.g. symptoms related to the refugee experience) most closely associated with PTSD criteria (Mollica *et al.*, 1991). Unfortunately, many clinicians prematurely reduce the potential clinical usefulness of describing torture symptom typologies by simply determining the presence or absence of PTSD criteria. While some PTSD criteria related to the torture experience may occur, other PTSD criteria such as 'survival guilt' and 'psychic-numbing' may not be relevant to the torture response. Certain features of PTSD are presumably 'core' to all torture responses while other symptoms may only be associated with specific types of torture events (Klerman, 1987). Since enormous variations exist in the types of torture administered and the human responses to these abuses, the latter conclusion if proven, would not be surprising.

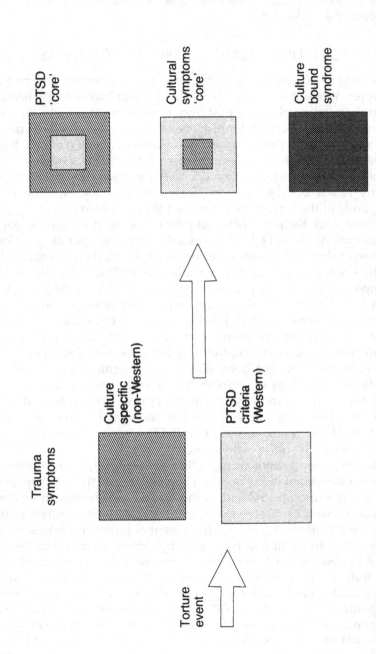

Fig.11.1 The possible relationships between PTSD criteria, culture specific symptoms and a torture induced culture bound syndrome.

Furthermore, the high prevalence of torture in many non-Western cultures and the entry of ethnically diverse survivors into torture treatment centers world-wide raise additional problems as to the cultural validity of the PTSD criteria. What constitutes a 'disease' entity in one culture is not necessarily viewed as a disease in another (Englehardt, 1975). Cross-cultural research suggests that assessment of psychiatric illness should begin with local phenomenological descriptions of folk diagnoses which then can be compared to Western psychological criteria. Westermeyer (1981) demonstrated this method in his study of the folk diagnoses of psychosis and depression in Laos. While he found a close overlap between Western and Laotian criteria for psychosis, little agreement existed between the two world views for depressive disorders. Whether PTSD (or its equivalent) is a meaningful disease category in other cultures is unknown. A culture bound syndrome or folk illness with traditionally defined symptoms and folk treatments for trauma or torture induced illnesses have not been demonstrated. While many culture-bound syndromes such as 'Amok', in the Philippines and 'Susto' (or 'soul loss') in Latin America (Simons & Hughes, 1985) have been defined, a culture bound illness associated with torture remains elusive. For example, in spite of extensive knowledge of the torture response of Indochinese patients (Mollica *et al.*, 1987), ethnographic studies have still to determine if a folk illness caused by torture exists in these cultures, and whether it is similar or vastly different from Western derived PTSD criteria (Eisenbuch, unpublished observations).

Whether a folk illness equivalent for PTSD exists or not, clinicians working with torture survivors need to be able to recognize culture specific symptoms associated with torture. Recent cross-national studies by WHO investigating depression have suggested a potential model for achieving this goal (Sartorius, 1987). WHO conducted a study in five countries for the purpose of identifying those clinical features shared by depressed patients, regardless of their cultural background. This study demonstrated the existence of a 'common core' of depressive symptomatology across the cultures studied. However, the results also revealed that while core depressive symptoms may be present across cultures, they may not be the symptoms most strongly endorsed by the patient. Similarly, cultural reactions will most likely also modify presumably 'core' PTSD criteria. Cross-cultural investigation of torture survivors will help determine those trauma symptoms that are culture specific for PTSD. Figure 11.1 summarizes the possible relationships between PTSD criteria, culture specific symptoms and a torture induced culture bound syndrome. Until both sides of this diagram are clarified within different cultures, clinicians must be aware of the important diversity of cultural reactions associated with torture.

Finally, the diverse cultural backgrounds of torture survivors raise the problem of bicultural communication for treatment centers which treat survivors from linguistic groups different from the host country. Modern methods in cross-cultural research have provided well-proven and useful approaches for translating the meaning of psychiatric terms from one language and culture into another (Westermeyer, 1985). Translation back-translation approaches using bilingual mental health clinicians who know the mental health concepts of both cultures can facilitate this process.

The following is an example of establishing in Laotian the linguistic equivalent for a torture experience – lost or kidnapped – commonly experienced by Laotian refugees (Manual for Harvard Trauma Questionnaire, unpublished manuscript).

> First, it was difficult to translate 'lost' into Laotian since some Laotians interpreted it in the sense of 'a lost object', and others as 'losing one's way'. The words chosen for lost were 'long thang', which means 'lost' in the sense of losing one's way. The relevance of the item to the refugee situation in the United States was also at issue. While this question was intended to solicit information on the migration experience, the bicultural consultants thought it was more relevant to the situation of the refugee in the United States. One translator thought the term 'kidnapped' should include 'for ransom' since this is the only context for kidnapping in Laos. 'Kidnapped' was translated as 'lak toua pay', literally 'steal person disappear'. 'For ransom', 'pheunrhatay' was used which literally means 'for price repayment'.

Clinicians should strive to accurately establish the proper culture terms for all events and symptoms related to the survivor's torture experience. This is a difficult and time consuming task even when translating commonly used psychiatric concepts such as anxiety and depression. Finally, clinicians must be aware when using new checklists developed for interviewing non-Western torture survivors (e.g. Indochinese versions of the HSCL-25) (Mollica et al., 1987) that although item by item validity for each symptom of the checklist has been established in the survivor's native language, the construct validity for the Western disease, which is associated with the sum of all of the original checklist symptoms, may not have been achieved in the new cultural setting. While the Western symptom items in these checklists have been demonstrated to be associated with Western disease criteria, such as depression, the translated checklist items may not add up to a disease or folk diagnosis in the culture represented by the translation (Flaherty *et al.*, 1988). Clinical sensitivity to translation and the cultural meaning of psychiatric terms can help guarantee that significant knowledge be shared between patient and therapist in spite of the limited ability of each to know fully the other's language and world view.

MEASURING TRAUMA EVENTS AND SYMPTOMS

Clinicians should be aware of the scientific development of standardized instruments with acceptable psychometric properties capable of measuring traumatic events and symptoms associated with PTSD. The majority of these instruments have focused on the assessment of American combat veterans. Recent validation and development of instruments for assessing the torture survivor have been influenced by the latter. A brief description of the most important and commonly used instruments from each category follows.

Combat Exposure Scale

In an effort to systematically assess the trauma events veterans experienced in the Vietnam war, Foy *et al.* (1984) developed *The Combat Exposure Scale*, a 7-item cumulative scale that describes in a hierarchical order the combat experiences of American Vietnam veterans. In developing this checklist, the authors attempted to:

- determine those items which cover a broad range of trauma events;
- assess the accuracy of retrospective reporting and allow a meaningful clinical picture to emerge;
- determine if the war histories reflected a continuum of trauma.

The authors helped to resolve these issues by developing a checklist which used a Guttman scaling method which orders traumatic events on a hierarchy according to frequency. It was assumed that less frequent events were also more traumatic. Findings indicated that combat veterans experienced more of the lower scoring events (i.e. less frequent and more traumatic) than non-combat veterans. Men who saw heavy combat also had more experiences that were less traumatic than others with lighter combat. Accuracy of reporting was assessed by comparing the original items which were drawn from the military history of the subjects. The association between scores on the scale and current PTSD diagnosis and symptom intensity was established. PTSD diagnoses were assigned according to DSM-III criteria based on interview responses; subjective symptom intensity was determined by summing up veterans' own ratings of the 15 DSM-III items describing PTSD related symptoms. Results demonstrated that war experiences measured by the Combat Exposure Scale were related to PTSD (i.e. the less frequent the event and the higher it was on the scale, the higher percentage of veterans with PTSD reporting it).

The Mississippi Scale for Combat Related PTSD

The Mississippi Scale (Keane *et al.*, 1988) is one of the most widely used and well validated instruments for identifying symptoms associated with PTSD in American combat veterans. The Mississippi Scale is a 35-item scale that includes PTSD symptoms defined in the DSM-III. Ratings allow for a range of response, from 'not at all true' to 'extremely true', and therefore permits assessment of PTSD symptom severity. Findings show that veteran ratings are stable over a 1-week period with repeated administrations; validation studies reveal that the scale is highly accurate for identifying PTSD in American combat veterans.

The Impact of Event Scale (IES)

The IES (Zilberg, Weiss & Horowitz, 1982) is a 15-item self-rating questionnaire, assessing current subjective distress for a specific traumatic life event, allowing for a response range from 'not at all' to 'severe'. Developed prior to the DSM-III guidelines for PTSD, the scale was derived from Horowitz's (1976) theoretical model of stress response which emphasized two common qualities found in the patient's response to a traumatic life event: intrusion/reexperiencing and numbing/avoidance. Intrusion was defined as unbidden thoughts and images, troubled dreams, strong pangs or waves of feelings and repetitive behavior; avoidance was defined as ideational constriction, denial of meaning and consequences of the event, blunted sensation, behavioral inhibition, counterphobic activity, and awareness of emotional numbness. Intrusion and avoidance were seen as alternating phases during the course of the post-traumatic experience (Zilberg *et al.*, 1982) due to their respective assumed functions of reintroducing the stressful perceptions (intrusion) and defending against them (avoidance). The 15 IES items describe the intrusion and avoidance phenomena. Although widely used in PTSD research and clinical practice, the validity of the theory underlying the IES and the IES correlation with PTSD criteria still remain unsettled.

The Allodi Scale and Harvard Trauma Questionnaire (HTQ)

In October 1974, the Danes created the first medical group within Amnesty International and initiated the first comprehensive medical assessment of torture survivors. A comprehensive review of their methods and findings have recently been presented (Rasmussen, 1990). Until 1980, their initial medical and psychiatric evaluation of the torture experience consisted of an examination procedure which utilized open-ended questions. Direct questions, such as 'Have you been tortured by electricity?' were not used. The Danish investigators attempted to obtain the history of the person who had been tortured by having the patient state it in their own words. When it came to torture methods, all details were requested from the patient. Eventually, patients were asked to pantomime the torture sessions. By 1980, the Danish group had abandoned this open-ended approach and adopted a standardized method using the instruments of Allodi and his colleagues in Toronto (Allodi, 1985).

The Allodi Trauma Scale

The Allodi Trauma Scale (Allodi, 1985) is one of the first semi-structured interview schedules developed to document the torture experience. It is a 41 item questionnaire which assesses traumatic experiences associated with political persecution, imprisonment, disappearance and death of individuals and families. It includes seven parts: 1) non-violent persecution; 2) arrest history; 3) physical torture; 4) deprivation during imprisonment; 5) sensory manipulation; 6) psychological torture and ill treatment, and 7) violence to family members. A respondent can receive a subtotal score for each section (except for trauma to family which is not graded) as well as a total score between 0 and 40 measuring his/her total trauma/torture experience.

The Harvard Trauma Questionnaire (HTQ)

The HTQ was designed to measure the trauma events and symptoms of Indochinese refugees, most of whom had survived torture and the trauma of mass violence (Mollica *et al.*, 1991). This instrument was developed in three Indochinese languages using rigorous translation back-translation methods of cross-cultural instrument development (Westermeyer, 1985). It includes three sections. The first section includes 17 trauma events historically accurate for assessing the Indochinese refugee experience. The second section consists of an open-ended question which asks the respondent to describe the most terrifying event(s) that have happened to him/her. The third section includes 30 symptoms related to the torture and trauma experience. Sixteen of these symptoms were derived from the DSM-IIIR criteria for PTSD; 14 were derived from clinical studies of Indochinese torture survivors. Initial validation of the questionnaire revealed the ability of the HTQ to correctly classify Indochinese patients with PTSD. The accuracy of diagnosis was enhanced by the addition of the 14 refugee items. These preliminary findings indicate that symptoms unique to Indochinese cultures may be associated with PTSD criteria. The HTQ was primarily developed as a clinical tool to assist the screening of refugee patients. It provides a culturally sensitive instrument for measuring torture and trauma events and symptoms which can be adapted for use with other non-English speaking populations.

CONCLUSION

The accurate assessment of torture events and symptoms and the proper classification of this information into a diagnostic system is fundamental to the effective treatment of torture survivors. Accomplishing this goal is a difficult task. Extensive clinical experience with torture survivors has revealed that many factors exist which interfere with the health provider's ability to obtain knowledge of the survivor's traumatic life experiences and symptoms. A commonly recognized definition of torture does not exist because torture has many unique forms and cultural meanings in different geopolitical regions. Variations in physical and psychological responses to torture are therefore enormous. Scientifically documented associations between torture events and medical sequelae have not been established. High emotional arousal, neuropsychiatric impairments, special coping mechanisms and culturally prescribed sanctions against revealing the torture experience, influence accuracy of reporting and stability of memory over time. Therapist/patient interactions, including the bicultural relationship also seriously affect the quality of assessment and patient care.

Categorizing and assembling torture symtoms into a diagnostic system pose concern as to the usefulness and validity of the diagnoses.

While a torture syndrome has not been demonstrated, the usefulness of DSM-IIIR post-traumatic stress disorder (PTSD) criteria remains questionable. Torture specific (i.e. based upon type of events) and culture specific (i.e. unique to the survivor's culture) symptoms still need to be identified. It is unknown whether culture bound or folk diagnoses exist for the torture response equivalent to Western derived PTSD disease category. While many PTSD criteria may presumably be 'core' to the torture experience, the 'core' PTSD symptoms associated with torture across cultures have not been established. Advances in cross-cultural research and the recent development of instruments with suitable psychometric properties capable of measuring trauma and torture events and symptoms will help identify a valid diagnostic system useful for treatment.

REFERENCES

Allodi, F. (1991). Assessment and treatment of torture victims: a critical review. *Journal of Nervous & Mental Disease*, **170(1)**, 4–11.

Allodi, F. (1985). Physical and psychiatric effects of torture: Canadian study. In E. Stover and E. O. Nightingale, eds. *The Breaking of Bodies and Minds: Torture, Psychiatric Abuses and the Health Professions*, pp. 66–78, New York: W. H. Freeman & Co.

American Psychiatric Association (1987). *Diagnostic and Statistical Manual of Mental Disorders* (3rd edn-revised). Washington, DC: American Psychiatric Association.

Amnesty International Report (1991). *Women in the Front Line*. New York: John D. Lucas Printing.

Bartlett F. C. (1932). *Remembering: A Study in Experimental and Social Psychology*. England: Cambridge University Press.

Başoğlu, M. & Marks, I. (1988). Torture. *British Medical Journal*, **297**, 1423–4.

Ring, R. & Vischer, A. L. (1919). Some remarks on the psychology of internment based on observations of prisoners of war in Switzerland. *Lancet*, 696–7.

Brett, E. A. & Ostroff, R. (1985). Imagery and posttraumatic stress disorder: an overview. *American Journal of Psychiatry*, **142**, 417–24.

Cienfuegos, A. J. & Monelli, C. (1983). The testimony of political repression as a therapeutic instrument. *American Journal of Orthopsychiatry*, **53**, 43–51.

Eich, J. E. (1980). The we dependent nature of state dependent retrieval. *Memory and Cognition*, **8**, 157–73.

Eitinger, L. & Strom, A. (1973). *Mortality and Morbidity after Excessive Stress: A Follow-up Investigation of Norwegian Concentration Camp Survivors*. New York: Humanities Press.

Engelhardt, H. T. (1975). The concepts of health and disease. In H. T. Engelhardt and S. F. Spicker, eds. *Evaluation and Explanation in the Biomedical Sciences*, pp. 125–141. Holland: D. Reidel Publishing Co.

Flaherty, J. A., Gaviria, F. M., Pathak, D., Mitchell, T., Wintrob, R., Richman, J. S.

& Birz, S. (1988). Developing instruments for cross-cultural psychiatric research. *Journal of Nervous & Mental Disease*, **176(5)**, 257–63.

Fogarty, S. J. & Hemsley, D. R. (1983). Depression and the accessibility of memories: a longitudinal study. *British Journal of Psychiatry*, **142**, 232–7.

Foy, D., Lund, M., Sipprelle, C. & Strachan, A. (1984). The combat exposure scale: a systematic assessment of trauma in the Vietnam war. *Journal of Clinical Psychology*, **40(6)**, 1323–8.

Freud, S. (1984). *Civilization and its Discontents* (standard edn, 21), pp. 57–145, New York: Norton.

Goldfeld, A. E., Mollica, R. F., Pesavento, B. & Faraone, S. (1988). The physical and psychological sequelae of torture: symptomatology and diagnosis. *Journal of the American Medical Association*, **259(18)**, 2725–9.

Horowitz, M. (1976). *Stress Response Syndromes*. New York: Aronson.

Jensen, T. S., Genefke, I. K., Hydlebrandt, N. *et al.* (1982). Cerebral atrophy in young torture victims. *New England Journal of Medicine*, **307**, 1341.

Keane, T. M., Caddel, J. M. & Taylor, K. L. (1988). Mississippi Scale for combat-related posttraumatic stress disorder: three studies in reliability and validity. *Journal of Consulting and Clinical Psychology*, **56(1)**, 85–90.

Kellner, C. H., Boy-byrne, P. P., Rubino, D. R. *et al.* (1983). Cerebral atrophy in torture victims. *New England Journal of Medicine*, **308**, 903.

Keshavan, M. S., Channabasavanna, S. M. & Narayan-Reddy, G. N. (1981). Posttraumatic psychiatric disturbances: patterns and predictors of outcome. *British Journal of Psychiatry*, **138**, 157–60.

Kinzie, J. D., Boehnlein, J. K., Leung, P., Moore, L. J., Riley, C. & Smith, D. (1990). The prevalence of postraumatic stress disorder and its clinical significance among Southeast Asian refugees. *American Journal of Psychiatry*, **147(7)**, 913–17.

Klerman, G. L. (ed.) (1987). Book review: culture and depression. *Social Science & Medicine*, **24(9)**, 785–90.

Kolb, I. L. & Multipassi, I. R. (1982). The conditioned emotional response: a subclass of the chronic and delayed posttraumatic stress disorder. *Psychiatric Annals*, **12**, 979–87.

Miller, T. W. (1988). Advances in understanding the impact of stressful life events on health. *Hospital & Community Psychiatry*, **39**, 615–22.

Mollica, R. F. (1988). The trauma story: the psychiatric care of refugee survivors of violence and torture. In F. M. Ochberg, ed. *Post-Traumatic Therapy and Victims of Violence*. New York: Brunner/Mazel.

Mollica, R. F. (1989). What is a Case? In M. Abbott, ed. *Refugee Resettlement and Wellbeing*. Auckland, New Zealand: Mental Health Foundation of New Zealand.

Mollica, R. F. & Caspi-Yavin, Y. (1991). Measuring torture and torture related symptoms. *Journal of Consulting and Clinical Psychology*, in press.

Mollica, R. F., Caspi-Yavin, Y., Bollini, P., Truong, T., Tor, S. & Lavelle, J. (1991). The Harvard trauma questionnaire: validating a cross-cultural instrument for measuring torture, trauma and posttraumatic stress disorder in Indochinese refugees. *Journal of Nervous & Mental Disease*, **180(2)**, 111–16.

Mollica, R. F. & Jalbert, R. R. *Community of Confinement: The Mental Health Crisis in Site Two (Displaced Persons Camps on the Thai-Kampuchean Border).* World Federation for Mental Health, February 1989.

Mollica, R. F. & Lavelle, J. (1988). Southeast Asian Refugees. In L. Comas-Diaz and E. F. H. Griffith, eds, *Clinical Guidelines in Cross-Cultural Mental Health.* New York: Wiley & Sons.

Mollica, R. F. & Son, L. (1989). Cultural dimensions in the evaluation and treatment of sexual trauma: an overview. *Psychiatric Clinics of North America,* **12(2)**, 363–79.

Mollica, R. F., Wyshak, G., de Marneffe, D., Khuon, F., Lavelle, J. (1987). Indochinese versions of the Hopkins Symptom Checklist-25: A screening instrument for the psychiatric care of refugees. *American Journal of Psychiatry,* **144(4)**, 497–500.

Mollica, R. F., Wyshak, G. & Lavelle, J. (1987). The psychosocial impact of war trauma and torture on Southeast Asian refugees. *American Journal of Psychiatry,* **144**, 1567–72.

Petersen, H. (1989). The controlled study of torture victims. *Scandinavian Journal of Social Medicine,* **17**, 13–20.

Rasmussen, O. V. (1990). Medical aspects of torture. *Danish Medical Bulletin,* **37**, 1–88.

Sartorius, N. (1987). Cross-cultural research on depression. *Psychopathology,* **19(2)**, 6–11.

Silver, J. M., Yudofsky, S. C. & Hales, R. E. (1987). Neuropsychiatric aspects of traumatic brain injury. In R. E. Hales, S. C. Yudofsky, eds, *Textbook of Neuropsychiatry.* Washington, DC: American Psychiatric Press, Inc.

Simons, R. C. & Hughes, C. C. eds, (1985). *The Culture-Bound Syndromes.* Holland: D. Reidel Publishing Co.

Sluzki, C. E. (1990). Disappeared: semantic and somatic effects of political repression in a family seeking therapy. *Family Process,* **29(2)**, 131–43.

Stuker, P. B., Winstead, D. K., Goist, K. C., Malow, R. M. & Allain, A. N. Jr (1986). Psychopathology subtypes and symptom correlates among former prisoners of war. *Journal of Psychopathology & Beh Assessment,* **8**, 89–101.

Stuker, P. B., Winstead, D. K., Galina, Z. H. & Allain, A. N. (1991). Cognitive deficits and psychopathology among former POWs and combat veterans of the Korean conflict. *American Journal of Psychiatry,* **148(1)**, 67–72.

Thygesen, P., Hermann, K. & Willanger, R. (1970). Concentration camp survivors in Denmark: persecution, disease, disability, compensation. *Danish Medical Bulletin,* **17**, 65–108.

Tulving, E. (1983). *Elements of Episodic Memory.* New York: Oxford Press.

United Nations Convention Against Torture and Other Cruel, Inhuman or Degrading Treatment of Punishment (1985). GA Res. 39/46, 39 GAOR Supp. (No. 51) at 197, UN Doc. A/39/51, *opened for signature* 4 February 1985, *entered into force,* 26 June 1987.

Westermeyer, J. (1981). Lao Folk diagnoses for mental disorder: comparison with psychiatric diagnosis and assessment with psychiatric rating scales. *Medical Anthropology,* **5**, 425–43.

Westermeyer, J. (1985). Psychiatric diagnosis across culture boundaries. *American Journal of Psychiatry*, **142**, 798–805.

Wolfe, J. & Keane, T. M. (1990). The diagnostic validity of posttraumatic stress disorder. In M. E. Wolfe and A. D. Mosnaim, eds, *Posttraumatic Stress Disorders: Etiology, Phenomenology, and Treatment*. Washington, DC: American Psychiatric Press, Inc.

Zilberg, N. J., Weiss, D. S., Horowitz, M. J. (1982). Impact of event scale: a cross-validation study and some empirical evidence supporting a conceptual model of stress response syndromes. *Journal of Consulting and Clinical Psychology*, **50**, 407–14.

Part IV

REHABILITATION PROGRAMMES FOR
TORTURE SURVIVORS

12
ORGANIZATION OF CARE AND REHABILITATION SERVICES FOR VICTIMS OF TORTURE AND OTHER FORMS OF ORGANIZED VIOLENCE: A REVIEW OF CURRENT ISSUES

Loes van Willigen

INTRODUCTION

Torture is one of the most cruel forms of organized violence. In 1986 a working group of the WHO regional office for Europe defined organized violence as 'The interhuman infliction of significant, avoidable pain and suffering by an organized system of ideas and attitudes. It comprises any violent action that is unacceptable by general human standards, and relates to the victim's feelings. Organized violence includes, *inter alia*, "torture, cruel, inhuman or degrading treatment or punishment" as mentioned in Article 5 of the UN Universal Declaration of Human Rights (1948). Imprisonment without trial, mock executions, hostage taking or any other form of violent deprivation of liberty fall under the heading of organized violence' (van Geuns, 1987, p. 9). According to the working group 'organized violence must be considered as an important health hazard' and 'since uprooting and exile is closely associated with organized violence, it must be relevant to consider all refugees victims of organized violence'.

As indicated in previous chapters, torture and other forms of organized violence entail both physical and psychosocial consequences for the victim which affect not only the victim but also his/her family, relatives, friends, party members and the community as a whole. Both the victim and his/her family may have to face legal problems. In addition, the victims living in exile are often exposed to a painful process of uprooting. If they arrive in a host country seeking asylum they often undergo a traumatizing asylum procedure (see Baker, this volume). Such problems have necessitated the formation of various care and rehabilitation services to provide medical, psychosocial, psychiatric and legal help for those in need. Since the 1970s efforts have been paralleled by an increasing awareness of, and interest in, organized violence sufferers among health care professionals throughout the world.

This chapter will review the various forms of care and rehabilitation services available to organized violence victims in different countries, giving a brief account of their historical development and considering aspects of their organization and the fundamental principles and concepts behind their approach. As most care and rehabilitation centres help not only victims of torture but also victims of organized violence in general, the discussion will cover health care services for all organized violence victims. To highlight certain aspects of the current approaches in the field, reference will be made to the history of the care services for survivors of the Second World War. The chapter will conclude with a discussion on the need for specific help for organized violence victims and on the importance of participation by the national and international governmental and non-governmental organisations in this field.

As so much depends on the specific political and economic conditions in which the centres have to operate, it is clearly difficult to assess, and indeed unfair to judge, the effectiveness of any particular type of approach used. However, given the rapidly increasing interest in this area, it is both necessary and timely to review the current situation to determine where we stand in relation to the goals set by the WHO definition of health.

A BRIEF REVIEW OF THE HISTORICAL DEVELOPMENT OF CARE AND REHABILITATION CENTRES

After the *coup d'état* in Chile by Pinochet on September 11, 1973 and the murder of Allende together with thousands of Chileans, citizens who were persecuted, or who had relatives imprisoned, tortured or missing, set out to seek legal and medical assistance. Mostly under cover, networks were formed and, later, centres and organizations were founded by health professionals for the care of victims of organized violence and of other human rights violations. Some of these organizations, such as the Fundación de Ayuda Social de las Iglesias Cristianas (FASIC) and Vicaria de la Solidaridad, were closely connected with the Church while others, for example Equipo de Denuncia, Investigación y Tratamiento al Torturado y su Nucleo Familiar (DITT) of the Comité de Defensa de los Derechos del Pueblo (CODEPU), were affiliated to a political opposition party. In the 1970s similar developments took place in Argentina and Uruguay. These groups started offering medical and especially social and psychotherapeutic help to victims of political repression.

In the early 1970s Danish and Dutch physicians in Amnesty International started research in Europe into the consequences of torture.

Initially, their interest was focused on victims of torture in Ireland and Greece, but when Latin American exiles began arriving in Western Europe countries, mostly in response to the invitation of the European governments, they began research and counselling work with tortured refugees. This experience later led to the foundation in the early 1980s of centres in Denmark, France, Canada and the Netherlands for medical and psychosocial help for refugees and victims of torture.

Meanwhile, independent of this development, two centres, one in Brussels (Colectivo Latinoamericano de Trabajo Psicosocial – COLAT) and the Psychosoziales Zentrum fur Fluchtninge in Frankfurt were founded in 1976 by Latin American physicians and psychiatrists concerned for the welfare of their exiled compatriots. In 1978, the Social Psychiatric Service for Latin American Refugees was set up in The Netherlands to meet the demands for help made by Latin American refugees. The service was mainly undertaken by Latin American health professionals who were themselves living in exile.

The interest in medical and psychosocial help for victims of torture and other forms of organized violence gradually increased in Europe and in other parts of the world.[1] At the end of the 1970s and the beginning of the 1980s centres were founded in the USA for psycho-social and psychotherapeutic help for refugees from South-East Asia. National Red Cross organizations, particularly those in the Scandinavian countries, turned their attention to the problems of the incoming refugees. As a result of the combined efforts of the Church, university groups, political groups and human rights and refugee organizations, centres appeared in Germany, England, Norway, Sweden, Denmark, France, Spain and outside Europe in the Philippines, South Africa, Uganda, Pakistan, Turkey, Australia, Canada, the USA and in many Latin American countries.

There has also been a surge of interest in scientific communications and exchange of information in this area. In 1989 a total of 151 professionals representing 91 centres throughout the world attended the Second International Conference of Centres, Institutions and Individual Professionals Concerned with the Care of Victims of Organized Violence in Costa Rica. It should be borne in mind that these figures by no means reflect the total number of workers in the field since many professionals currently working under a repressive

---

[1] The interest in the medical and psychosocial problems of refugees was not a new development. Already in the fifties articles had appeared (e.g. by Eitinger in Norway and Tyhurst in Canada) about the psychological and psychosocial problems of refugees – mostly concentration camp survivors – fleeing from Eastern Europe to the West after World War II.

regime have to work underground (as was the case in Chile, Argentina, and Uruguay in the past) and therefore can have no access to such international conferences.

CURRENT MODELS OF ORGANIZATION OF CARE AND REHABILITATION SERVICES

Due to constraints of space this review deals only with selected group of care and rehabilitation centres chosen to show, as far as possible, the diversity of approach in the field. The information presented here is by no means a comprehensive account of their work since the descriptions are limited to their most important activities.[1] The centres will be reviewed under three broad categories: those based in the home country of the victims where there is a present or past history of political repression, those based in Western host countries, and those situated in host countries that are in the same region of the world as the refugees' home country. In this brief survey, no account has been taken of the professionals who work in various refugee camps throughout the world.

Centres based in the home country of victims

The help offered in countries which have a past or present history of political repression (e.g. in Chile, Argentina, Uruguay, Colombia, El Salvador, Guatemala, the Philippines, Pakistan, South Africa) is generally multidisciplinary and not restricted to the care of somatic or psychological problems. These institutions often also offer legal help and social support. Some centres have adopted a clear political position and have not restricted themselves solely to care. They regard torture as one of the many forms of political repression or 'state terrorism' and consider it as part of their task publicly to impeach the repressive regimes for their violations of human rights.

In general, the multidisciplinary teams in these centres largely consist of psychiatrists, psychologists and social workers who focus on the social and psychological problems resulting from organized violence. Some of them (e.g. DITT/CODEPU) visit prisons to offer political prisoners support and counselling. Similar help is offered to the

---

[1] The information is obtained from a 'List of Treatment and Rehabilitation Centres Worldwide' of the Medical Foundation for the Care of Victims of Torture, London, from the 'Presentation de quelques centres participants aux travaux' of the First World Meeting of Medical and Psychosocial Centres specialized in the Treatment of Victims of Organised Violence in Paris 1987 and information from the centres themselves.

inhabitants of the 'poblaciones', which are often most severely hit by political repression. The organization FASIC in Chile, for example, has formed medical teams in co-operation with the inhabitants of the slum districts of Santiago. These teams give help to the victims either during or immediately after violent attacks and systematic house searches by soldiers and the police.

Other groups too (e.g. Medical Action Group (MAG), Philippine Action Concerning Torture (PACT) in the Philippines, Organization for Appropriate Social Services in South Africa (OASSSA), an organization of psychologists, psychiatrists, psychiatric nurses and social workers, and National Medical and Dental Association (NAMDA), a national association of health professionals in South Africa) have focused their activities particularly on the inhabitants of marginalized districts – prime targets for repressive regimes and 'apartheid.' They train nonprofessional people in these areas to provide direct medical and psychosocial help to the victims.

The workers in some centres (e.g. Centro de Estudios Legales y Sociales (CELS) in Argentina) not only offer psychosocial support to the victims of the so-called dirty war but also participate in the search for the children of disappeared people or of ex-prisoners – children given away by the military police for adoption by foster parents during the imprisonment of their real parents. They also offer legal help to facilitate the recovery of the children by their families. The members of the Psychosocial Team of the Madres de la Plaza de Mayo still hold weekly demonstrations with the mothers in the square now well known throughout the world. The Rehabilitation and Health Aid Centre for Torture Victims (RAHAT) of the Voice Against Torture (VAT) in Pakistan not only provides treatment for torture victims, but also fights against the abuse of the medical profession as under Pakistani laws doctors are sometimes required to participate or assist in cruel punishments and torture (see chapter on Pakistan).

In addition to medical and various forms of psychosocial care, most of these centres concentrate also on rehabilitation of violence survivors, organizing, among other activities, various handicraft workshops as occupational therapy.

Since the transition to democracy in Argentina, Uruguay and Chile the centres in these countries have also been offering help to their compatriots returning from exile. Another important aspect of their work is the fight against 'impunity' which involves putting pressure on the present governments to ensure that the acts of human rights violations during the dictatorial regime are made public and the culprits brought to trial. For them truth and justice are essential not only for the psychological repair of the individual violence survivor, but also for the restoration of the whole society[1] (Neumann *et al.*, 1990, p. 151; Lira *et al.*, 1989, p. 198).

Thus, although these teams mainly consist of psychologists and psychiatrists, their work covers practically all consequences of organized violence. With the exception of one or two centres which offer help to refugees from neighbouring countries[2] they cater mainly for their own compatriots. Most of these centres rely on financial support particularly from European funds and the UN Fund for Torture Victims. Those that are affiliated to religious institutions are supported by the Church (e.g. the World Council of Churches).

It is important to note that quite often these workers themselves become the victims of organized violence and suffer multiple imprisonments and even torture. The Vicaria in Santiago de Chile is a case in point. In 1989 the members of this institution were interrogated about their clients and the documentation of their work was seized.

Centres based in host countries – Europe, Canada, USA and Australia

Compared with the centres discussed above, those based in Europe, Canada, USA and Australia show a greater diversity in the structure of their teams, the forms of assistance provided, targeted groups and financial resources. The first centres established in Europe for medical and psychosocial assistance for refugees were COLAT in Brussels and the Psychosocial Team for Refugees in Frankfurt.

COLAT (nowadays called COLAT/EXIL) was founded with a clear political position. Its services are not restricted to the individual refugee but cover also the family and the Latin American refugee community. The team organizes a summer camp for the children every year, and offers workshops and other services such as a general practitioner's consulting hour and psychotherapeutic help. For the last few years they have opened their doors to refugees of other nationalities. The team members are of Latin American or Belgian descent. They receive a minimal amount of financial support annually from the Belgian government.

The Frankfurt Psychosocial Team for Refugees consists of one psychiatrist, psychologists and social workers. Originally made up

[1] As the priest and psychologist Ignacio Martín Baró, brutally killed in El Salvador in November 1989, put it: 'the people who cannot confront themselves with their historical past are condemned to repeat it' (Martín Baró, 1989, p. 13).
[2] Two such centres are the Centro Medico Psicosocial in Mendoza, Argentina which helps Chilean refugees and RAHAT in Pakistan which helps refugees from Iran, Afghanistan and India.

only of Latin Americans whose work was restricted to their compatriots, the team has for some time now had members from various countries and offers help to refugees from all countries. They give social and psychotherapeutic help and organize workshops and discussion meetings. They are financed by, among other bodies, the Evangelic Church and the Federal Government. Both these centres help not only tortured refugees but all victims of violence.

The centres which have their origins in the activities of the medical groups within Amnesty International (the Rehabilitation Centre for Torture Victims (RCT) in Copenhagen, the Canadian Centre for Victims of Torture (CCVT) in Toronto, Comité Medical pour les Exilés (COMEDE) in Paris and the Centrum Gezondheidszorg Vluchtelingen (CGV) in The Netherlands) concentrated originally on the physical consequences of torture and organized violence; most of the founding members of these centres were physicians. Only later were the teams expanded with the recruitment of psychologists and social workers. These four centres show fundamental differences from one another.

The RCT is a highly specialized team which deals only with victims of torture and their families. Asylum seeking torture victims who have not yet received refugee status are excluded. It consists of a multidisciplinary team of Danish professionals although occasionally Latin American psychologists have also been members of the team. The centre administers a standard form of intake and treatment. The multidisciplinary approach involves specialist medical and psychotherapeutic help, social services, and physiotherapy, and the team has initiated a workshop for ex-patients and also run a documentation centre. Considerable weight is given in promoting its model of services to other countries and the RCT has organized many international symposia and seminars. It also trains physicians from within the general Danish health care system. The centre receives financial support from the Danish government, the UN Fund for Victims of Torture and many other private funds and individuals.

The CCVT consists of a relatively small team of workers from different nationalities but operates with a large network of volunteers. Although its intake was originally restricted to torture victims, the centre now offers medical, psychosocial and legal help to all refugees from different nationalities. It trains professionals and offers guidance to volunteers who help refugees with their integration into Canadian society. The centre is financed by the Canadian government and private funds.

COMEDE specializes in medical and psychosocial help to asylum seekers, especially to those who, not having yet gained refugee status, are denied access to the French health care system. The team consists of general practitioners, psychiatrists, psychologists and social workers backed-up by an extensive network of medical specialists in Paris. The team provides medical care, medicines, and psychosocial help. No discrimination is made between torture victims and victims of other forms of organized violence nor between different nationalities. The centre is financed partly by the French government and partly by private funds.

The CGV in The Netherlands originally set out to offer a preliminary medical examination to quota refugees. Subsequently the work was extended to medical and psychosocial help for all asylum seekers and refugees. The emphasis in the work of the CGV is on the initial reception (medical examination, information, referral) in the reception centres for refugees and asylum seekers to prevent the importation of diseases and the long-term consequences of violence, and on medical and psychosocial assistance in the municipalities where the refugees are housed. The CGV also emphasizes the dissemination of expertise to regular health care institutions, in connection with which it runs a documentation centre. The team consists of physicians, social workers and nurses specially trained in (psycho-)social work. It is a 'baseline' and primary health care centre. The team co-operates closely with the SPD-V, a social psychiatric service for refugees (previously only for Latin Americans), which provides ambulatory psychological health care for the refugees in The Netherlands. The CGV also has access to a team of medical specialists at the Academic Hospital in Leiden (the AZL/CGV-team) for specialist medical examination and treatment. The CGV and the SPD-V do not make a distinction between clients with regard to nationality, the type of traumatic events experienced (e.g. torture or other forms of organized violence) or whether refugee status has, or has not yet, been granted. Both teams consists of professionals of different nationalities. The CGV is part of the Ministry of Welfare, Health and Cultural Affairs and has a fixed budget. The SPD-V is financed by the regular medical insurance system and also subsidized by the government.

The Red Cross Centre for Victims of Torture in Stockholm was originally modelled on the RCT in Copenhagen. Soon after the centre came into existence, however, the team distanced itself from the RCT model and developed its own. The team includes medical specialists, psychologists, psychiatrists, social workers, physiotherapists, and nurses, mainly Swedish and some Latin Americans. They admit only tortured refugees and refer asylum seekers to a team of volunteer specialists. They are financed by medical insurance companies, the Red Cross and by various Swedish governmental bodies.

The Centre for Psyko-socialt Arbejde for Flygtninge (CEPAR) in Copenhagen is a team of psychologists, a social worker and a physiotherapist of various nationalities who provide transcultural, psychosocial and psychotherapeutic help for asylum seekers and refugees and act as advisors to volunteer groups and refugee organisations. They are financed by the medical insurance system.

The Psychosocial Team for Refugees in Oslo is part of the Department of Psychiatry of the University of Oslo. The team consists of Norwegian psychiatrists, psychologists and social workers who provide psychosocial and psychotherapeutic help for refugees and they pay a great deal of attention to training general health care workers, particularly those in primary health care. They are financed by the University and the government.

The Psychiatric Referral Centre for Spanish Speakers in Stockholm provides social, psychotherapeutic and psychiatric help for all Spanish-speaking inhabitants of Stockholm, whether they are migrants or refugees. The team consists of mainly Latin American psychiatrists, psychiatric nurses, psychologists and social workers.

The Medical Foundation for Victims of Torture in London gives help to refugees and asylum seekers. It consists of a small team which can call on a large network of English physicians, psychologists and psychiatrists for voluntary help. A large part of the team's work involves examination of asylum seekers and preparation of medical statements for asylum procedures. Furthermore, the team offers medical, social and psychotherapeutic help, organizes workshops, and publicizes the consequences of torture and political repression.

The Indochinese Psychiatry Clinic in Boston is based in a primary health care setting. The team consists of psychologists, psychiatrists, psychiatric nurses, social workers, and South-East Asian cross-cultural workers. They offer psychiatric help and social services and function as 'family doctors' for the South-East Asian community in Boston. They are financed by the government of Massachusetts.

The Service for Treatment and Rehabilitation of Torture Trauma Survivors (STARTTS) in Australia is a small team of psychotherapists and bilingual counsellors derived from various refugee groups. They offer psychotherapeutic help and social services and refer their clients to physicians, physiotherapists and other specialists for medical help whenever necessary. They co-operate closely with refugee communities. An integral part of their work is informing the public about the nature of activities.

In addition to the centres not mentioned here, there are many individual psychologists, child and adult psychiatrists, and social workers in the West who have taken up work with refugees. These workers are usually employed by regular institutions. Other workers in the field include physicians in the Scandinavian and other European countries who perform an initial medical examination of refugees and asylum seekers to prevent imported diseases, those who provide psychosocial help in reception centres for refugees and/or asylum seekers, and volunteer organizations in many countries helping refugees with allowance, housing, employment and language problems.

Centres for refugees from regional countries

In addition to the medical and psychosocial services for refugees living in refugee camps there are centres which are based independently in their own regions serving refugees either from the neighbouring countries or from the same region of the world. Only a few of them will be reviewed here.

In Bolivia Centro de Estudios y Servicios Especializados sobre Migraciones Involuntarias (CESEM) provides psychotherapeutic help and psychosocial services, including economic aid to and medical care for Latin American refugees. The centre supports projects which provide employment for refugees in rural areas. The team consists of a psychologist, a physician, an agro-technician, and social workers. It is financed by the UNHCR.

In Costa Rica various centres are involved in the work with refugees. The Equipo Centroamericano de Trabajo Psicosocial (ECPT) is a small team of one psychiatrist, two psychologists and a social worker. It provides social and psychotherapeutic help for refugees from the region. One of the psychologists is also employed by El Productor, a centre which helps refugees in starting various agricultural and labour projects such as cattle breeding, carpentry workshops and so on. These projects are initially funded for some years but thereafter must be self-supporting. The team consisting of social workers, a psychologist, an agro-technician and an economist provides support – technical as well as psychological – for the refugees involved in these projects. Both the ECTP and El Productor operate with funds from Europe.

In Pakistan the Psychiatric Centre for Afghans was founded to provide psychotherapeutic and psychiatric help to Afghan refugees – victims of war and repression. They offer both ambulatory and clinical psychiatric treatment and train refugee camp residents in self-help.

SIMILARITIES AND DIFFERENCES BETWEEN CARE AND REHABILITATION CENTRES

The differences between various care and rehabilitation centres world-wide concern mainly the nationalities of their clients and the nature of the violence they have suffered (e.g. torture as opposed to other forms of organized violence), the composition of their teams in various disciplines, and their proclaimed goals (e.g. political as opposed to purely humanitarian). Some centres are supported by the government or are part of it, while others are not approved of or even persecuted by their government.

Centres in countries with a past or present history of political repression show more similarities to each other in their aims, their organizational models, and the type of help offered than do the centres in the Western countries. The former group of centres are multidisciplinary in the sense that they focus on training and counsell-ing of non-professionals in areas most severely hit by repression as well as providing psychosocial and sometimes medical and legal help for organized violence victims and their families. Their work is mostly based on political solidarity with their clients, which is often manifes-ted by public condemnation of the repressive regimes, demonstrations and other forms of action. However, despite the apparent similarities between these centres, fundamental differences in methods and aims may arise. Debate over these issues appears mainly to stem from differences in political ideologies – a critical factor in defining methods and aims. Most of these centres are financially insecure having to rely on liberal-minded private or international funding bodies in Western countries.

The centres in Western countries are more heterogenous in their policies for diagnostics and client intake criteria. The controversy between them in fact largely centres around these issues (see discuss-ion) and is connected to a much lesser extent with their methods and organizational models, despite the fact that these differ considerably among the various centres. Their work is mostly based on humanitar-ian solidarity with the victims of organized violence. The centres differ in their organization as to whether they use a uni- or multidisciplinary approach, whether they take refugees from only one or more regions, or whether they employ only indigenous professionals. Some admit only tortured refugees while others do not make this distinction. Some limit their activities to those who have been granted refugee status only whereas others also include those still seeking asylum. These centres also differ in the nature of their work. Some provide only one form of help while others have undertaken a wide variety of services. Some centres give priority to training medical professionals in general health care institutions and/or informing the public about their work while others concentrate on specialist medical care and/or research. Some centres work in collaboration with a network of specialists in the general health care system. Some centres, but not others, have adopted a community-oriented approach, making domiciliary visits and maintaining contact with other volunteer and refugee organizations.

As they are dependent on yearly contributions from government bodies and private and international funds, most of these centres are financially unstable. Only a few centres such as the RCT and the CGV can rely on an adequate annual budget. The CGV and the Psychosocial Team for Refugees in Norway are apparently the only centres which do not have to raise funds or subsidies every year.

DISCUSSION: ISSUES IN CARE AND REHABILITATION OF ORGANIZED VIOLENCE VICTIMS

Political repression, disappearances, imprisonment and torture are designed to break the opposition to a regime. Subjecting individuals to violence, depicting them in the media as terrorists or communists threatening prosperity or as capitalists prospering at the expense of others, and exposing them to solitary confinement and other forms of torture during imprisonment all serve to terrorize and thereby pacify political opponents and isolate them from the rest of the society. Political repression is thus a means of maintaining a dictatorial system and has profound effects on the individual, the family and on the society as a whole. Systematic violations of human rights are often denied by the regimes concerned or are often justified as being a defence against terrorist actions or threats to the State.

Given the fact that political repression can take so many different forms, torture as an act of violence cannot be taken in isolation from organized violence in general. Likewise, tortured people cannot be regarded solely as individual victims, as they have often undergone other forms of repression prior to their torture trauma, such as threats to life and family, loss of employment or opportunities for study, having to go into hiding and so on. Moreover, their plight usually does not end with imprisonment and torture; they often have to face similar repressive acts after their traumatic ordeal. Consequently, flight may be seen as the only means of physical and psychological survival. However, flight may entail yet more traumatic events for the refugee including the process of uprooting and settlement in a new country.

The relative impact of this process depends partly on the personality, coping skills, education, degree of familiarity with the new culture, and language skills of the individual and partly on various character- istics of the host country (e.g. mono-ethnic versus multi-ethnic) which determine how easily a newcomer can be integrated into the society, housing, employment, and education (Berry *et al.*, 1987). In many Western countries, refugees either live alone or in ghettos, isolated from the native population. Asylum seekers have to acquire refugee status through a tortuous, lengthy and often traumatizing asylum procedure. In many countries, they are neither allowed to work nor study during this period. After asylum is granted, they are confronted with other problems. They are often either unable to find employment or forced to work in jobs for which they are far too highly qualified. Most of them have to live in a vacuum in the absence of a family and/or a social network. Living in exile thus means a continuation of often traumatic stress. Moreover, refugees remain confronted by the repress- ion in their country of origin through the media and letters from relatives and friends. Feelings of doubt, guilt and impotence may be intensified by both good and bad news from their country. Refugees who have left their country because of a civil war may suffer from feelings of impotence and be further traumatized particularly if they find themselves, as sometimes is the case, in between two fighting parties both of which accuse them of collaboration with the other. Furthermore, organized violence victims often have to cope with the stigma of being a 'victim' and deal with the conscious or unconscious tendency of the society to ostracize them – a problem that arises in their own culture as well as in a host country. Clearly, organized violence is not a single, isolated incident but often entails a sequence of physical and particularly psychological traumata over time. Despite the enormity of the problem for individuals concerned, help is only available from a small number of professionals, some of whom may themselves be persecuted and victimized by their government.

The tendency to deny the existence of the problem of organized violence and to avoid confronting its consequences – sometimes called the 'conspiracy of silence' – is probably due to a reluctance to face a gruesome reality which is liable to provoke feelings of complicity and guilt. Such a conspiracy of silence over war victims existed in some Western countries such as The Netherlands after the Second World War. When the war ended, governments and society alike turned their attention to the future leaving behind the painful memories of the past. Thus, perhaps not surprisingly, little attention was paid to the relief of concentration camp and war survivors, resistance fighters and other people who had suffered severe psychological traumas. The war victims were generally unable to find people with whom they could talk about the violence they had suffered and consequently learned to suppress their painful memories. In The Netherlands it was not until the 1950s that Dutch society and the medical world took an interest in relieving the suffering of concentration camp survivors and resistance fighters. It was eventually realized that civilians, too, might have medical and psychological problems resulting from war violence. Similarly, it was only towards the end of the 1970s that attention was turned to the psychological suffering of people who had been kept in Japanese concentration camps in Indonesia.

A consequence of this delayed interest was the emergence of a notion that certain types of war trauma were more serious than others, thus creating a hierarchy of degree of victimization. This in turn led to rivalry between the survivors, expressed during group therapy sessions for example, when solidarity, not rivalry, was most needed. Another ill-conceived belief was that only highly specialized professionals could handle the psychological problems of war victims. At a time when society had begun to pay attention to the consequences of the war, unearthing of painful memories and facing reality was so harrowing and difficult that only specialized centres seemed able to help.

There are important lessons to be learned from experience with war victims and Vietnam veterans as well as with the hijack victims in The Netherlands in the 1970s. First, early recognition of the problems caused by war and organized violence may be important in the prevention of their long-term serious medical consequences (Van Der Ploeg *et al.*, 1985, p. 188–9; Kleber, 1986, p. 247). Similarly, experience with the children of war victims has shown the need for early attention in the care of the children of victims of organized violence (Keilson, 1985). In some countries, there is as yet no systematic attempt to ensure this early recognition and care. Secondly, it is essential to avoid a hierarchical approach in determining the seriousness of victimization to prevent secondary victimization. Too great an attention to or emphasis on those with a history of torture may, by relegating other forms of organized violence and their psychological impact on the individual to a position of secondary importance, inadvertently result in the neglect of people who, though not tortured, are nevertheless highly traumatized. Moreover, such a distinction may lead to the exclusion of individuals possibly unaware of the connection between their torture experience and their medical and psychological complaints. Professionals must take into consideration the complex and multicausal nature of the problems of organized violence sufferers and counteract any marginalization of victims which may result from failure to recognise the importance of their problems. Recent studies have shown the importance in the coping process of support from social networks directly after the trauma (Dasberg, 1986; Kleber *et al.*, 1986, p. 247) and the need for recognition, not only by the medical world but also by the society as a whole, of the effects of organized violence, in order to prevent serious long-term consequences (Begemann, 1987, p. 87; Leliefeld, 1985, p. 79).

The current debate concerning etiology and diagnostic issues in post-violence problems is similar to that which existed in the post-war era. The psychological problems of war victims were then attributed, particularly in the Scandinavian countries, to organic causes such as nutritional deficiency, brain atrophy, and other somatic factors. In the USA, on the other hand, the search for causes took place mainly in the field of psychiatry (Thorvaldsen, 1986, p. 44). A diagnostic distinction was made between the problems of concentration camp survivors (KZ syndrome) and those manifested by victims of other types of war trauma. Similar differences in approach still exist today. The RCT and the Danish group of Amnesty International physicians conduct research into physical causes of post-torture problems and have published articles implicating brain atrophy and hormonal insuffi-ciencies as etiological factors (Kosteljanetz, 1983; Lunde *et al.*, 1980; Rasmussen, 1990, p. 28, 35). They also maintain that a 'torture syn-drome' may exist, distinguishable from problems following other types of organized violence. Until now, however, they could not confirm this hypothesis (Rasmussen, 1990, p. 43).

A further issue of debate arises from the classification of the psycho-logical complaints resulting from traumatic stress in organized vio-lence victims under the heading of Post-Traumatic Stress Disorder. For a number of reasons the DSM–IIIR classification is rejected by many workers dealing with organized violence victims[1], the first and fore-most reason being that the term *post*-traumatic stress cannot be applied to most victims. As indicated earlier, traumatic stress is not, for most organized violence sufferers, usually an isolated incident, many victims undergoing a sequence of traumatic events and continuing to experience traumatic stress even when in exile. Secondly, the DSM–IIIR is based on Western concepts of illness and health. Given the fact that culture is an important factor in determining the manifes-

[1] In: Synthesis of conclusions from the First World Meeting of Medical and Psychosocial Centres specialized in the treatment of Victims of Organized Violence, held in Paris, 1987, published by COMEDE, Paris, and CGV, Rijswijk.

tation of psychological complaints, it may not be applicable in non-Western cultures. Thirdly, with a strict diagnostic approach of the kind proposed by the DSM–IIIR, there is the risk of overlooking other important psychiatric problems that may result from organized violence as well as of giving the false impression that psychological problems related to the trauma which cannot be diagnosed as PTSD or torture syndrome are not serious (Lansen, 1989). This, in turn, may deprive those equally in need of the necessary care and treatment. Finally, the psychological complaints of organized violence victims are mostly normal and recognizable reactions to abnormal and inhuman situations. The term 'disorder' is thus not appropriate in their case since it implies pathology. DSM–IIIR or any other categorical approach reduces normal reactions to non-normal and transforms what is essentially a socio-political problem into medical pathology.

The influence of social and cultural factors on the presentation of psychological complaints is of great importance in work with refugees, as has been recognized for years by professionals in this field. For the work among refugees to be effective, professionals trained in cross-cultural work, trained interpreters, and members of the target group must be recruited. A plea has been made at various international meetings for the recruitment of such staff. So far, however, remarkably little progress has been made, despite the fact that there are medical professionals and social workers among the refugees. Whether this is due to ethnocentrism or paternalism on the part of the organizations which help organized violence victims or due to Western governments blocking the employment of allochtonous helpers, by, for example, refusing to accept non-western qualifications, is not clear.

Although it is often recognized that psychosocial problems, particularly in non-Western cultures, are mainly expressed in somatic complaints, this recognition is not usually reflected in the structure of the staff in rehabilitation centres. General practitioners are often the first to be consulted for somatic complaints, particularly in Western countries, but they are involved in the work in only a few centres.

Moreover, it is questionable whether the kind of help offered to refugees corresponds to the kind of help they think they need. In many non-Western countries, being treated by a psychologist or psychiatrist is considered as a taboo subject. Such treatment means being declared insane and causes loss of face in the family and in the circle of friends. Similarly, in many countries, social service as a form of help is unknown. A refugee may thus find it difficult to trust a profession he/she is not familiar with. Some refugees are used to consulting a specialist and receiving medicines for their (psycho-somatic) complaints. Thus referral to, or treatment by, a psychologist may not meet the expectations of the client.

As regards the help offered by centres with a political aim, the question is whether this aim always corresponds to the needs of their clients. If the political stance is too dominant, clients may be put off and thereby deprived of help. Conversely, clients who expect political solidarity from those caring for them may not be satisfied with humanitarian help alone. Trust in the carer is of particular importance for victims of organized violence. Often this also means trust in his or her political stance. The question is whether a professional helper can be as effective in counselling clients with totally different political backgrounds.

As stated earlier, the organizational models of care and rehabilitation services in various countries will be shaped by the structure of the general health care systems in those countries. For instance, in The Netherlands and in Norway the family doctor plays a central role in the system of health care and has been trained not only to deal with somatic complaints but also with psychosocial problems, often in co-operation with other disciplines within the primary health care system. Accordingly, the CGV in The Netherlands consists of general practitioners, social workers and social nurses. In both countries the government's health care policy is designed to make the regular health care services accessible to all groups in the society. Therefore the emphasis of work in the CGV and in the Psychosocial Team for Refugees in Norway is on dissemination of information to and stimulation of the necessary expertise in the regular health care system, particularly in baseline and primary health care (Lycke Ellingsen & Hauff, 1988). In countries where primary health care does not receive much emphasis, the care and rehabilitation centres are more likely to be founded by medical specialists and psychologists. In countries where there are highly developed psychosocial and psychiatric services in general health care, the organizational structure of the centres follow the same pattern. On the other hand, in countries where there is a strong biological orientation in the study of human behaviour, care and rehabilitation teams mainly consist of medical specialists. The political situation and public awareness in a country are also important factors that determine whether attention is paid to the consequences of organized violence and whether a distinction is made between refugees and asylum seekers, torture victims and victims of other forms of organized violence, and between refugees of various nationalities. Finally the health professionals' own concept of health and illness and their perception of their own role in dealing with problems caused by organized violence will affect their approach (e.g. multidisciplinary as opposed to uni-disciplinary, transcultural as opposed to ethnocentric).

EXCHANGE OF KNOWLEDGE AND EXPERIENCE

The growth in efforts world-wide to help victims of organized violence has led to an increase in the need for exchange of information between the professionals concerned. The centres founded in Europe by the physicians in Amnesty International maintained regular contact with each other since the 1980s. Contact was also sought with other centres in Europe and elsewhere. Similarly, in Latin America regional meetings were organized with a view to exchanging knowledge and experience. Occasional and often personal contacts between professionals in Europe and Latin America ultimately developed into major international conferences. In 1987 in Paris and in 1989 in San José, Costa Rica, the first and second international conference of centres, institutions and individual professionals concerned with the care for victims of organized violence took place. It was concluded that these conferences are of great importance in facilitating the exchange of experience and expertise and helping to break down the isolation of many professionals in the field. It was also suggested that there is a need to formalize the network of professionals helping victims of organized violence. It is expected that the third conference in 1991 will put this idea into operation.

Further activities in the field include the organization of three work group meetings from 1980 onwards under the auspices of the WHO regional office for Europe and by the initiative of the Dutch government. These groups have made recommendations on work with refugees and the research needed in the field.

In 1985 the International Commission of Health Professionals for Health and Human Rights (ICHP) was founded. One of its aims is to support and defend health professionals engaged in the protection of Human Rights and to denounce the perpetrators of human rights violations. It co-operates with the UN and has national sections in various countries including Argentina, the Philippines, South Africa, the USA and The Netherlands.

RECOMMENDATIONS

As organized violence appears to threaten all aspects of health (defined by the WHO as an optimum of physical, mental and social well-being), not only of the individual but also of the family and of the community, it is of great importance to adopt a multidisciplinary approach to the consequences of organized violence.

As important as primary prevention of organized violence is the secondary prevention of its long-term major consequences. Early identification and acknowledgement of the problems can help prevent them. For this the public must be kept informed and early support and care actively offered to the victims, as well as to their relatives. Experience and scientific studies suggest that initial reception often need not go further than giving advice, information and social services (Kleber *et al.*, 1986, p. 252; Van Der Ploeg, 1985, p. 190). But this form of assistance should be offered actively, as it seems that victims of violence are reluctant to seek help themselves when they need it (Van Der Ploeg *et al.*, 1985, p. 127–128). With support from their social network, many victims seem able to cope with the violence they have undergone. What is essential is the opportunity to talk to others about their experiences and express their emotions, either in a group setting or individually (Kleber *et al.*, 1986, p. 254).

Sometimes support and counselling are necessary to help the victims reconstruct their social network. Such help need not always be provided by professional helpers. Medical help may be needed for the (psycho)somatic consequences of torture and other forms of organized violence and with refugees in general a medical check-up for imported diseases (e.g. tuberculosis) can be very important (Hondius & van Willigen, 1989; van Willigen, 1988). It is equally important to provide support for the victims' integration into a new society – support which often involves helping them learn about the new society and its health care structure and find language lessons, housing, study and work (Begemann, 1987). For asylum seekers, legal help and advice is indispensable. Specialist help in the form of psychotherapy and psychiatric care is only necessary when there is no progress in the coping process or when psychiatric problems arise (Kleber *et al.*, 1986, p. 255).

As long as regular health care and welfare institutions in various countries are not sufficiently accessible to those victims of organized violence who need them, special care and rehabilitation services will be necessary for early and adequate care and help. Moreover, these institutions have a symbolic value for the victims for whom their existence implies a recognition of their problems and signifies solidarity with them – a recognition and solidarity often not demonstrated by society. At the same time such institutions are at risk of being marginalized in society together with their target groups (Begemann, 1987).

Breaking the conspiracy of silence still remains confined to a small group of professional helpers.

The WHO work group mentioned above proposed in 1986 that persons who suffered organized violence should be legally entitled to equity in access to health services. Equity in access implies not only removing financial and organizational barriers but also the availability of the necessary knowledge and expertise in regular health care to ensure early recognition within that system of the consequences of organized violence. This recommendation is in keeping with the WHO motto of 'health for all' by the year 2000. In attempts to realize this aim more emphasis is being given to primary health care, health promotion, preventive measures and to closer involvement of target groups in health programmes (WHO Regional Office for Europe, 1985).

In order to break through the conspiracy of silence and to facilitate access to regular health care, the existing special centres and institutions must disseminate their expertise to other health professionals. Only then can adequate reception and care services be made more easily accessible to the target group and provided more quickly. Furthermore, the reception and help offered should be planned in closer co-operation and consultation with the target groups. In particular, attention needs to be paid to children and second generation victims of organized violence. So far Norway and The Netherlands seem to be the only countries where the government has clearly adopted a policy of supporting the growth of expertise in this field and its dissemination to regular health care institutions. In other countries, dissemination of expertise still largely depends on the financial resources available and on the willingness and facilities to that end of individual institutions. Active support of and stimulation from governmental health care organizations, international organizations such as the WHO and other relevant sections of the UN are necessary, while the network of care and rehabilitation services for victims of torture and other forms of organized violence could play a stimulating role.

ACKNOWLEDGEMENTS

I am grateful to the editor who stimulated me to write this chapter and especially to my colleagues who were helpful in supplying information.

REFERENCES

Begemann, F. A. (1987). *Reacties op geweld.* Utrecht, Stichting ICODO.

Berry, J. W., Kim, U., Minde T. & Mok, D. (1987). Comparative studies of acculturative stress. *International Migration Review*, **21**(3) 491–511.

Dasberg, H. (1986). Social aspects of trauma following war, genocide and terror. In *Health Hazards of Organized Violence.* Rijswijk, Ministry of Welfare, Health and Cultural Affairs.

Geuns, H. A. van (1987). The concept of organized violence. In *Health Hazards of Organized Violence.* Rijswijk, Ministry of Welfare, Health and Cultural Affairs.

Hondius, A. J. K. & Willigen, L. H. M. van (1989). Base line health care for refugees in the Netherlands. *Social Science and Medicine*, **28**(7) 729–33.

Keilson, H. (1985). Sequentiele traumatisering bij kinderen. *Nederlands Tijdschrift voor Geneeskunde*, **129**(18) 832–4.

Kleber, R. J., Brom, D. & Defares, P. B. (1986). *Traumatische ervaringen, gevolgen en verwerking.* Lisse, Swets en Zeitlinger.

Kosteljanetz, M. & Aalund, O. (1983). Torture: A challenge to medical science. *Interdisciplinary Science Review*, **8**, 1–9.

Lansen, J. (1989). Een kritische opinie over het begrip posttraumatische stress-stoornis. *ICODO-info.*, **89–4/90–1**, 11–18.

Leliefeld, H. J. (1985). Van KZ-syndroom tot post-traumatisch stress syndroom. In: J. Smeulers, ed., *Martelingen, medische en psychosociale aspecten.* Lochem, De Tijdstroom.

Lira, E., Becker, D., Kovalskys, J., Gómez, E. & Castillo M. I. (1989). Daño Social y Memoria Colectiva: Perspectivas de Reparación. In D. Becker and E. Lira, eds, *Derechos Humanos: Todo es segun el dolor con que se mira.* (s.n.) Instituto Interamericano de Salud Mental y Derechos Humanos.

Lunde, I., Rasmussen, O. V., Lindholm J. & Wagner, G. (1980). Gonadal and sexual functions in tortured Greek men. *Danish Medical Bulletin*, **27**(5) 243–5.

Lycke Ellingsen, I. & Hauff, E. (1988). Psychosocial rehabilitation of refugees in Norway. *International Journal of Mental Health*, **17**(3) 38–45.

Martín Baró, I. (1989). Democracia y Reparación. In D. Becker and E. Lira, eds, *Derechos Humanos: Todo es segun el dolor con que se mira.* (s.n.) Instituto Latinoamericano de Salud Mental y Derechos Humanos.

Neumann, E., Monreal, A. & Macchiavello, C. (1990). Violacion a los Derechos Fundamentales – Reparación Individual y Social. In H. Riquelme U., ed., *Era de Nieblas.* Venezuela, Editorial Nueva Sociedad.

Ploeg, H. M. van der (1985). *Late gevolgen van gijzelingen: Een psychologisch onderzoek bij slachtoffers van gijzelingen in Nederland (1974–1977).* Lisse, Swets & Zeitlinger.

Ploeg, H. M. van der (1985). *Psychologisch onderzoek naar (het ontbreken van) de hulpvraag van slachtoffers van geweld; Deel 2: Gevolgen, hulpvraag en hulpverlener.* Lisse, Swets & Zeitlinger.

Rasmussen, O. V. (1990). Medical aspects of torture. *Danish Medical Bulletin*, **37**(1) 1–88.

Summary report of a working group on Health Hazard of Organized Violence (1987) In *Health Hazards of Organized Violence*. Rijswijk, Ministry of Welfare, Health and Cultural Affairs.

Thorvaldsen, P. (1987). Health Hazards of Organized Violence. In *Health Hazards of Organized Violence*. Rijswijk, Ministry of Welfare, Health and Cultural Affairs.

Willigen, L. H. M. van (1988). De lichamelijke en geestelijke conditie van vluchtelingen in Nederland. *Nederlands Tijdschrift voor Geneeskunde*, **132(27)** 1251–5.

World Health Organisation, Regional Office for Europe (1985). *Targets for Health for All*. Copenhagen.

MULTIDISCIPLINARY APPROACH IN THE TREATMENT OF TORTURE SURVIVORS

Søren Bøjholm and Peter Vesti

INTRODUCTION

Most refugees go into exile unwillingly, hoping that it is only temporary, but this hope often evaporates. The loss of hope, combined with exposure to a new culture, may have a profound effect on the psychological state of the refugee, often leading to behavioural changes such as severe reactions to relatively slight strains. These crisis reactions are described elsewhere in the literature (Melamed *et al.*, 1990).

It is difficult to make reliable estimates of the proportion of torture survivors (a term we prefer to victims) among refugees. Survivors often deny any past experience of torture, while some refugees may make unfounded claims about having been tortured in the hope of obtaining asylum more easily. Nevertheless, it has been estimated that no less than 20–30% of refugees up to 1990 have been tortured. Torture survivors suffer from many of the same severe psychological problems as do other refugees (Melamed *et al.*, 1990), but have also other distinguishing characteristics which make it possible for experienced medical personnel to identify them among refugees. The dissemination of our knowledge on the sequelae of torture beyond the medical profession has enabled professionals from other disciplines to become more efficient in identifying tortured refugees.

REFERRAL PROCEDURES AND SELECTION OF PATIENTS

The survivors referred to the Rehabilitation and Research Centre for Torture Victims (RCT) for treatment constitute a selected group among torture survivors, due to various screening factors. Referrals are usually made by the Danish Refugee Council, general practitioners, or hospital departments, although self-referrals or referrals by independent individuals are also accepted. Because of its limited capacity, the RCT now has a waiting list.

The demographic characteristics of the patients referred to the RCT vary from one year to the next. During the first years of the Centre, the client population consisted mainly of Latin Americans who had come to Denmark with their families. Today, the patients are often single men from the Middle East.

Sometimes a survivor who has been granted asylum in Denmark prefers not to be referred for treatment to the RCT or other similar institutions. He or she may be unwilling to talk about traumatic experiences, either because of the pain involved or because of the suspicion that the treatment centres have ulterior motives in seeking this information. This lack of openness reflects areas of conflict within the individual, as well as the current refugee policy in Denmark.

Some of those on the waiting list never start treatment, or may not want treatment when it is finally offered, or may already have left Denmark. Some may never, in fact, have been exposed to torture, and a few may have been admitted to psychiatric wards because of severe psychoses which we consider best not handled by the RCT. Some survivors may suffer in later life from psychiatric disturbances, such as major depression, which will require proper psychiatric treatment. Such delayed effects are not uncommon and are particularly evident in concentration camp survivors. Detailed data on such delayed effects, however, are still lacking (Winnick, 1967).

RATIONALE FOR SPECIALIZED TREATMENT

Torture survivors, due to the sequelae of torture, have greater difficulty in coping with the problems of living in exile than do other refugees (Vesti & Genefke, this volume). Furthermore, they often have certain psychological problems related to torture that distinguish them from other refugees. Typically these include low self-esteem, lack of trust in others and a chronic state of fear with intense anxiety reactions to apparently harmless words, sounds or events which evoke memories of past torture experience (Juhler & Vesti, 1989; Kastrup *et al.* 1988; Rasmussen, 1990). This is indeed the objective of systematic torture (Somnier & Genefke, 1986).

Following release or escape from prison, the survivors have often had to go in hiding for some time and then face the dangerous and chaotic circumstances of flight into exile. Furthermore, they may still be pursued by the authorities from their home country and live in fear of being sent back. Under such circumstances, their mistrust of other people as well as of authorities may make them reluctant to seek help from public institutions.

PRINCIPLES OF TREATMENT

The principles of treatment at the RCT which were formulated in 1974, are still being developed as part of an ongoing collaboration with individuals and treatment centres in other countries.

Initially, the torture survivors were treated in a ward at the University Hospital in Copenhagen, but it soon proved unsatisfactory to regard them as ordinary patients. They sometimes showed severe anxiety reactions when exposed to hospital surroundings and various examination methods, which all too often resembled the setting in which their torture took place. Most survivors are now treated as outpatients. Hospital admission is occasionally necessary when, for instance, general anaesthesia is required for surgery or other investigations such as colo-rectoscopy.

Previous experience with survivors, particularly concentration camp survivors, indicated a need for a treatment centre with specialized treatment programmes undertaken by specially trained personnel. Similarly, work with torture survivors requires a wide knowledge of torture methods and their effects.

Rehabilitation at the RCT is based on the following main principles:

1 securing the patient's trust and confidence,
2 respect for the individual,
3 avoidance of situations which remind the patient of interrogation or torture,
4 strict adherence to appointment times, and
5 carefully informing the patient about special medical examinations or treatments such as ECG, EEG, or surgery before these procedures are carried out. Professional confidentiality must also be strictly observed during treatment.

In accordance with these principles, the following treatments are administered concurrently:

1 psychotherapy,
2 physical examination and treatment, including ordinary physiotherapy as well as specialized therapy for specific dysfunctions,
3 social advice, and
4 legal advice, when required.

Care is also offered to spouses and children, because the survivor's imprisonment, torture and consequent suffering has often had a traumatic impact on the family. Furthermore, the family may have shared the extremely stressful experience of flight into exile. The family's inability to understand the survivor's excessive emotional reactions such as irritability, anger outbursts, night terrors, etc may cause further problems within the family.

Should the patient prove to be a torturer who has been tortured, his treatment must take place elsewhere, and not at the RCT, because of the other patients.

Treatment starts with an in-depth history-taking which involves an exploration of the ways in which overt symptoms relate to the particular forms of torture sustained.

PRELIMINARY PHYSICAL EXAMINATION

A thorough medical examination is necessary to establish whether the survivor's complaints are due to somatic disease or dysfunction. Many torture survivors present with psychosomatic symptoms and believe that their complaints are of organic origin. Whatever their origin, these complaints should be taken seriously and the patient's right to a full medical examination respected. The therapist should bear in mind that not all symptoms are psychological consequences of torture and avoid the potentially serious mistake of making inferences without full investigation (Juhler, in press). Moreover, these presenting complaints provide an opportunity for the therapist to establish a trusting relationship with the patient which is essential for later psychotherapy.

It is important to enquire about the survivor's state of health before, during, and after torture. During this process, care must be taken not to remind the patient of his or her past experience of interrogation. Because survivors have often been tortured naked, undressing for an examination may trigger severe distress. Certain procedures, such as taking blood for laboratory tests, may recall unpleasant memories of injections of unknown drugs, or of situations in which people were covered with blood. Electrical procedures such as ECG may recall electrical torture; X-ray apparatus, refined torture instruments and confinement in small rooms; examination of mouth and teeth, torture of the teeth; otoscopy, blows to the ears or electrical torture; gynaecological examinations, sexual torture; anascopy and rectoscopy, anal torture. Therefore, the physical examination must be explained to the patient very carefully, and carried out in an atmosphere of trust. If anxiety reactions such as sweating, strained respiration and mydriasis occur, the examination must be discontinued and postponed.

Once the forms of torture and their sequelae suffered by the survivor have been adequately explored, a programme for further physical examinations can be arranged. All survivors undergo standard laboratory tests: haemoglobin, liver function, serum creatinin, routine urine tests, and ECG. These tests usually yield normal results, but they are nevertheless considered necessary as part of a thorough examination, which also serves to reassure the patient that complaints are being taken seriously. The standard programme includes an examination at the School of Dentistry – which often reveals poor dental hygiene and sometimes direct sequelae of torture. Also included in the programme is a rheumatological examination. Most survivors have musculoskeletal symptoms, either due to direct trauma such as blows to the feet or suspension by the limbs, or to chronic stress (Skylv, this volume).

Many survivors believe that the functioning of their internal organs, muscles, bones and joints has been damaged as a result of torture. The standard programme is usually reassuring in this respect. Specialist examinations are occasionally necessary, for example, in cases of eye injuries due to prolonged blindfolding, of ear injuries due to blows or electrical torture to the ear, of injury to sexual organs, anus, or rectum, or of musculoskeletal injuries due to blunt beating. Except when they require anaesthesia, these additional examinations can usually be carried out without hospital admission. When surgery is required, the patients will always be admitted to the special ward at the University Hospital, for treatment by staff experienced in dealing with torture survivors.

Medical examination under anaesthesia may release repressed traumatic material during the pre- or post-anaesthetic phase, a process similar to that which occurs during narcoanalysis. The survivor may then relive past torture experiences and become very agitated. A nurse from the RCT, well known to the patient, will therefore always be present during such procedures. It is also important, particularly in patients previously exposed to asphyxia-inducing torture procedures, not to start artificial ventilation before the patient is deeply asleep.

RCT TREATMENT IN PRACTICE

While the treatment of exiled torture survivors includes established physical and psychological methods, it has also been necessary to develop new methods (Roth *et al.* 1987; Ortmann *et al.* 1987). Post-torture psychological problems often include complaints without apparent organic cause. The psychological treatment of these psychosomatic problems is described elsewhere (Vesti & Genefke, this volume).

Medical treatment

Conditions such as tuberculosis, eczema, high blood pressure, and epilepsy are treated according to established medical practice (Lunde et al. 1981).

Surgical treatment

When surgical treatment is necessary, care needs to be taken that the hospital staff is adequately orientated about the patient's history as a torture survivor. The surgery itself should involve as little pain as possible. Plastic surgery may have to be performed to remove disfiguring scars or to correct fractured noses.

Physiotherapy

Torture survivors may have suffered injury to the musculoskeletal system, depending on the form of torture used. Any sequelae are treated with additional physiotherapy but an understanding of the particular forms of physical torture the patient has suffered is required so as to avoid excessive pain which may evoke memories of past experience. Thus, survivors who have been subjected to suspension by the limbs should not be treated with traction, and therapy in swimming pools should be avoided when treating patients whose torture has involved water.

Most survivors suffer from tension headache. The headache may be due to direct blows on the head, sometimes severe enough to cause loss of consciousness, or to chronic anxiety. Such cases are treated with heat and massage to the galea aponeurotica, the neck, and the shoulder girdle.

Another prominent symptom is painful feet. The chronic condition is often caused by falanga (beating of the soles of the feet), during which the pads of the feet may have been destroyed and the small bones fixed and is treated with mobilization of the joints of the foot, ultrasound, and active movements of the joints to just below the pain threshold. Plaster bandages and special footware may also be used.

A few items of technical equipment are kept in the physiotherapy department. These include a couch, an ultrasound apparatus, an exercise bicycle, and a mattress on the floor with pillows of different sizes. A large mirror may be used in situations where the patient cannot bear the presence of the therapist behind him or her, and needs to know what the therapist is doing. The mirror can also be used to help the patient regain body perception. This is particularly useful in patients who deny and neglect parts of their body – a problem which may prevent a normal sexual life. Physiotherapy usually has a beneficial effect, but many 1-hour sessions may be required. The sessions end with active exercises to build up strength. Physiotherapy is often given either before or after psychotherapy sessions, sometimes with both therapists present (Bloch, 1988).

Nursing care

In addition to their regular duties, the nurses at the RCT are expected to complete a nursing programme for each patient, based on the theory of self-care. Health care is encouraged through training and guidance in nutrition and personal hygiene (Jacobsen & Vesti, 1990).

Dental care

The dentist must be aware that the normal discomfort experienced by most people during dental treatment may be intensified for survivors and even attain phobic proportions. Survivors may fear being constrained in a dentist's chair, as this may evoke memories of torture to their teeth, and such fears may lead to a total avoidance of dentists for many years. Thus, local anaesthesia is often required, together with a very thorough explanation of what the treatment involves. In addition to regular dental care, cosmetic treatment may be needed, especially in younger patients with missing teeth. Treatment with a dental occlusal splint is often needed for patients who complain of myogenic headaches.

Social counselling

Torture survivors' social problems do not differ from those of other refugees, but their treatment can be more difficult. The survivors often have serious language problems, and also suffer from a loss of social status resulting from not being able to work in jobs suited for their professional qualifications. Furthermore, their living conditions are often very poor.

Most survivors have difficulty in contacting authorities (e.g. when pursuing legal matters) because of their social disability. The social worker will often make the contact with relevant authorities and inform them about such difficulties.

Those who cannot cope with classes are offered private lessons in Danish for some time. The teaching is undertaken by a language teacher using the facilities at the Centre where the survivors feel comfortable. After some time they are usually able to attend ordinary classroom teaching.

Housing problems affect nearly all torture survivors. Small rooms or cubicles remind them of the prison cell. The social worker often needs to invest a lot of energy and show creativity in solving the housing problems.

It is often difficult to find a job suited to the patient's original qualifications, mainly because of the differences between vocational training or education in Denmark and that in the patient's home country. The social worker, in co-operation with the authorities, tries to help the survivor obtain additional qualifications.

Many survivors have distressing financial difficulties as most of them live on social security. It is sometimes possible for the social worker, as part of the treatment at the RCT, to obtain supplementary benefit for the survivor on important occasions (Jacobsen & Vesti, 1990).

Social support should be aimed at improving the social conditions of the family, helping them to get acquainted with and integrate into a new society and its institutions. The social advisor should assume the role of a helper and not of a guardian.

Legal issues

The therapist should avoid a judgmental attitude towards the survivor for any past actions. His/her concern should be to help the survivor as much as possible. However, all treatment procedures will be conducted in accordance with the laws and regulations of the country of asylum, including those ratified by international conventions.

Professional confidentiality

Treatment of survivors is built on trust. The patient must feel assured that the therapist will observe strict confidentiality. No one outside the treatment centre should be allowed access to information about the patient without the patient's consent. Even when consent is obtained, the therapist should warn the patient about possible harmful consequences of an oral or written statement.

Liability

The RCT assumes no liability in cases where the patient is not psychotic since the patient is responsible for his or her own acts. Psychotic patients are subject to the relevant Danish laws.

Matters concerning asylum

Patients under treatment at the RCT have already received asylum in Denmark. We sometimes have to help our clients understand certain Danish procedures, for instance those concerning reunion of family members. In such cases, we advise the patients on current regulations and ensure that the law is adhered to.

Matters concerning international law

The United Nations Convention Against Torture was adopted in 1984 and came into force in June of 1987 when it was ratified by 20 countries. At present the Convention has been ratified by more than 50 countries (Council of Europe, 1989). Three aspects of this Convention are of particular relevance to the treatment of torture survivors. First, the Convention clearly states that any form of torture is illegal according to standard laws, both national and international. During treatment it may be useful to stress this point to show the patient that the treatment to which he or she was subjected during imprisonment was a criminal act. Second, under the same Convention, it is possible to punish torturers wherever they might be, even in countries other than the one in which the act was perpetrated. This is important to survivors, who often cannot understand how torturers can go free, either at home or in the same country of exile as themselves. Finally, the Convention states that people cannot be sent back to the country in which they were tortured and where there is a possibility that they may be tortured again. In some cases, this has been of practical value in connection with asylum applications in Denmark, either for close relatives in Denmark who had not yet obtained asylum, or for relatives living in another country where they were insecure and at risk of being sent back to their homeland. Avoiding such expulsions often resulted in a breakthrough in psychotherapy.

CONCLUSION

Torture is a combined and physical and psychological attack on an individual. Our experience has consistently shown that torture leaves scars on both the body and the mind. Therefore, physical treatment, especially physiotherapy, is necessary in conjunction with psychotherapy.

Until now we have chosen a policy to raise public awareness regarding acts of torture and its sequelae. We find it unethical to conduct controlled studies on torture survivors. Last year the RCT completed an investigation on children of torture survivors, which has led to a treatment project on affected children. An evaluation study on psychotherapy outcome in torture survivors is in progress.

REFERENCES

Bloch, I. (1988). Physiotherapy and rehabilitation of torture victims. *Clinical Management in Physical Therapy*, 8, 26–9.

Council of Europe (1989). Explanatory Report on the European Convention for the Prevention of Torture and Inhuman or Degrading Treatment or Punishment. *Council of Europe, Strasbourg, France*.

Jacobsen, L. & Vesti, P. (1990). *Torture Survivors – A New Group of Patients*. Copenhagen: Danish Nurses' Organisation.

Juhler, M. & Vesti, P. (1989). Torture: diagnosis and rehabilitation. *Medicine and War*, 5, 69–79.

Juhler, M. (1991). Physical complaints and findings in torture survivors. In *The International Handbook of Traumatic Stress Syndrome. New York: Plenum Press*. (In press).

Kastrup, M., Genefke, I. K., Lunde, I. & Ortmann, J. (1988). Coping with the exposure to torture. *Contemporary Family Therapy*, 10, 280–7.

Lunde, I., Rasmussen, O. V., Wagner, G. & Lindholm, J. (1981). Sexual and pituitary–testicular function in torture victims. *Archives of Sexual Behavior*, 10, 25–32.

Melamed, B. G., Melamed, J. L. & Bouhoutsos, J. C. (1990). Psychological consequences of torture – a need to formulate new strategies for research. P. Suedfeld, ed. *Psychology and Torture*. Hemisphere Publishing Corporation.

Ortmann, J., Genefke, I. K., Jacobsen, L. & Lunde, I. (1987). Rehabilitation of torture victims: an interdisciplinary treatment model. *American Journal of Social Psychiatry*, 7, 161–7.

Rasmussen, O. V. (1990). Medical aspects of torture. *Danish Medical Bulletin*, 37 (suppl. 1), 1–88.

Roth, E. F., Lunde, I., Boysen, G. & Genefke, I. K. (1987). Torture and its treatment. *American Journal of Public Health*, 77, 1404–6.

Somnier, F. E. & Genefke, I. K. (1986). Psychotherapy for victims of torture. *British Journal of Psychiatry*, 149, 323–9.

United Nations Convention Against Torture and Other Cruel, Inhuman or Degrading Treatment or Punishment (1984). *United Nations, Geneva.*

Winnick, H. Z. (1967). Further comments concerning problems of late psychopathological effects on Nazi persecution and their therapy. *Israel Annals of Psychiatry and Related Disciplines,* **5,** 1–16.

14
SEXUAL TORTURE AND THE TREATMENT OF ITS CONSEQUENCES
Inge Lunde and Jørgen Ortmann

INTRODUCTION

Although numerous investigations have been conducted on torture, relatively little has been written on sexual torture. In publications about concentration camp survivors (Thygesen et al., 1970; Eitinger, 1969; Strøm, 1968; Kral, 1951; Kral, Pazder & Wigdor, 1967), or the Korean (Beebe, 1975) and Vietnam War veterans (Golub, 1985; Rosenheck, 1985), sexual torture is either not mentioned or referred to indirectly as, for example, 'mental torture of a very sadistic type'. These articles, however, often acknowledge the existence of sexual problems resulting from severe stress or torture.

In 1974, the Danish Medical Group within Amnesty International, of which the first author (IL) was part, initiated and systematised the examination of torture survivors. Although the prevalence of sexual torture was not reported in our initial publications (Amnesty International, 1977; Rasmussen, Dam & Lunde, 1977; Amnesty International 1978a; Amnesty International, 1980; Rasmussen & Lunde, 1980), we were aware of the fact that both physical and psychological torture involved sexual assaults. However, sexual problems were reported for subsamples (Amnesty International, 1978b; Lunde et al., 1981). A later survey (Lunde, 1981) found that 53% of 135 torture survivors had been subjected to sexual torture. Other studies do not include information on the total prevalence of sexual torture, but some give prevalence figures on specific forms. Allodi & Cowgill (1982) noted that 43% of 41 survivors had been tortured by 'sexual molestation' defined as touching, stripping and attempted rape, and 15% had been raped. Domovitch et al. (1984) found that 23% of 104 survivors had been subjected to blows to the genitals, 41% to electrical torture to the genitals and/or anus, 12% to sexual abuse and 53% to forced undressing. An official report by the Salvadorian Human Rights Organization (1986) on 434 male prisoners indicated that 19% had received blows to the testicles, 58% had been stripped naked, 5% were raped and 15% were threatened with rape. No data on the total prevalence of sexual torture were given. Based on these figures, Agger and Jensen (1988) estimated the prevalence of sexual torture in the Salvadorian sample to be 62%. In a review article Goldfeld *et al.* (1988) concluded that the true prevalence of sexual torture is unknown.

Between 1975 to 1987, the present authors took part in the clinical examination of 283 torture survivors. 135 survivors were examined from 1975–1979 (Rasmussen & Lunde, 1980), while 148 survivors were examined (and treated) in 1984–1987 (Lunde, Boysen & Ortmann, 1987; Ortmann & Lunde, 1988). As scientific literature on sexual torture as well as on sexual problems was very sparse, we set up a project to analyse our accumulated findings (Lunde & Ortmann, 1990). In the first group of 135 torture survivors (109 male, 26 female, mean age 31 years, range 17–59, 85% in the age range 20–39) each examination was carried out by two doctors and consisted of a semi-structured interview about the survivor's former state of health, imprisonments, methods of torture and after-effects, and a clinical assessment. An interpreter was present during almost every examination. The torture survivors were examined in their native country, in Denmark as refugees, or in a third country. In the second group of 148 torture survivors (119 male, 29 female, mean age 35 years (19–67), 74% 20–39) the examinations were carried out by doctors and psychologists according to a structured interview and examination form. The main questions were about previous state of health, imprisonments, methods of torture applied, and current after-effects. An interpreter was present during almost every examination. The prevalence of sexual torture in the sample (283) was analysed in elation to gender, framework of examination (group 1 vs group 2), and ethnic groups. In the analysis of sexual difficulties subsequent to torture the non-sexually tortured victims were used as controls. The prevalence of sexual difficulties was analysed in relation to age, sex, framework of examination, ethnic groups and sexual torture. The group 2 population was used to estimate the prevalence of sexual difficulties in relation to age, gender, ethnic groups, sexual torture, anxiety, low self-esteem and depression. The chi-square test was applied in the analysis of the relationship between sexual torture and ethnic groups. Logistic regression was applied in all other analyses.

Of the 283 torture survivors from 21 different countries, 198 were refugees with asylum in Denmark, 16 had asylum in other countries and 69 were examined in their home countries. The following discussion is based on data from this study.

SEXUAL TORTURE

We defined and categorised sexual torture as 1) violence against the sexual organs; 2) physical sexual assault, i.e. sexual acts involving direct physical sexual contact between victim and torturers, between victims, between victim and an animal, or all three; 3) mental sexual assault, i.e. forced nakedness, sexual humiliations, sexual threats and witnessing others being sexually tortured; 4) a combination of the three. Within each of these principal groups there is a wide range of sexual torture methods. Furthermore, sexual torture is often carried out in conjunction with other torture, both physical and psychological.

These definitions are based on what the individual survivor reported as being for him or her sexual torture. Clearly, the perception of what is or is not sexual torture depends on the cultural background, education and social status of the survivor and may vary from nationality to nationality. No scientific studies have been carried out on this, but it appears that, independent of nationality, assaults against sexual organs and physical abuse by rape and other forms of direct sexual physical contact, as well as forced sexual contact with animals, are generally experienced as sexual torture by most people. The important issue is that the victim is subjected to *involuntary* sexual acts which, precisely because they are involuntary, are very painful.

Regardless of the survivors' individual sexual preference or individual manner of sexual outlet, it is the torturers' purpose to destroy the survivors' sexuality. The forms of sexual torture are gleaned from the individual's reactions while subjected to torture or while observing others being tortured and/or torture inferred. The survivors' background history can also be used to determine the vulnerable points for sexual torture. It is within this area that doctors and psychologists are able to refine torture methods.

From our results (Lunde & Ortmann, 1990) we have set out what in different cultures is experienced as sexual torture. In western, Christian and in some Islamic countries, it would not be experienced as sexual torture if torturers removed a woman's headscarf, thereby exposing her hair to a foreign male; however, for some Iranian, religious women (after the Islamic revolution in that country), it is not only sexually degrading, but also a reason for the authorities to put that woman into prison. Some would argue that it is not sexual torture, but religious. In the principal religions such as Islam, Buddhism, Hinduism and Christianity, male and female sexual morals and behaviour are defined. Even in countries where people are not very religious, it is characteristic that, in some way, the norms and morals are in compliance with former religious beliefs. That is to say, in different countries one might observe different aspects of what is considered effective in implementing sexual torture.

Never having been exposed to a torture situation, people from the West cannot imagine that to be exhibited naked is torture at all. Of course, it might be humiliating, but not sexually so. This is not the viewpoint of the torture survivors. They all, independent of culture, had experienced forced nakedness as not only humiliating, but also as a sexual assault. This is emphasized by the illustration of torture in Iran, where after execution the sexual organs of the dead prisoners were exposed to be viewed by their remaining fellow prisoners. The dead body as such was not enough to intimidate the prisoners. Only those who have been subjected to sexual torture can tell us what it is.

As part of physical and psychological sexual torture, it is characteristic for torturers to attack sexual identity and/or reproductive abilities. When torturers torture a man in his anus, they proclaim him gay or 'no longer a man'. Coupled with physical violence against sexual organs, regardless of whether the victim is male or female, the torturers say that now it will no longer be possible to have children or should offspring be produced, then the child will be deformed. In general, the torturers attempt to indoctrinate torture survivors with the belief that they will never be able to tell anyone of the activities within the torture chamber, and this applies especially to sexual torture.

CONSEQUENCES OF SEXUAL TORTURE

To show the specific consequences which are a direct result of sexual torture is complicated, not least because all the examined torture survivors have been subjected to other, non-sexual, physical and psychological torture.

Physical

With certain types of physical and sexual torture it is, however possible to describe resultant physical consequences. *Immediately after* electrical torture and/or blows to the genital region, one may find haematuria due to injuries to the urethra and bladder. Blows to the scrotum can result immediately in severe swelling while use of cutting, burning implements and caustic agents results in scar tissue wounds on genital organs and consequent scar transformation. The introduction of objects into the vagina and rectum can result in injury to these organs. During direct sexual contact, whether vaginal or rectal, venereal infection, including AIDS, can be transmitted and can, just as other urogenital infections, be passed on. In women, acute vaginal bleeding often occurs. Blows to the uterus of a pregnant woman can cause aborting, coupled with severe complications, as is often the purpose. Rape by the torturers can impregnate the female victim.

Later, other physical signs are evident: in men atrophy of testes and alteration in epididymis, hydrocele, changes in the spermatic cord, prostate as well as sterility. In women, vaginal scar changes are in evidence and injury of the uterus which can obstruct full-term pregnancy. Moreover, menstrual disorder and infertility is ascertained. In addition, destruction of breast tissue is found with resultant necrosis of the papillae so that a mother cannot breastfeed her infant. In both sexes, changes of the anus are evident by fissure, vascular change and splitting of the sphincter muscle. Additionally, changes in the rectum are found, such as injury to the mucus membranes and vascular tissue. The prevalence of later signs in the genital organs as a result of sexual torture is only described in a single study of 61 torture survivors (Lunde *et al.*, 1988). Signs were registered in 31%.

Psychological

A psychological symptom is the reliving of sexual torture triggered by certain situations such as sexual intercourse or in dreams. In daily life, seeing a person who resembles the torturer, a newspaper article, a television program, or pictures in a magazine may recall memories of past torture and evoke intense fear, anger or even panic.

If degrading and insulting comments were made about the sexual appeal or ability of the survivor or his/her sex or sexual preference was called into question, this might result in a rejection of, and disgust, for the survivor's own body, and anxiety over sexual involvement, and over a dubious sexual identity and preferences. The destruction of the survivor's sexual identity might result in an experience of being asexual despite the survivor intellectually knowing him/herself to be male or female. This feeling of being asexual causes great uncertainty. A male survivor stated: 'I was at a gathering where I felt one of the men present "made eyes at me" and made a sexually inviting gesture. I remembered the torture situation where the tormentors forced a large bottle into my anus and said that I was no longer a man; then they laughed. I thought perhaps I had changed or maybe that was what I was supposed to feel. I was terribly uncertain. But I feel no sexual desire or attraction either toward men or women – I am sexually dead.'

The torturers' statements that the victim will be unable to have children later on, or should this occur, then the children will be deformed, can lead to the fear of sterility or the fear of bearing deformed children. A married, female torture survivor with two children explained: 'My oldest daughter is growing up and wants to talk to me about sex, but I withdraw and rudely reject her because I am angry, angry with my tormentors, I am discouraged because of that which happened to me. I don't feel like a woman any longer and I hate my body, particularly my womb. Therefore, I agreed to sterilisation, because I am certain that if I gave birth to a child now, after being tortured, it would not only be physically deformed but also psychologically marred. I have guilt feelings enough in respect of the children I already have – particularly my daughter.'

Sexual problems

Another consequence of sexual torture is sexual problems. However, these problems can also occur in survivors who are not sexually tortured.

Few studies have examined the prevalence of post-torture sexual problems. Lunde *et al.* (1981) found that 29% of tortured men suffered from sexual dysfunction. In another study (Allodi & Cowgill, 1982) 12% of the patients suffered from severe sexual dysfunction, but no definition of sexual dysfunction or severity was given. A third study (Domovitch *et al.*, 1984) reported a figure of 51%, but this was based on a subgroup of patients for whom some information on sexual problems was available (26% in the entire sample).

In our study of 283 torture survivors (Lunde & Ortmann, 1990), 32% reported sexual problems. A higher incidence of sexual problems was noted in survivors from Turkey, the Middle East and the Orient. The problems included reduced libido, erectile dysfunction, ejaculatory dysfunction (premature ejaculation, retarded ejaculation, oozing of seed), orgastic dysfunction, painful intercourse, disgust with sex, fear of sexual involvement, and concern over permanent injury to sexual organs, infertility or having deformed children. Uncertainty and anxiety concerning one's self and own body were pronounced.

In the same study, we examined the relationship between the prevalence of sexual problems and sexual torture. Of the sexually tortured survivors 40% reported sexual problems in comparison with only 19% of non-sexually tortured survivors. The difference was statistically significant and independent of age, sex, country of origin and clinical variables such as depression.

Social and cross-generational consequences

The physical and psychological influences of sexual torture listed above often have serious social consequences such as divorce and ostracization of raped women and of homosexually raped men.

An important consequence is the influence on the next generation. The effects of torture in general on the second generation are described in several publications (Allodi, 1980; Kestenberg, 1980; Axelrod, Schnipper & Rau, 1980; Danieli, 1981; Grubrich-Simitis, 1981; Cohn *et al.*, 1985). The most common consequences are psychological and psychosomatic symptoms such as anxiety, insomnia, introversion, behaviour difficulties, enuresis, headache and stomach ache. Parents with uncertain sexual identity, uncertain sexual preferences and problematic sexual functioning cannot help but affect the sexual development and later sexual functionability of their children.

TREATMENT OF THE CONSEQUENCES OF TORTURE

Background

As the foundation for any endeavour to treat illness and trauma, it is mandatory to establish a method for examination as well as treatment. The descriptions of Methods and Results of the preliminary investigations relevant to torture survivors have been previously published (Evidence of Torture, 1977; Rasmussen *et al.*, 1977; Report of an Amnesty International Mission to Northern Ireland, 1977; Report of an Amnesty International Mission to Spain, 1980; Report of an Amnesty International Medical Seminar, 1978; Amnesty International Manual for Medical Groups, 1979). As a result, investigative methods were further developed and a treatment model evolved (Lunde *et al.*, 1985; Agger *et al.*, 1985; Somnier & Genefke, 1986; Lunde, Boysen & Ortmann, 1987; Ortmann *et al.*, 1987; Roth *et al.*, 1987; Kastrup *et al.*, 1986, 1987, 1988; Ortmann & Lunde, 1988; Lunde *et al.*, 1988; Rasmussen & Lunde, 1989).

Treatment of the consequences of sexual torture will always constitute a part of *our total general treatment programme for torture survivors*. This includes general medical treatment, psychotherapy, physiotherapy, dental treatment, social counselling and treatment of the family (Lunde *et al.*, 1987). As the basis for describing the more specific treatment of the consequences of sexual torture, we have found it important to summarize two areas.

Psychotherapy[1] and physiotherapy – general principles

In psychotherapy we use a wide spectrum of treatment modalities: psychoanalytical psychotherapy, Gestalt therapy, behavioural therapy, cognitive therapy and pharmacotherapy. Within the above methods auxiliary techniques of dream analysis, psycho-drama and role-playing are used.

Psychotherapy focuses on the trauma of torture. Theoretically it can be divided into the following stages:

Establishing contact and confidence

This is obviously a prerequisite for any form of therapy. In the case of torture survivors, however, this process is more difficult and takes longer than with other patients. Most survivors typically explore and test the therapist's credibility and capability during this phase. This is due to a lack of confidence in others arising from their past torture experience.

The cognitive stage

The survivor is encouraged to reconceptualize what actually happened during torture. We ask the survivor to recount the torture down to the minutest detail. The therapist then tries to make the survivor understand the real aim of torture, and to understand that all responsibility and guilt must rightly be placed on the torturers. The therapist must clarify that during torture the survivor was faced with a series of impossible choices, and that his or her answers to the interrogators' questions made no difference whatsoever; other people would have been endangered and/or hurt regardless of what he/she said. Such a situation is best illustrated thus. When taken into custody, the authorities demand the names of friends. Should the detainee refuse to give the requested information, he is told that his wife or another family member will be imprisoned, tortured or worse, shot. However, if names are given then these persons will be imprisoned, tortured or even shot. No matter whom the detainee chooses to defend, the consequences of his choice will be unacceptable to him – a double bind situation – 'The impossible choice'.

---

[1] This method was developed by the first author in 1985. It has been presented in Denmark in 1985, Turkey in January 1988, Norway in March 1988 and in Australia in May 1988.

The emotional stage

Here there is a further development from the cognitive phase. Often the survivor's defense mechanisms function well and even while describing torture with his intellect he does not relate all that happened, he eliminates emotion in the telling to avoid reliving the experience. In the emotional stage the therapist encourages the torture survivor to act out repressed emotions of anger, sorrow, hatred and rage.

The torture experiences are returned to the past

Many torture survivors feel that torture is a perpetual state and experience it as in the present tense. To reach the point where torture is placed in the past, and is now finished, is a difficult process. Naturally, the process starts with the initial treatment session and continues concurrently throughout, yet it is characteristic that one must first go through the above stages before any radical improvement is evident.

Restoring of identity

To destroy the survivor's personality is an important aim of torture. Many torture survivors later complain of changed identity (72%) as well as low self-esteem (70%) including a negative perception of their own bodies (Ortmann & Lunde, 1988). During stages 1–4 some reinstatement of identity occurs, and in stage 5 concentrated emphasis is placed on this; the therapists also actively focus on issues of self-esteem and body perception.

Plans for the future

If the therapy has been successful, the survivor will now be able to conceive a plan for his/her future.

Certain auxiliary techniques can help facilitate progress during psychotherapy. For example, the survivor may be asked to use a tape recorder to express his/her feelings or thoughts as they occur, typically at night, when the therapist is not present. Then the tape is reviewed during the next therapy session, and in that way the survivor is in control of how much is to be 'processed' at any one time. Therapeutic drawing is used where the torture situation can be depicted. Visual material is an important element in helping stimulate memory and/or breaking down resistance. This material can be newsclippings, photographs, dias/slides or videotapes. As a special form of teatment use is also made of aquarelles painted by an artist, who had himself been subjected to torture. This material consists of 12 plaques which depict torture situations as well as the victim's inner feelings during and after torture.

Physiotherapy

Physiotherapy will also proceed in a series of steps. It starts with an interview during which the physiotherapist's treatment is explained and where initial contact and confidence begins. The psychotherapist is normally present during this first meeting. An important prerequisite for selecting the relevant forms of physiotherapy is that the physiotherapist is acquainted with the torture form to which the survivor has been subjected. It is particularly important during the initial phase that the physiotherapist does not inflict pain; quite the opposite, the therapist must alleviate pain. At the first meeting, one must evaluate the extent to which it will be possible to ask the patient to undress. It will often be the case that the first treatment must be carried out on fully clothed patients.

The physiotherapy we use is based on traditional methods and techniques such as massage, thermotherapy, ultrasound, posture correcting exercises, pool treatment, physical training in general, laser and TNS (trancutaneous nerve stimulation). With regard to massage, it is important that the initial treatment is only gentle massage and not tapotement. Common mechanical traction on columna cannot be used, it being mandatory that manual traction is applied. In addition, grounding, touching, confidence-body training and training in front of a full-figure mirror are used.

SPECIFIC TREATMENT OF CONSEQUENCES OF SEXUAL TORTURE

As a rule, examination and treatment follow the principles outlined above, but additional and special measures and techniques can be employed.

Considerations in selecting interpreter and therapist

Age, sex and cultural background are generally important factors to be considered, and when speaking of sexually tortured survivors it is vital. Moreover, the therapist's educational background is also of importance. With clinical experience from examinations and treatment of torture survivors who came from a variety of cultures, we (IL and JO) generally found that all of them wanted common medical treatment. Many had difficulty in accepting the necessity for psychological treatment, even though psychic symptoms were acknowledged. When the torture survivor did accept psychotherapy, persons from Latin America often preferred a psychologist as therapist. Survivors from other countries were frequently suspicious of psychologists as well as psychiatrists, but after learning that a psychiatrist is first trained as a physician, then most preferred a psychiatrist. In general, they preferred a therapist older than or the same age as themselves, as they felt that such a therapist would be more experienced than someone younger.

In ETICA Treatment Centre, we have the following general guidelines. The interpreter and therapist should be older than (or possibly contemporaries of) the torture survivor. For women who have been sexually tortured, both interpreter and therapist must be female. In respect of sexually tortured men, it is preferable that the interpreter and therapist be male. However, we have experienced that some male torture survivors have difficulty in speaking freely to men, but find it easier to relate to women.

With regard to cultural background, it is often advantageous if the interpreter is from the same cultural environment but not the same country, as the torture survivor may be suspicious of fellow countrymen. The same guidelines should apply to the therapist, but in treating torture survivors in exile, this is seldom possible.

To date, no experience is available concerning physiotherapists as all of our clients are treated by female therapists, who are Danish and about 40 years of age.

In addition to the specific guidelines listed above, it is of the *utmost* importance that both the interpreter and the therapists have a well-defined and harmonious view of their own sexuality. This is necessary to minimize the risk of ambigious sexual signals being given during treatment. Therapists should have knowledge (e.g. education) of sexology and also be responsible for the education of the interpreter in this specific area.

The initial interview

Here, one usually receives clear information on the physical, violent sexual torture and on its direct physical consequences. Information on other, more specific sexual torture, as a rule, usually comes later, while other consequences of a more psychological character emerge during subsequent treatments.

Treatment of the physical sequelae

The treatment of the physical consequences of sexual torture is conducted along the lines of current medical practice. The specialists who will undertake the patient's medical treatment should be adequately informed regarding the nature of torture suffered, so that measures can be taken to avoid situations likely to evoke intense emotional reactions in the patient during medical procedures such as gynaecological examination or surgery. In the likelihood of such events full anaesthesia would normally be used. Often the male client will be afraid that sexual torture has caused injury to the sexual organs during homosexual rape, e.g. injury to anus or rectum, along with damage to testes. In females a similar fear is present of damage to vagina, ovaries and uterus, as well as to anus/rectum if raped that way. In this connection, it is immensely important to have specialists undertake thorough examinations either to confirm or reject the need for corrective treatment and, if needed, to establish the extent of treatment required. Completion of such examinations has a therapeutic value in itself in that it clarifies the situation.

Psychotherapy/physiotherapy – parallel treatments

In psychotherapy one considers sexual torture in depth and the feelings connected with it, while parallel treatment is given with physiotherapy to the bodily areas affected by the sexual torture. Quite often, it is at this point one first receives information regarding special forms of sexual torture. Further, it does sometimes happen that clients, who previously had not mentioned sexual torture, now come forward with such information. It can occur during the general review of torture experiences – in psychotherapy; in physiotherapy it may happen when the physiotherapist simply touches the client and so releases a reaction. Moreover, the physiotherapist may have ascertained a stiff pelvis and from that alone have become suspicious that sexual torture has taken place, and so consciously provoked the client to relate the experience.

In psychotherapy, use is made of picture material with sexual torture situations. These pictures have been produced by an artist who is also a torture survivor. The material is used partly to provoke and wear down resistance, and partly as proof that others have also been victims of that particular form of sexual torture, the latter being extremely important, as the majority of clients believe that he/she is the only one who has been subjected to precisely that particular form of sexual torture.

In psychotherapy the therapist is often confronted with the information that the torturers used 'swear words'. Although meeting with great resistance from the client, it is vitally important that the therapist discovers what lay behind these 'swear words'; it is mandatory that the therapist is active in taking the lead, even provoking the client. Our experience shows that underneath these words often lurks psychological sexual torture which the client felt was the worst torture: 'Your mother is a whore, you are not a man, you are homosexual, everyone will be disgusted with you'.

In psychotherapy one can observe short-lived reactive psychoses with deterioration of consciousness (micropsychoses), provoked by using certain words, pictures or other techniques. Equally so, the physiotherapeutic treatment can affect a state in which the torture survivor is remote and without contact with the therapist, and where he/she finds him/herself returned to the torture situation. Reactions of this type can be consciously or unconsciously called forth; in both circumstances, the reaction can be used therapeutically. It demands a close co-operation between the physiotherapist and the psychotherapist because, as is quite obvious, the client must not be abandoned in a therapeutic void.

An illustration of this is provided by the case of a young man, 17 years old, who was arrested and tortured, exposed to many different forms of physical and psychological torture, and who, in consequence, had severe difficulties. In physiotherapy as well as psychotherapy he was very co-operative, and as a result his health improved greatly within a few months. The psychotherapist had been informed that among other things he had been tortured by a female torturer and that she had been the worst of all. She employed the good/bad technique: She was first caring, solicitous and friendly towards him, but when he did not confess to his alleged deeds, she was completely different the next day scolding and hitting him very hard with, among other things, a rifle butt. The psychotherapist had a suspicion that this torture was central to his case and should be clarified. But, in spite of all the efforts of the psychotherapist to reach this core, there was no progress. One day, when the physiotherapist asked the survivor to carry out certain arm exercises where he was to say 'get out' (to signify that the pain should go away), the client suddenly was distant. It was impossible for the phyisotherapist to get through to him despite persistent attempts. That condition lasted only a few minutes. The client slowly returned to awareness, to the fact that he was physically in Copenhagen. Thereafter, he was able to explain that he had been on a trip to his homeland and had been in a certain torture situation. It was the torture situation in which the female torturer had used degrading words which sounded the same as the Danish therapist's 'get out'. The day following this episode, the client was treated by the psychotherapist who had, in the meantime, been informed of the above occurrence. Once again, the psychotherapist asked the client what had happened in the actual torture situation. It was only now that the client was able to relate what he had previously withheld. The female torturer, in addition to subjecting him generally to humiliating and physical torture, had administered psychological sexual torture as well in that she had called him gay and yelled at him degradingly that he was nothing and that he should *'get out'* (or what in his language sounded the same), he was horrible and no one could respect him any longer. This information could be utilized by the psychotherapist, the greatest torture trauma had now been revealed.

Some sexually tortured survivors relive the sexual torture while having sexual intercourse with their partner, and react by using the same defence mechanisms which would have been appropriate when they were being subjected to sexual torture, but which are destructive in the present circumstances. A commonly used defence mechanism is 'cut off the head from the body and think of something beautiful'. The following illustrates that reaction. One of our clients, when she saw herself in the mirror, could only see her face even though the mirror was large enough to reflect her whole body. A particularly negative body awareness is connected with this. At times there is no body awareness at all.

In psychotherapy, the sexual trauma is revived, analysed, dealt with, and in that way the inappropriate defence mechanisms are slowly removed. The therapist strives to re-establish a normal, realistic perception and general, realistic self-awareness within the sexual area, and this includes reestablishing self-awareness of one's own body. Obviously, this therapy demands a very close co-operation between the physiotherapist and the psychotherapist. In this context, it is useful if common treatment sessions are held with both therapists present. This is the time that a full-figure mirror and physiotherapy exercises among other things are utilized; also, the physiotherapist and the psychotherapist participate to some extent in the session so that the client can form a realistic body awareness by comparison with the therapists' bodies and body language(s). The circumstances are also conducive to making the client understand that it is not a torture situation where sexual attack is imminent, but, on the contrary, he/she is in a treatment session where he/she can move freely about and where there are no torturers.

As long as the torture survivor is living within a stable relationship, sex therapy can be used, such as the Masters and Johnson method with individual modifications, while also taking into consideration the sexual torture the individual survivor has been subjected to as well as the cultural group to which he/she belongs. It is important to ensure that the survivor's spouse knows which type of sexual torture the survivor has been subjected to before commencing the actual sexual therapy. Quite often it is true that the survivor has never told the spouse anything about the torture. Such information could be introduced during an interview where both partners are present; the therapist makes the proposal, but it is the torture survivor who decides wheher he/she finds it acceptable. As part of the treatment, it may prove necessary to give sex education. Here we use pictures showing the male and female inner and outer sexual organs; also given are descriptions of intercourse, impregnation, pregnancy and birth. The visual material must be of a high professional quality so that it does not appear pornographic – a good deal of the available visual material in books in western countries might be experienced as pornographic. Quality drawings are preferable to photographs.

If the torture survivor has children, it is generally important that the therapist be aware of where they are, how they live and their general situation. When it comes to the children of families where one or both parents have been sexually tortured, it is vital for the therapist to have these facts.

Should the torture survivor be alone with children, his/her sexual torture and its consequences usually affect the children. As far as couples are concerned, the above also applies, with the additional effect of the parents' mutual sexual problems. The children learn to reject their own bodies, they have problems in developing a sexual identity as well as having a remoteness from later sexual functioning.

Thus, it is important that the therapist takes the initiative to help the children and, if necessary, establish family therapy.

TREATMENT RESULTS

Publications concerning treatment results are very few and preliminary. Larsen and Lopez, 1987, had positive results in a pilot project on relaxation treatment in connection with psychotherapy. In a retrospective study of 148 torture survivors, we found that 74% felt better and 18% were cured (Ortmann & Lunde, 1988, Lunde & Ortmann, 1990).[1] The treatment results are registered on the basis of a total evaluation of the torture survivors' psychological and physical condition, as well as ability to function socially.

We stress that our design was retrospective, and so far no follow-up examinations have been undertaken. It remains unknown whether, after what period, a relapse occurs.

In regard to this, one naturally queries whether torture survivors are not cured spontaneously with the passage of time? With this in mind, it could be justifiable to allow enough time to elapse without giving professional treatment, presuming the result would be exactly the same whether treatment had been given or not.

It would be most desirable, and an appreciable saving of public funds, if 'time cured all wounds'. However, previous experiences with concentration camp survivors and POWs has shown that time alone is not sufficient to bring about a cure. It was generally believed that the only treatment necessary for a former concentration camp prisoner was to re-establish the proper level of nourishment. But 25 years after prisoners' release, Danish scientists, among others, found that quite the opposite was true. An advancing condition of deroute occurred physically as well as psychologically and this was described scientifically as the concentration camp syndrome (Thygesen et al., 1970).

It has also been found in our examinations that there is no indication of spontaneous recovery of torture survivors. The majority of torture survivors, who are included in the study under review, have been subjected to torture between 8 and 10 years before being examined and tested.

Therefore, it is important that the professionals within the health and welfare sectors are aware that the torture survivor cannot cure him/herself, so that use can be made of the experiences gained from previous wars' torture survivors: both give treatment for the actual injuries and guard against eruption of latent consequences.

In our opinion, to be able to determine the type and degree of

[1] *Cured* is defined as: the torture survivor feels healthy and has a normal ability to socialize, regardless of possible residual symptoms due to permanent injuries, and has, after clinical examination and evaluation, proved capable of adjusting to his/her own psychological and physical limitations.
  Improved is defined as: the sequelae of torture are reduced but the client is still impaired physically, psychologically and socially. This is evaluated by clinical examination in which reduced symptoms and fewer objections are found than when treatment started.

torture consequences as well as their extent, and to evaluate treatment methods and treatment effect, it is mandatory that prospective research in this area be undertaken on a global plan, anywhere and everywhere where work with the treatment of torture survivors is carried out. Research should, in our opinion, be carried out following various designs so that it is possible to attain maximum knowledge.

Generally, the epidemiological model should be utilized in this respect. Also the prospective design should be used; likewise the causistical method could be employed for a qualitative analysis of treatment results.

Intervention and action research methods are also serviceable. A traditional method such as the controlled clinical test can be used as long as pharmacological treatment is used.

Another controlled method is that of continuous EEG registering during sleep with a view to controlling the effect(s) of treatment. The description of design and preliminary results are found in Åstrøm *et al.*, 1989.

Finally, there is the consensus method. This must be carried out by impartial, professionally qualified persons, and on the basis of anonymous, blind descriptions of health and treatment. A suggestion for prospective research projects have been described by Lunde *et al.*, 1987.

Accumulation of knowledge could be enhanced and achieved more speedily if multicentre research were to be conducted in accordance with a common protocol. This should involve professionals from different countries with different cultural backgrounds and experiences in the examination and treatment of torture survivors. Such a project might result in knowledge as yet non-existent. This applies not least to the area of sexual torture where research so far is sparse.

REFERENCES

Åstrøm, C., Lunde, I., Ortmann, J., Boysen, G. & Trojaborg, W. (1989). Sleep disturbances in torture survivors. *Acta Neurologica Scandinavica*, **79**, 150–4.

Agger, I., Duarte, A., Genefke, I. K. & Lunde I. (1985). Torture victims – on the psychotherapy of refugees who have been submitted to torture. *Nordisk Psykologi*, **37**, 177–92.

Agger, I. & Jensen, S. B. (1988). Den potentielle ydmygelse – seksuel tortur af mandlige politiske fanger: nedbrydningsstrategier overfor mandling potens. *Nordisk Sexologi*, **6**, 31–54.

Allodi, F. (1980). The psychiatric effects of political persecution and torture in children and families of victims. *Canadian Mental Health*, **28**, 8–10.

Allodi, F. & Cowgill, G. (1982). Ethical and psychiatric aspects of torture. *Canadian Journal of Psychiatry*, **27**, 98–102.

Amnesty International (1977). *Evidence of Torture: Studies by the Amnesty International Danish Medical Group.* London: Amnesty International Publications.

Amnesty International (1978a). Report of an Amnesty International Mission to Northern Ireland, 28.XI–6.XII, 1977. London: *Amnesty International Publications.*

Amnesty International (1978b). Report of An Amnesty International Medical Seminar: Violations of Human Rights: Torture and the Medical Profession, Athens 10–11.III, 1978. London, *Amnesty International Publications.*

Amnesty International (1979). *Manual for Medical Groups.* Copenhagen. Amnesty International Publications.

Amnesty International (1980). Report of an Amnesty International Mission to Spain, 3–28 October 1979. London, *Amnesty International Publications.*

Axelrod, S., Schnipper, O. L. & Rau, J. H. (1980). Hospitalized offspring of Holocaust survivors. Problems and dynamics. *Bulletin of the Menninger Clinic,* **44,** 1–14.

Beebe, G. W. (1975). Follow-up Studies of World War II and Korean War Prisoners. *American Journal of Epidemiology,* **101,** 400–22.

Cohn, J., Danielsen, L., Holzer, K. I. M., Koch, L., Severin, B., Thøgersen, S. & Aalund, O. (1985). A study of Chilean refugee children in Denmark. *The Lancet,* **331,** 437–8.

Comisión de Derechos de El Salvador (CDHES). (1986). Torture in El Salvador. The 'La Esperanxa' ('HOPE') Prison, Ayutuxtepeque, San Salvador, El Salvador: Stencil.

Danieli, Y. (1981). The group project for Holocaust Survivors and their children. *Children Today,* **5,** 11 and 33.

Domovitch, E., Berger, P. B., Waver, M. J. et al. (1984). Human torture: description and sequelae of 104 cases. *Canadian Family Physician,* **30,** 827–30.

Eitinger, L. (1969). Rehabilitation of concentration camp survivors (following concentration camp trauma). In Th. Spoerri, Bern, W. Th. Winkler, Gütersloh, eds, *Proceedings of the 7th International Congress of Psychotherapy, Wiesbaden 1967, Part V: Rehabilitation Psychotherapy and Psychosomatics.* Basel/New York, S. Karger.

Goldfeld, A. E., Mollica, R. F., Pesavento, B. H. & Faraone, S. V. (1988). The physical and psychological sequelae of Torture. Symptomatology and Diagnosis. *Journal of the American Medical Association,* **259,** 2725–9.

Golub, D. (1985). Symbolic expression in posttraumatic stress disorder: Vietnam combat veterans in art therapy. *The Arts in Psychotherapy,* **12,** 285–96.

Grubrich-Simitis, I. (1981). Extreme traumatization as cumulative trauma. Psychoanalytic investigations of the effects of concentration camp experiences on survivors and their children. *The Psychoanalytic Study of the Child,* **36,** 415–50.

Kastrup, M., Genefke, I. K., Lunde, I. & Boysen, G. (1986). Die Rehabilitation von Volteropfern. Internales Zentrum zür Rehabilitation von Volteropfern. In G. Feuser and W. Jantzen, eds, *Jahrbuch für Psychopatologie und Psychoterapie VI/1986.* Köln, Pahl-Rugenstein.

Kastrup, M., Lunde, I., Ortmann, J. & Genefke, I. K. (1987). Victimization inside and outside the family: families of torture – consequences and possibilities for rehabilitation. *PsychCritique*, 2, 337–49.
Kastrup, M., Genefke, I. K., Lunde, I. & Ortmann, J. (1988). Coping with the exposure to torture. *Contemporary Family therapy*, 10, 280–7.
Kestenberg, J. S. (1980). Psychoanalyses of children of survivors from the Holocaust: case presentations and assessment. *Journal of the American Psychoanalytic Association*, 28, 775–804.
Kral, V. A. (1951). Psychiatric observations under severe chronic stress. *American Journal of Psychiatry*, 108, 185–92.
Kral, V. A., Pazder, L. H. and Wigdor, B. T. (1967). Long term effects of a prolonged stress experience. *The Canadian Psychiatric Association Journal*, 12, 175–81.
Larsen, H. & Lopez, J. D. (1987). Stress-tension reduction in the treatment of sexually tortured women – an exploratory study. *Journal of Sexual Marital Therapy*, 13, 210–18.
Lunde, I., Rasmussen, O. V., Lindholm, J. & Wagner, G. (1981). Sexual and pituitary–testicular function in torture victims. *Archives of Sexual Behaviour*, 10, 25–32.
Lunde, I. (1981). Les Aggressions Sexuelles et la Torture. *20th Congress French Criminology, Lille*. Amnesty International Regie Stencil.
Lunde, I., Boysen, G., Genefke, I. K., Agger, I., Bloch, I., Duarte, A., Jakobsen, L. & Svendsen, G. (1985). Presentation of the International Rehabilitation and Research Center for torture victims. *Ugeskrift for Læger*, 147, 2407–12.
Lunde, I., Boysen, G. & Ortmann J. (1987). Rehabilitation of Torture Victims: Treatment and Research. In H. van Geuns, ed., *Health Hazards of Organised Violence*. The Hague: Ministry of Welfare, Health and Cultural Affairs. Distribution Centre of Government Publications.
Lunde, I., Foldspang, A., Hansen, A. H. & Ortmann, J. (1992). Monitoring the Health of Torture Victims. A Pilot Study. In L. van Willigen, ed., *Health Situation of Refugees and Victims of Organized Violence*. The Hague: Ministry of Welfare, Health and Cultural Affairs.
Lunde, I. and Ortmann, J. (1990). Prevalence and sequelae of sexual torture. *The Lancet*, 336, 289–91.
Ortmann, J., Genefke, I. K., Jakobsen, L. & Lunde, I. (1987). Rehabilitation of torture victims: an interdisciplinary treatment model. *American Journal of Social Psychiatry*, 7, 161–7.
Ortmann, J. & Lunde, I. (1988). Mental and sexual disturbances in 148 torture victims treated at the RCT. Treatment results and transcultural aspects. Personal communication. *World Psychiatric Association Regional Symposium*, May 4–6, 1988, Sydney.
Ortmann, J. & Lunde, I. (1992). Changed identity, low self-esteem and anxiety in 148 torture victims treated at the RCT – in relation to sexual torture. In L. van Willigen, ed., *Health Situation of Refugees and Victims of Organized Violence*. The Hague: Ministry of Welfare, Health and Cultural Affairs.
Rasmussen, O. V., Dam, A. M. & Lunde, I. (1977). Torture: an investigation of

Chileans and Greeks who had previously been submitted to torture. *Ugeskrift for Læger*, **139**, 1049–53.

Rasmussen, O. V. & Lunde, I. (1980). Evaluation of investigation of 200 torture victims. *Danish Medical Bulletin*, **27**, 241–3.

Rasmussen, O. V. & Lunde, I. (1989). The treatment and rehabilitation of victims of torture. *International Journal of Mental Health*, **18**, 122–30.

Rosenheck, R. (1985). Maligant post-Vietnam stress syndrome. *American Journal of Orthopsychiatry*, **55**, 166–76.

Roth, E. F., Lunde, I., Boysen, G. & Genefke, I. K. (1987). Torture and its treatment. *American Journal of Public Health*, **77**, 1404–6.

Somnier, F. and Genefke, I. K. (1986). Psychotherapy for victims of torture. *British Journal of Psychiatry*, **149**, 323–9.

Strøm, A., ed. (1968). Norwegian Concentration Camp Survivors. Oslo, Universitetsforlaget.

Thygesen, P., Hermann, K. & Willanger, R. (1970). Concentration camp survivors in Denmark. Persecution, disease, disability, compensation. A 23-year followup. A survey of the long-term effects of severe environmental stress. *Danish Medical Bulletin*, **17**, 65–107.

M

Part V

PSYCHOTHERAPY

15
PSYCHODYNAMIC APPROACHES IN THE TREATMENT OF TORTURE SURVIVORS
Enrique Bustos

The psychotherapy of the torture survivor is in its infancy

RICHARD MOLLICA

THE TREATMENT OF TORTURE SURVIVORS

Despite the efforts of the UN to get its members to act according to the Article 5 of the United Nations Universal Declaration of Human Rights (United Nations, 1948) and the Convention against Torture (United Nations, 1984), individuals are still being subjected to torture in many countries (Amnesty International, 1991). Torture is characterized as an intentional, planned activity which is often systematically executed. It is a fierce attack on the individual's integrity with the aim of humiliating and depriving the person of his/her identity, willpower, and commitment and leads to physical damage and pain. The goal is to break down and destroy the individual's personality. Ultimately, it serves to terrorize the entire population and end any opposition to the regime.

In the last ten years a number of institutions working with survivors of torture have emerged (see, e.g. Chester, 1990; Gruschow & Hannibal, 1990; Sirett, 1985 for a selected directory). The rehabilitation of torture survivors has become a new field and communication between teams of professionals has opened the way for discussions about their treatment orientation. The search for an effective treatment approach still continues.

A careful medical and psychiatric examination is necessary not only for obtaining information about the atrocities suffered by the survivor but also for planning psychotherapy in accordance with the range and severity of the physical and psychological symptoms (Goldfeld *et al.* 1988; Jensen *et al.* 1989). The psychotherapeutic intervention is often the most significant aspect of the treatment. The restoration of basic trust during psychotherapy enables the individual to develop a working alliance with the therapist, which in turn facilitates a partial or total resolution of the past trauma and the restoration of personal dignity and the ability to find effective solutions to new problems.

Most of the existing psychiatric and psychological literature on torture survivors concerns phenomenological descriptions of the methods of torture and its short- and long-term effects. A few authors have provided guidelines for a therapeutic intervention and a discussion of its theoretical framework (e.g. Agger & Jensen, 1990; Allodi, 1982; Bustos, 1990b; COLAT, 1983; Foighel & Jørgensen, 1990; Lira, Becker & Castillo, 1990; Lunde, Boysen & Ortmann, 1987; Mollica, 1987; Santini, 1989; Schlapobersky & Bamber, 1988; van der Veer, 1990; Vieytes & Barudy, 1985; see also Başoğlu, this volume). Some of these authors, particularly those from Argentina, Chile, The Netherlands, Scandinavia, and the United Kingdom use a psychodynamic approach in the treatment of torture survivors.

THE PSYCHODYNAMIC VIEW ON EXTREME TRAUMATIZATION

The concept of psychic trauma since Freud's first formulations in 1895 (Freud & Breuer, 1895) has had a considerable, yet varying, importance within psychoanalytic theory. In the original theory of trauma, the focus was on the external event. Freud, however, turned the focus away from the field of human interaction towards the intrapsychic problem. In the intrapsychic view, the objects of reality were transformed into mental representations, and the conflict was reduced to inner conflicts between the different parts of an individual's mental apparatus. Metapsychologically the trauma was now described, in terms of the drive theory, as the intensity of the libidinous strivings and defensive battle of the ego against these conflicts. More recently, cases of extreme traumatization have helped dramatically in further theoretical elaborations of the concept (e.g. Bettelheim, 1979; Furst, 1967; Horowitz, 1976; Kardiner, 1941; Kelman, 1945; Krystal, 1968, 1971, 1978, 1988; Krystal & Niederland, 1970; Ulman & Brothers, 1988). The authors cited above are some of the psychoanalysts who have developed this concept in relation to extreme traumatization in children and adults. Bettelheim showed the disintegrating effects on personality of being imprisoned without previous support systems and being subjected to torture and degradation (Bettelheim, 1943, 1979). Horowitz has focused attention on the role of intrusive and repetitive thoughts in traumatized individuals and considered such thoughts as the mind's effort to process new information. He has developed the theory of stored, split-off traumatic memories which set off an intrusion-denial cycle in which the organism tends to seek equilibrium. Krystal has made a critical analysis of how this view has been used in theoretical and clinical work with traumatized people. According to Krystal (1988, p. 142) the trauma causes 'a paralyzed, overwhelmed state, with immobilization, withdrawal, possible depersonalization, and evidence of disorganization'.

As noted earlier, extreme traumatic situations in adults have often been reported in the psychoanalytic literature in terms of external, behavioural and after-effect-related data. Krystal has developed a theory in which traumatization is a process that starts with a virtually complete blocking of the ability to feel emotions and pain and progresses to a major inhibition of other mental functions.

THE THERAPEUTIC MODEL

The psychopathology in torture survivors varies in nature and severity. The characteristics of psychodynamic psychotherapy with survivors of torture will be determined by the nature of the problems facing the patient and the dynamic interaction between the after-effects of the trauma and other traumas the patient may have experienced in the earlier years. As Fanon (1983) made clear in his analysis of torture in Algeria, traditional psychiatry gives more importance to the event than to the biological, psychological, and emotional background of the individual. Therefore, in a psychodynamic diagnosis of a survivor of torture, the following variables are of major importance:

- degree of motivation
- psychological and physical after-effects of torture
- type of trauma
- degree of psychopathology
- personality structure
- repertoire of defensive manoeuvers
- family dynamics
- social network
- degree of political awareness
- presence of other traumatic experiences in the past
- if the treatment takes place in exile, the different phases of the adaptation process and the importance of a future repatriation.

The core of the psychodynamic approach is the intrapsychic processing of the trauma. The aim is 'to enable our patients to be masters of

themselves and of their emotions' (Amati, 1976). Through a psychotherapeutic process, it is possible for a survivor of torture to undergo
a psychic recuperation, regaining the emotional strength to recover
from broken expectations of life. Lira and her colleagues (Lira, Weinstein & Kovalskys 1987) describe the psychotherapy as a process of
obtaining insight into the past trauma. Schlapobersky (1990) views
the goal of rehabilitation as being 'centered on the purpose of freeing
victims rather than "curing them"'. They all point to the importance
of working through the trauma and the obstacles that hinder a
healthy psychological functioning. The importance of the working
through the trauma should be seen in relation to the individual's
emotional responses to unbearable stimuli and overwhelming affects.
These responses usually produce a disorganization of all psychic
functions. Therefore, the psychodynamics of the trauma in the survivor of torture (or other traumatized individuals) are seen as being
directly related to the individual's capacity to organize and integrate
the intrapsychic processes in relation to the outer traumatic event
(Krystal, 1971).

Regression is an important aspect of human response to trauma and
crucial in understanding the intrapsychic recovery processes of the
individual. The relationship that is established between the torturer
and the tortured through regression 'deconstructs' the primary basic
unit of human civilization in the internal world of the individual
(Scarry, 1985). Such relationships in the external world are internalized
in the psychic world of the survivor and associated with pain, degradation, and dehumanization. This often reduces the survivors'
capacity for human relatedness in the future. This aspect of the
problem is of great importance in terms of future interactions between
the patient and the therapist during psychotherapy. The symptomatology presented by tortured survivors should also be seen as related to
extreme regression during torture and a reduced capacity for
relatedness.

The main objectives of psychodynamic treatment are generally
formulated in the following terms: relief from distressing symptoms,
working through of the traumatic experience, reconstruction of new
expectations of life, and resolution of family and social problems. A
Chilean group used to include the restoration of a 'life project' as the
main objective of the psychotherapeutic process (Weinstein, 1984; Lira
et al., 1987).

Most descriptions of therapy models for torture survivors have
followed the tradition of classifying the various phases of treatment.
These descriptions are outlined below.

The opening phase

This phase involves the linking of the survivor's traumatic memories to the symptoms and the corresponding affective states. The mapping of the core conflict and the associated psychopathology is one of the important processes of this phase. Attaining the basic confidence of the patient is necessary for the challenges with which the patient and the therapist will be confronted in the therapy process. The therapist's ability to understand the individual's regressive behavior during this phase is essential for the establishment of a therapeutic relationship and the patient's recovery of his/her sense of identity and basic trust in humanity. Mollica, Wyshak & Lavelle (1987) state how difficult it is to obtain a detailed description of the trauma in a research interview and stress the importance of developing a trusting relationship before eliciting the patient's trauma story. Chilean psychologists have developed a special method for obtaining information during this phase. This method involves the use of testimony as a therapeutic technique. The aim of this technique is to facilitate the integration of the traumatic experience and the restoration of self-esteem, while also providing symptomatic relief in certain patients (Cienfuegos & Monelli, 1983; Lira & Weinstein, 1984b; Weinstein, 1984). Agger & Jensen (1990) have adapted this method for political refugees living in exile but have included concepts and techniques outside the framework of psychodynamic approach.

The working-through phase

This phase is characterized by the formation of the therapist-patient unit or, in classical terms, the working alliance. This alliance initiates the working-through of the trauma. During this phase the therapist helps the patient to verbalize the chaotic, frightening, life-threatening, and incomprehensible experiences, receives such anxiety-charged psychological material without being overwhelmed by uneasiness and fear, and takes care to distinguish between resistance and inability to give a coherent narrative. The expression of the traumatic experiences during torture and imprisonment is usually encouraged by means of verbal and non-verbal methods of reconstruction. Santini's (1989) eight-year-long treatment of a survivor illuminates the significance of the psychotherapeutic process in the construction of a reparative link, whereby the patient, by externalizing conflicts and fantasies, can achieve insight and integration of the trauma into his/her personal history.

The termination phase: establishment of a new equilibrium

Termination of therapy will be determined by the patient's life circumstances as well as by the circumstances of the therapy situation. The emergence of new problems during the course of the therapy often requires a reconsideration of the objectives and lines of action. In the final stage, the patient should have gained a satisfactory level of psychological, personal, and social functioning. Giving a new meaning to, and regaining control over, the trauma help gain mastery over traumatic memories and new related stimuli. The drama of separation at this phase tests the patient's ability (and the effectiveness of the psychotherapeutic process) to cope with an irretrievable loss of a human relationship involving solidarity, attachment, and affection.

The fundamental difference between the traditional psychodynamic model and others concerns the issue of therapist neutrality. Many psychodynamically oriented professionals argue that neutrality has to be put aside during treatment (Guinsberg, 1984; Jensen & Agger, 1990; Lenhardtson *et al*. 1990; Lira *et al*. 1987). Many mental health professionals who are aware of the adverse effects of political repression on society and individuals have taken up Human Rights campaigning in addition to their treatment work with survivors of torture. Schlapobersky (1990), in describing the rehabilitation work carried out by the Medical Foundation in the United Kingdom, points to the importance of advocacy for the rights of asylum seekers and refugees. He states that, for therapists, working with torture survivors is 'a part of a broader human rights commitment'. Bonano (1986) also emphasizes this view in his analysis of the work undertaken by the Group of Psychological Assistance to the Mothers of Plaza de Mayo in Argentina.

THE PSYCHOTHERAPEUTIC PROCESS

The experience of torture leads to an extreme use of psychological defences in order to avoid depression, guilt, shame, and helplessness. The affective regression and the impoverishment in cognition lead to an increased use of primitive defenses like denial, splitting, and projective identification (Krystal, 1988; Ogden, 1982). Also observed are a breakdown in the interactional patterns of the patient with the family members and an alteration of the relationship between the individual and social reality (Lira, Becker & Castilo, 1990).

Regression

The survivor of torture has gone through extremely traumatic experiences during which human relationships were associated with danger, anxiety, and fear of annihilation. The internal world of the survivor has been altered by pathologically internalized external objects. Splitting or denial are the common defenses against pathological internalizations related to traumatic situations, and they prevent the formation of accurate representational memories. Amnesia and numbing serve to prevent the repetitive and intrusive flooding of painful memories and to block affects related to the internalized relationships. In some cases, this leads to a psychological shutting-off. Torture leads to an overwhelming of the self-preserving functions and diminution of problem-solving abilities. This creates a regressive state with a disorganization of feelings, thoughts, and behaviour (Amati, 1990; Krystal, 1988). The incidence of such disorganization after torture is variable. Because of associative processes and the defensive use of regression, disorganization may persist and even become worse. In some individuals, protective defences such as derealization, depersonalization, and other states of altered consciousness may arise, leading to a severe constriction, desymbolization, and fragmentation of mental functioning (Krystal, 1988).

Human relatedness

The experience of helplessness and total dependence on others constitutes a psychological bedrock for all subsequent emotional events in the life of the traumatized refugee. Apitzsch (1987) has defined torture as a psychological construction where the individual is forced into a state of extreme infantile helplessness, faced with the absolute mercilessness of an omnipotent persecutor. Gómez (1985), based on her experience with tortured Chileans in Chile, has outlined five aspects of the relationship between the torturer and the tortured

1 extreme inequality in the exercise of power
2 exercise of highly irrational aggressive behaviour
3 sadistic qualities in the torturer's behaviour
4 constant dehumanization of the tortured
5 intense emotional involvement during torture.

According to Foighel & Jørgensen (1990), torture undermines the ability to develop and maintain confidence and basic trust in others. This view is also expressed by Müller (1990), who stresses the importance of focusing on the issue of trust and confidence in the therapist-patient relationship. The need for and dread of human relatedness in the therapeutic setting should be considered as a consequence of regression during which the survivor comes into contact with his/her painfully internalized relationships, memories, and blocked emotions and is reminded of the experience of helplessness and total dependence on others. Since torture takes place within the context of human interactions the interactional nature of psychotherapy may facilitate regressive behaviour and absolute dependence on others and ultimately bring the traumatic experience onto the stage of the therapeutic process. This may lead to psychic disintegration and inability to relate to other human beings.

Transference

In 1905 Freud had already spoken of transference as 'a whole series of psychological experiences that are revived, not as belonging to the past, but as applying to the person of the physician at the present moment' (Freud, 1905). This influence of the past on the present, an active dynamic force within the present, is of particular importance in all psychotherapies. The exploration and interpretation of the transference responses, including resistance to transference, are considered essential by many therapists (Schwaber, 1985). The phenomenon of transference makes it possible to work with internalized human relationships, and bring to the surface unresolved conflicts and emotions generated by traumatic experiences. The therapeutic role of transference relies on its interpretation. The interpretation of transference has a positive effect only if the therapist is first internalized as a real, benign object into the patient's internal world. The resolution of transference is thus not only an informative interpretation that says 'I am not the torturer, I am not the one that you think I am', but also an act of engagement and caring. Consequently, the relationship between patient and therapist acquires a deeper form of communication whereby human relatedness is heightened and a more emphatic understanding of the patient's traumatic experiences is facilitated. In more severe cases, therapists deal with a kind of maternal transference where the central psychic conflict is related to survival (Krystal, 1988) and the therapist assumes the role of the primary object, the mothering parent that lends organizing, life-maintaining powers to the patient. The dread which these patients feel for the union with a maternal love object is the consequence of the helplessness and dependence experienced during an extreme regression to earlier states of development. A traumatic disappointment concerning the mothering object impedes the process of affect development (emotional bonding) in new relationships. The transference makes it possible to start working with a silent communication of emotions. The intense anxiety and helplessness inhibits verbal communication, but stimulates the therapeutically necessary process of object seeking. The extreme dependency and vulnerability experienced during the trauma is repeatedly disclosed during the transference, heightening the importance of emphatic relatedness which later gives way to a more direct communication of differentiated and verbalized affects associated with the trauma.

Verbal and non-verbal communication

Gómez (1985) has observed a relationship between the duration of the trauma and the capacity to share verbally this experience. A progressive verbal inhibition takes place together with a blocking of the emotions and projections are intensively used as a communication. Being in the room, sharing the experience through awareness of the countertransference reactions, and feeling the new introjected object and its effect on our psychic world rather than making premature verbal interpretations can help facilitate pre- and non-verbal ways of communication. The somatic manifestations, the body language, externalization of the traumatic experience through non-verbal support, acting, and playing help reach a level of psychic functioning that later allows the establishment of a verbal communication within a state of controlled regression. Helping the patient to verbalize the chaotic, life-threatening and incomprehensible experiences, while still being able to receive such anxiety-charged material without being overwhelmed by uneasiness and fear is a major task for the psychotherapist.

Countertransference

Countertransference, as described by Freud, involves conflict-laden reactions that interfere with the therapist's role as a sensitive receiver of emotions. Through the years there have been many discussions and divergent opinions about this concept (Gorkin, 1987; Racker, 1968). Some believe that countertransference exists because of neurotic traits in the therapist that disturb the therapeutic process whilst others see it as the key that allows the internal object world of the patient. For the purposes of this article, countertransference is defined as all antitherapeutic interventions by the therapist which tend to satisfy his/her own unconscious needs evoked by the patient, thereby creating a situation in which he/she is incapable of maintaining the limits of the therapy and dealing with projections of the patient's internal object world. Thus transference and countertransference are viewed as being closely interrelated in a transactional psychic process.

   Multiple forms of countertransference may be encountered in therapeutic work with survivors of torture (Bustos 1989, 1990a). Many of these are directly related to different phases of the therapeutic process and are therefore common to all patients. However, other countertransferential reactions exist which are specific to work with torture survivors and traumatized refugees. Imprisonment, sexual abuse, persecution, and torture, together with a history of pathogenic conditions for psychosocial development in some survivors may generate strong countertransferential reactions in the therapist when these experiences are conveyed by verbal and nonverbal communication. The 'conspiracy of silence' (Danieli, 1980; Krystal, 1971), a phenomenon studied in depth in relation to the Holocaust survivors, is a clear example where the therapist and the patient together, symbiotically attached, avoid discussing, either altogether or in sufficient detail, the material relating to the trauma because of its incomprehensible, unbelievable or unbearable nature. Being overwhelmed by the nature of inhuman cruelty during torture may lead the therapist to see the therapeutic setting as a defiant arena and stimulate the use of 'warding off' or 'disarming' techniques when he/she meets the patient. While acknowledging the importance of the physical sequelae of torture and other somatic complaints in survivors, an undue emphasis on the patient's somatic symptoms can be a sign of another form of countertransference which impedes progress in therapy.

   In work with refugee torture survivors, three additional major forms of countertransference should be noted: culturally determined, colonial, and ethno-identificative countertransference.

The culturally determined countertransference

This form of countertransference appears in work with refugees or migrants. The therapy is adversely affected by the therapist's value system which is a product of a socialization process different from that of the patient. Such culturally determined countertransferential reactions are also strengthened by generic myths about ethnic groups.

The colonial countertransference

The lack of a common language may lead to the rejection of a client as not being 'sophisticated' enough for insight therapies. A colonialist paternalism on the part of the therapist stimulates a 'supporting environment' which allows acting out or other situations that conspire against the therapeutic contract. This is often justified by a counter-transferential rationalization in terms of the patient's inability to play by the rules of insight or analytic therapy.

Ethnoidentificative countertransference

This form of countertransference occurs in therapists belonging to the same ethnic group as the patient (or other groups with similar experiences) and is brought about by previous unresolved traumatic experiences or their revival by the new trauma material presented by the patient. The interaction of common needs allows a mutual projective identification whereby both the patient and the therapist avoid verbalization of affects related to traumatic situations. A non-declared alliance is formed, which involves use of signals, gestures, sounds to avoid a clear expression of the traumatic material. Identity and self-esteem conflicts, and narcissistic outrages displayed during therapy by most refugees can be reactivated in the therapist. A kind of conspiratorial, ethnocentric alliance against other groups is developed which leads to a splitting on a macrosocial level. 'We and They' becomes the framework for future therapy, thereby violating the norms of the therapeutic neutrality.

CONCLUSION

New theoretical and clinical findings concerning torture trauma necessitate a revision of the traditional psychodynamic therapy strategies in the treatment of torture survivors. Regression, human relatedness, verbal and non-verbal communication, transference and countertransference are some important therapy variables that acquire a different dimension because of the specificity of torture as a traumatic experience. Emotional blocking in torture survivors is a consequence of experiencing total defencelessness, together with hopelessness and fear of dying. Verbal inhibition impedes the traditional method of verbally working-through the traumatic experience and leads to pre- and non-verbal ways of communication.

The importance of the interactional processes that are established in the psychotherapeutic process needs to be stressed. Man is intrinsically social and human nature is realized only through interaction and participation with others. The nature of the relationship established during the therapy will determine the success of the working-through process necessary to resolve the traumatic disappointments concerning other human beings.

REFERENCES

Agger, I. & Jensen, S. B., (1990). Testimony as ritual and evidence in psychotherapy for political refugees. *Journal of Traumatic Stress*, **3**(1), 115–30.

Allodi, F. (1982). Psychiatric sequelæ of torture and implications for treatment. *World Medical Journal*, **29**(5), 71–75.

Amati, S. (1976). Some thoughts on torture to introduce a psychoanalytical discussion. Paper reproduced from International Psychoanalytic Students Organisation, Newsletters, April.

Amati, S. (1990). Aportes psicoanaliticos al conocimiento de los efectos de la violencia institucionalizada [Psychoanalytical contributions to the knowledge about the effects of the institutionalized violence]. In H. Riquelme, ed., *Era de Nieblas*, pp. 17–30, Caracas: Nueva Sociedad.

Amnesty International (1991). *Arsrapport 1991*. [Annual Report 1991]. Stockholm: Amnesty International.

Apitzsch, H. (1987). Tortyrens psykologi. [The Psychology of Torture]. *Psykisk Hälsa*, **4**, 259–72.

Bettelheim, B. (1943). Individual and mass behavior in extreme situations. *Journal of Abnormal Social Psychology*, **38**, 417–52.

Bettelheim, B. (1979). Trauma and reintegration. In B. Bettelheim, ed., *Surviving and Other Essays*, pp. 19–37, New York: Alfred Knoff.

Bonano, O. (1986). Represión política y análisis institucional. [Political Repression and Institutional Analysis] In D. Kordon & L. Edelman, eds, *Efectos psicológicos de la represión política*. [Psychological effects of political repression], pp. 113–28, Buenos Aires: Sudamericana/Planeta.

Bustos, E. (1989). Reacciones contratransferenciales en el tratamiento a refugiados torturados. [Contratransferential reactions in the treatment of tortured refugees]. Paper presented at the Second Conference of the centres and Individuals concerned in the Assistance to the Victims of Organized Violence, November 1989. San José, Costa Rica.

Bustos, E. (1990a). Dealing with the unbearable: Reactions of therapists and therapeutic institutions to survivors of torture. In P. Suedfeld, ed., *Torture and Psychology* pp. 143–63, New York: Hemisphere Publishing Corporation.

Bustos, E. (1990b). Psychotherapy with tortured refugees. *Refugee Participation Network*, August, **9**, 15–17.

Chester, B. (1990). Because mercy has a human heart: Centers for Victims of torture. In P. Suedfeld, ed., *Torture and Psychology*, pp. 165–84, New York: Hemisphere Publishing Corporation.

Cienfuegos, A. J. & Monelli, C. (1983). The testimony of political repression as a therapeutic instrument. *American Journal of Orthopsychiatry*, **53(1)**, 43–51.

COLAT (1983) *Psicopatología de la tortura y el exilio*. [The psychopathology of torture and exile]. Madrid: Fundamentos.

Danieli, Y. (1980). Countertransference in the treatment and study of Nazi Holocaust survivors and their children. *Victimology*, **5(2–4)**, 355–67.

Fanon, F. (1983). *Los condenados de la tierra*. Mexico, D.F.: Fondo de Cultura Económica.

Freud, S. & Breuer, J. (1895). *Studies on Hysteria*. The Pelican Freud Library. vol. III, Penguin Books.

Freud, S. (1905). Fragment of an analysis of a case of hysteria. *Standard Edition*, vol. 7, p. 7–122. London: Hogarth Press.

Foighel N. & Jørgensen, U. (1990). The tortured refugee and the psychopathology of the self. Paper presented at the Second European Conference on Traumatic Stress, Noordwijjkerhout, Netherlands.

Furst, S. (ed.) (1967). *Psychic Trauma*. New York: Basic Books.

Goldfeld, A. E., Mollica, R. F., Pesavento, B. H. & Faraone, S.V. (1988). The physical and psychological sequelae of torture. *Journal of American Medical Association*, **18**, 2725–9.

Gómez, E. (1985) La tortura como experiencia traumática [The torture as traumatic experience]. Paper presented in the International Seminar 'La Tortura en América latina', Buenos Aires, Argentina, December, 1985.

Gorkin, M. (1987). *The Uses of Countertransference*. New York: Aronson.

Gruschow, J. & Hannibal, K. (eds.) (1990). *Health Services for the Treatment of Torture and Trauma Survivors*. Washington: AAAS.

Guinsberg, E. (1984). Latinoamericanos en Copenhague. [Latin Americans in Copenhagen]. *Le Monde Diplomatique en español*, **34**, julio No. 67.

Horowitz, M. J. (1976). *Stress Response Syndromes*. New York: Aronson.

Jensen, S. B. & Agger, I. (1990). Menneskerettighedsarbejdet i Chile [Human Rights work in Chile]. *Ugeskrift for Laeger*, **152(13)**, 949–52.

Jensen, S. B., Schaumburg, E., Leroy, B., Larsen, B.O. & Thorup, M. (1989). Psychiatric care of refugees exposed to organized violence. *Acta Psychiatrica Scandinavica*, **80**, 125–31.

Kardiner, A. (1941). *The Traumatic Neuroses of War*. New York: Hoeber.

Kelman, H. C. (1945). Character and traumatic syndrome. *Journal of Nervous and Mental Disease*, **102**, 121–53.

Krystal, H. (ed.) (1968). *Massive Psychic Trauma*. New York: International Universities Press.

Krystal, H. (1971). Trauma: Considerations of its intensity and chronicity. In H. Krystal & W. G. Niederland (eds.) *Psychic Traumatization*. pp. 11–28, Boston: Little, Brown.

Krystal, H. (1978). Trauma and effects. *The Psychoanalytic Study of the Child*. **33**, 81–116.

Krystal, H., (1988). *Integration and Self-Healing. Affect, Trauma, Alexithymia*. Hillside, New Jersey: The Analytic Press.

Krystal, H. & Niederland, W. G. (eds.) (1970). *Psychic Traumatization*. Boston: Little, Brown.

Lenhardtson, E., De Conte, L. J., Rudeman, M., Kestelboim, E., Calvo, A., Capelli, W. *et al.* (1990). Some reflections about torture. In J. Gruschow & K. Hannibal, eds, *Health Services for the Treatment of Torture and Trauma Survivors*. pp. 91–8. Washington: AAAS.

Lira, E., Weinstein, E. *et al.* (eds.) (1984a). *Psicoterapia y represión política*. [Psychotherapy and political repression], Mexico DF: Siglo Veintiuno Editores.

Lira, E. & Weinstein, E. (1984b). El testimonio de experiencias políticas traumáticas como instrumento terapéutico. [The testimony of traumatic political experiences as a therapeutic instrument]. In Lira and Weinstein eds, *Psicoterapia y represión política*. [Psychotherapy and political represion], pp. 17–36, Mexico DF: Siglo Veintiuno Editores.

Lira, E., Weinstein, E. & Kovalskys, J. (1987). Subjetividad y represión política: Intervenciones terapéuticas. [Subjectivity and political repression: therapeutical interventions]. In Montero, ed. *Psicología política latinoamericana* [Latin American Political Psychology], pp. 317–346. Caracas: Panapo.

Lira, E. B., Becker, D. & Castillo, M. I. (1990). Psychotherapy with victims of political repression in Chile: therapeutic challenge. In J. Gruschow & K. Hannibal, eds. *Health Services for the Treatment of Torture and Trauma Survivors*. (99–114). Washington: AAAS.

Lunde, I., Boysen, G. & Ortmann, J. (1987). In E. van Geus, ed. *Health Hazards of Organized Violence*. pp. 136–48, The Hague: Ministry of Welfare, Health and Cultural Affairs.

Mollica, R. (1987). The trauma story: The psychiatric care of refugee survivors of violence and torture. In F. M. Ochberg, ed. *Post-Traumatic Therapy and the Victim of Violence*. pp. 295–314, New York: Bruner/Mazel.

Mollica, R. F., Wyshak, G., Lavelle, J. (1987). The psychosocial impact of war trauma and torture on Southeast Asian refugees. *American Journal of Psychiatry*, **144(12)**, 1567–72.

Müller, O. (1990). Psykologisk behandling av tortureofre [Psychological treatment of torture victims] *Tidskrift for Norsk Psykologforening*, **27**, 511–19.

Ogden, T. H. (1982). *Projective Identification and Psychotherapeutic Technique*. New York: J. Aronson.

Racker, H. (1968). *Transference and Countertransference*. London, Maresfield Reprints.

Santini, I. (1989). Trauma, Tratamiento y Recuperation [Trauma, Treatment and Recovering]. Paper presented at the Second Conference of the Centres and Individuals concerned in the Assistance to the Victims of Organized Violence, San José, Costa Rica, November.

Scarry, E. (1985). *The Body in Pain. The Making and Unmaking of the World*. New World: Oxford University Press.

Schlapobersky, J. (1990). Torture as the perversion of a healing relationship. In J. Gruschow & K. Hanibal, eds. *Health Services for the Treatment of Torture and Trauma Survivors*. (51–72). Washington: AAAS.

Schlapobersky, J. & Bamber, H., (1988). Rehabilitation work with victims of torture. In D. Miserez, ed. *Refugees: The Trauma of Exile*. pp. 206–222, Vitznau: Martinus Nijhoff Publishers.

Schwaber, E. A. (ed.), (1985). *The Transference in Psychotherapy: Clinical Management*. New York: International University Press.

Sirett, H. (1985). Selected organizations concerned with torture and/or psychiatric Abuse. In E. Stover & E. O. Nightingale, eds, *The Breaking of Bodies and Minds* pp. 280–98, New York: Freeman.

Ulman, R. B. & Brothers, D. (1988). *The Shattered Self*. Hilldale: The Analytic Press.

United Nations (1948). *Universal Declaration of Human Rights*. Office of Public Information. New York: United Nations.

United Nations (1984) *Convention Against Torture and Other Cruel, Inhuman or Degrading Treatment or Punishment*. Office of Public Information. New York: United Nations.

van der Veer, G. (1990). *Political Refugees: Psychological Problems and the Consequences of Repression and Exile*. Amsterdam: Author.

Vieytes, C. & Barudy, J. (1985). El proceso terapeutico. [The therapeutic process]. In J. Barudy & C. Vieytes, eds, *El dolor invisible de la tortura*. [The invisible pain of torture]. Bruxelles: Franja Ediciones.

Weinstein, E. (1984). El testimonio de experiencias políticas traumaticas como instrumento terapéutico. [The testimony of traumatic political experiences as therapeutic instrument]. In E. Lira & E. Weinstein *et al.* (eds.) (1984). *Psicoterapia y represión política*. [Psychotherapy and political repression], (17–36). Mexico DF: Siglo Veintiuno Editores.

16
PSYCHOTHERAPY FOR TORTURE SURVIVORS
Peter Vesti and Marianne Kastrup

INTRODUCTION

Since the late 1970s, a group of medical doctors in Copenhagen has treated survivors of torture who have obtained asylum in Denmark. The knowledge gained laid the foundation, at the beginning of the 1980s, for the establishment of the Rehabilitation and Research Centre for Torture Victims in Copenhagen (RCT).

The model of psychotherapy that will be discussed in this chapter has been developed from the experience at the RCT with the help of collaborating centres in developing as well as industrialized countries of the world (Pagaduan-Lopez, 1987; Kordon *et al.*, 1988). Furthermore, valuable concepts have been borrowed from the treatment of concentration camp survivors and from modern crisis intervention therapy (Malt & Weisæth, 1989; Eitinger, 1969).

Certain issues concerning the treatment of torture survivors are of fundamental importance and thus deserve attention here:

1 Physical and/or psychological trauma evokes psychological reactions in anyone. Furthermore, these reactions are longer lasting and of greater severity if the trauma is of human design (Melamed, Melamed & Bouhoutsos, 1990; Gunderson & Rahe, 1974). There is no evidence to suggest that torture survivors have any excess premorbid psychopathology.
2 The torture endured by most survivors is often of sufficient severity and duration to cause psychological problems and impairment in social functioning.
3 No organic cerebral syndromes have been demonstrated in the majority of victims.
4 Survivors presenting at treatment centres are a selected few. There are various screening factors that need to be taken into account in comparing results across centres. These include deaths during torture, inability to leave the country and obtain asylum elsewhere, availability of access to the centres (e.g.

geographic distance, criteria for treatment priorities at the centres, etc), variable source of referral, waiting list at the centres, and refusal of treatment by the survivor.

5 Torture reflects the society in which it is perpetrated. Similarly, the treatment offered to survivors is a product of the culture and the circumstances of the individual rehabilitation programme (e.g. organizational model, hierarchy structure, dominant professional group, funding, etc). In countries with a European cultural background it is based on Western concepts and classification of psychiatric symptoms. These concepts have limitations, even when dealing with patients from our culture, and may be regarded with scepticism or rejected by refugees from different cultures.

6 The treatment of patients from different parts of the world need not be identical.

7 Finally, there are different approaches in the rehabilitation of torture survivors and these are not mutually exclusive. Because of its history, traditions, and possibilities for specialized medical intervention, the RCT in Copenhagen has chosen a psycho-social medical model.

INSIGHT THERAPY

Insight therapy is a treatment method used at the RCT for refugee survivors of torture who have been granted asylum in Denmark. It is based on the assumption that being able to confront the traumatic experience has a therapeutic effect. This is achieved by reliving and abreaction of trauma-related emotions and subsequent reintegration of the trauma as an event of the past (Somnier & Genefke, 1986).

Practical issues in treatment

Since torture often affects the body as well as the mind, it is necessary to deal with both physical and psychological sequelae of torture. Therefore psychotherapy should be carried out concurrently with the treatment of physical illnesses and dysfunctions.

The problem presented by the patient may concern five spheres of functioning:

Psychological

Somatic   Social

Legal   Spiritual

There may be signs of severe dysfunction in each sphere that need attention. The patient's level of functioning in each sphere should be carefully assessed and problems dealt with as much as possible, giving due consideration to the patient's cultural background (see Bøjholm & Vesti, this volume, for a discussion of basic principles of treatment).

It is important to conduct a thorough assessment interview with the survivor before starting psychotherapy. The interview should cover pre-trauma history in order to identify any premorbid psychopathology (e.g. major psychiatric disorder) which may be of importance for psychotherapy. The particular forms and circumstances of torture endured and how they relate to the subsequent symptoms need to be explored as far as possible. The nature of the treatment and how it is conducted should be explained to the patient in detail and the issue of professional confidentiality emphasized.

The first two or three sessions after the initial interview are explorative, serving to build up trust and confidence. These sessions also help determine whether insight therapy is possible. Only a proportion of survivors are capable of developing insight in the psychotherapeutic sense. For others, supportive therapy may be more appropriate.

Sessions, lasting from 45 minutes to 1 hour, are usually held twice a week, but may be more frequent if the survivor is very disturbed. Sessions are held, as far as possible, just before or after physiotherapy sessions. Individual rather than group therapy is used and an interpreter is present during the sessions, if necessary. The therapist may be a psychiatrist, psychologist or a medical doctor with some psychiatric training. Family therapy is not usually undertaken but spouses and children are offered individual attention and even psychotherapy, if needed. Social and legal counselling are also offered but such work is carried out separately by social workers.

The patient is informed during the initial sessions that the symptoms may get temporarily worse once the memories of the trauma are revived.

The aim of insight psychotherapy is to help the survivor to understand the real purpose of the torturers in doing what they did to him/her and how s/he reacted psychologically to the life-threatening situation. In addition, the psychological defences and coping strategies used by the survivor during and after the trauma are analysed. Many sessions may be necessary for the survivor to recall the traumatic events in detail and reexperience and abreact repressed emotions. When the suppressed emotions begin to surface, the survivor often abreacts, showing emotional reactions such as tears, anger, or guilt.

Insight therapy uses the same treatment principles as crisis management therapy (Ochberg, 1988). In torture survivors, however, the interval from trauma to therapy is much longer. Furthermore, torture is a systematic act that targets several areas and functions of the body as well as of the mind. The psychotherapy, therefore, should not focus on one particular trauma but on a multitude of traumas experienced by the survivor and his/her responses such as fear, anxiety, and guilt.

The five phases of insight therapy

Insight therapy consist of five phases:

The meeting

During this phase which may last several sessions, the patient's trust and confidence in the therapist are consolidated. As the trauma story is recollected, the therapist explains how the somatic and psychological symptoms may be related to the painful memories of the torture. The patient is told that names and addresses are not important for the therapeutic process and may be omitted or substituted, if necessary. The expression of emotions associated with the specific circumstances is, however, essential for the therapeutic process.

Initial setting

The survivor starts to recollect life as it was before torture and gradually moves on to the day of arrest. Alternatively, s/he may prefer to start with the most traumatic event which s/he thinks may be related to his/her symptoms. It may be helpful to review all incidents of arrest/detention and the specific forms of torture that followed.

Emotive phase

As the survivor recollects scenes from the torture setting, the presence of repressed emotions becomes more clear. For example, the survivor may become nervous, smoke excessively, or display other signs of anxiety. As mentioned earlier, repressed emotions are addressed in a non-chronological fashion, often starting with a major trauma. When repressed emotions are released, the patient may cry, yell, or walk about the room, and even enter a brief reactive psychosis with flashbacks. The emerging emotions are allowed to run their full course. In case of a psychotic reaction, it is important to stay with the patient and gradually bring him/her back to reality through questions relating to the surroundings and practical aspects of daily life. After the episode, the patient stays in the treatment centre, sometimes for hours, until full recovery takes place. These psychotic episodes are usually very brief, lasting less than a few hours, and do not require hospitalization.

Reintegration of trauma

As the process of recall is continued, the survivor gradually begins to see the traumatic experience in a new light, realizing that his/her psychological reaction to the trauma was a predictable, normal human response. The emotional impact of the memories of the trauma is attenuated after they are relived several times, and eventually the survivor will be able to relate the torture experience without incapacitating emotional upheaval. The therapist actively supports the cognitive restructuring process in this phase.

End of therapy

As the survivor gradually resumes normal functioning in important areas of life, treatment is tapered off and eventually ended, often after 20 to 80 or more sessions. The number of sessions required for an individual patient depends on factors such as resistance towards reexperiencing the trauma, motivation for treatment, the severity of symptoms, the verbal ability of the patient, the complexity of the case and particularly the presence of concomitant somatic or social problems.

Contraindications

It is necessary to decide during the first few sessions whether the survivor is capable of gaining insight. These assessment sessions may be compared to a clinical assessment interview prior to psychotherapy, during which patient characteristics such as premorbid personality, previous psychopathology, verbal ability, and level of motivation for treatment are evaluated. It is also important to assess whether the patient can tolerate the intense anxiety that will be released during the sessions. Survivors with weak ego boundaries may have to be excluded from this kind of treatment, since they would be at risk of longer psychotic episodes. Other survivors who should not be offered insight therapy are those with paranoid ideation since the therapist frequently becomes part of the patient's delusional system.

Resistance

Human beings resist talking about traumatic ordeals, particularly when certain aspects of their personality are involved. Yet once trust and confidence have been established and the therapist has demonstrated knowledge in the area, survivors usually show little resistance to talking about their torture. Allowing for names and places to be omitted facilitates this process.

A potential pitfall in therapy is the therapist's interpretation of political, ideological or religious views expressed by the patient as defense mechanisms or resistance to therapy. For example, the anger expressed by some survivors towards the authorities in the host country may be based on realistic reasons. Such emotional reactions are understandable given the difficult and stressful exile conditions with which most survivors are confronted.

Religious beliefs may be of great help for the survivors both during the torture and in the country of exile. These beliefs should be respected and their importance for the survivor acknowledged. On the other hand, the same beliefs, if carried to an extreme, may also be a drawback in the thepeutic process.

The following psychological mechanisms may block the psychotherapeutic process if they are not identified and clarified to the patient by the therapist:

1 Denying psychological impact of the trauma (e.g. maintaining that the pain and distress experienced are caused by physical rather than psychological dysfunctions).
2 Intellectualization (e.g. constantly arguing against a particular political regime, even to the point of denying acts of individual perpetrators).
3 Displacing the anger (e.g. constantly expressing anger at the country of asylum).
4 Day-dreaming, for example, about an immediate return to home country where nothing has changed. There is therefore no need to integrate into the new system.
5 Revenge fantasies (e.g. cutting up the torturers into a thousand pieces; nothing else is important).
6 religious preoccupation (e.g. the torture comes as a punishment or a lesson from God and thus should be accepted).

Supportive therapy

Supportive psychotherapy may be needed for survivors who are unable to gain insight into their psychological problems or for whom insight therapy may be contraindicated. This form of therapy deals with practical matters such as bodily diseases and dysfunctions and possible ways of living with the sequelae of torture. Also important in supportive therapy are social problems concerning issues such as housing, language training, and education. Sessions may also be used to help the survivor develop a basic understanding of the social system and culture in the new country of residence. Such supportive therapy sessions are also required in insight therapy and constitute about a fourth to a third of all sessions during therapy at the RCT.

Interpreters

When work with survivors of torture started at the RCT, treatment could only be given through interpreters. Interpreters are still indispensable for therapy if the patient and the therapist do not speak a common language. Contrary to initial concerns about the use of interpreters in working with survivors of torture, they may have a useful role in psychotherapy, provided the interpreter is 1) the same person throughout therapy, 2) approved by the survivor, 3) a national of the host country in cases where the survivor distrusts fellow citizens, and 4) not related to the survivor as a friend or a family member (Bentsen *et al.*, 1989).

A better understanding of the importance of cultural factors in therapy has transformed the role of the interpreter into that of a bicultural translator who not only translates from one language to another but who also helps the therapist understand the client's culture-specific non-verbal expressions during therapy.

Because of cultural differences between the survivor and the therapist, it may also be necessary to formulate concepts in a more symbolic manner. Drawings may be used to achieve this purpose. Figure 16.1 illustrates the psychological mechanism of intellectualization.

Survivors often have no difficulty talking in general terms about a regime or even about notorious tyrants who were ultimately responsible for their torture. When talking about the prison itself, they often describe what they heard or saw as witnesses, rather than relating to themselves as victims of brutal assault. Finally they put their names or 'I' on the suffering individual. As therapy unfolds, many patients begin to understand how they move up and down 'the staircase of

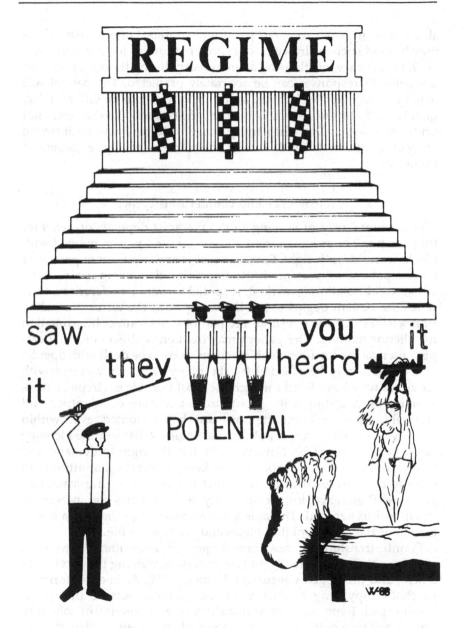

Fig. 16.1 The psychological mechanism of intellectualization.

abstraction' in order to avoid painful memories. Other artistic forms may be used such as drawings or representations of torture situations. Such pictures are worth using at an impasse during therapy, provided the patient's responses can be accurately predicted. The patient will usually claim that the situation in his/her case was quite different, e.g. guards and torturers were in civilian clothes, he/she was not undressed, but ... Drawings and pictures of torture may elicit strong emotional outbursts and should only be used by experienced therapists.

Transference and countertransference

The survivors' way of relating to the therapist depends on whether they see him/her as an ignorant 'do-gooder' or a person imbued with idealism and deep insight. Some form of friendship is often perceived by the patient as part of the therapeutic relationship, particularly when social isolation is marked. A special form of transference occurs when the patient begins to see the therapist as the torturer or when s/he believes that the questions are part of some form of interrogation for ulterior motives. The patient may frequently dream of the therapist, often as the torturer. Such reactions need to be dealt with openly.

Therapists may be affected by the many hours they spend with survivors who have lived through the most horrible of circumstances. Working in a setting with clients from a variety of countries and cultural backgrounds, the therapist may be confronted, even within the same day, with diverse political ideologies. Whatever the ideology of the patient might be, however, s/he has the right to demand and receive treatment. It is important to keep a professional attitude in therapy and always bear in mind that the work is on humanitarian grounds. Preference for, or solidarity with, a particular person or group is thus avoided. Therapists, however, may go through a reevaluation of their own political views and attitudes to life.

Countertransference reactions frequently encountered are rage, sadistic gratification, dread and horror, shame, viewing the survivor as a hero, and privileged voyeurism (Danieli, 1984). As in other forms of psychotherapy, any contact with the patients outside therapy is discouraged. Issues of countertransference and feelings of solidarity can be addressed through supervision of therapists, which may be offered individually as well as in a staff groups. Interpreters should also have the opportunity to work through their emotional reactions with an experienced therapist. Furthermore, intramural as well as extramural supervision through staff group meetings is necessary.

Extramural supervision may, for example, be accomplished by the participation of consultants from outside the treatment centre in the rehabilitation procedures in a supervisory capacity.

Aims of treatment

The evaluation of psychotherapy outcome has always been a controversial issue within psychiatry. It is thus not surprising that no consensus has yet been achieved regarding the goal of psychotherapy with torture survivors. In some forms of therapy 'the re-establishment' of political ideology has been emphasized as a treatment aim (Grupo Colat, 1982).

The aim of treatment may be an alleviation of symptoms in order to increase the survivor's social functioning in the country of exile. Treatment may include an in-depth psychotherapy for premorbid personality traits that may not be directly related to the torture or it may emphasize the importance of giving testimony and of the experience of political solidarity.

At the RCT the change measured in manifest symptomatology (e.g. a decrease in number of nightmares, improved ability to speak the language, less muscular dysfunction or pain, etc) has been accepted as a criterion of improvement in mental health status. An additional treatment goal is to help the patient improve his/her state of social functioning and regain control over life such that s/he is once again able to choose between the various options available. The therapist needs to take care not to influence the patient's decisions concerning these options.

It should be pointed out that the survivors do not seem to experience any prolonged change in their political awareness as a result of torture. In our experience the vast majority of survivors maintain their political views despite the fact that some of them may have sustained injuries severe enough to prevent them from fighting for their ideas. In some rare cases, however, the survivor may use the defensive strategy of conversion in order to cope with the extreme stress of the torture. This implies that s/he may no longer object to the rules and ideas expressed by the regime. Torture, as a means of breaking down the identity of the opponents of the regime, may thus occasionally act as a powerful deterrent.

In the years following the torture, survivors may also choose not to devote their lives to the same political ideas as before. This can be due to several reasons, including change with age, the emergence of problems related to the exile of a feeling of lethargy that is prevalent particularly in untreated survivors.

Patient attitudes to the therapeutic process

Survivors, when asked about their observations on the therapy process, often state that they were initially very distrustful of the therapy and of the therapists' knowledge about torture and its effects and sceptical about psychology in general. They often consider openness with respect to the treatment facilities, background, security, etc, as very important for the therapy process.

Subjective improvement is usually acknowledged when survivors can sleep better or when they are able to fight back or run away from danger in a nightmare. At the end of therapy, patients are often surprised that they are not transformed into new human beings, as some feared, and that they can still remember everything that happened during the torture. Memories, however, no longer affect daily life adversely.

OTHER TREATMENT FORMS

Other treatment centres and their methods are outlined elsewhere in this volume. Different approaches exist depending on the local circumstances of the treatment facility, the number of survivors waiting for treatment, the members of the staff, and the political views of the therapists at the facility, etc.

The main alternative methods of treating torture survivors are outlined below. A combination of the therapies described in the following is frequently used in order, for example, to deal with resistance to therapy.

Family therapy

Family therapy, involving young children, does not seem appropriate since it is unlikely that children would benefit from being exposed to the horrors experienced by the parents. Marital therapy, however, may be applied, particularly when communication between the spouses is at an impasse. There are only a limited number of therapists who are experienced in marital therapy where one or more members of a family are torture survivors, and reports of the outcome of such therapy are scant. It is questionable whether sexual abuse should be explored during such therapy unless explicitly desired by both husband and wife.

Non-verbal forms of treatment

Non-verbal therapy techniques may sometimes be needed since some survivors are not suitable for insight therapy. During the physiotherapy sessions at the RCT, significant amounts of repressed emotions are released. For example, manipulation of lower abdominal and back muscles in persons who have been subjected to sexual abuse is quite provocative and may lead to abreaction. Physiotherapy and psychotherapy sessions, therefore, always follow one another.

A somewhat different approach to the treatment of the body is relaxation therapy. Clients are taught to relax individual muscle groups as well as to lower the general level of muscular tension. This is a method employed by therapists in the Philippines (Larsen & Pagaduan-Lopez, 1987).

Group therapy

Individual therapy is the treatment of choice at the RCT because of the psychotherapeutic training and expertise available among the therapists, and the language barriers which require the use of interpreters during therapy. Even when patients speak the same language, they may belong to politically opposing groups, in which case direct confrontation in group sessions is inappropriate.

On the other hand, group sessions have been successfully used by the Plaza de Mayo Group in Argentina. The survivors treated by this group speak the same language and therapy focuses on the understanding of torture as a political instrument. The number of torture survivors that need help in Argentina also necessiatate large-scale treatment. Group therapy is also sometimes used at the Red Cross Centre in Malmö, Sweden.

Short-term therapy

There are obvious differences in treatment of torture survivors between countries where torture is being systematically perpetrated and 'peaceful rich distant countries'. In the treatment centres of the Philippines and South Africa, special short-term therapies have been developed (Foster, 1987). Each session is structured, as far as possible, as a complete therapy because of the uncertainty about further attendance. The Red Cross centre in Stockholm has used a form of short-term therapy, usually consisting of five sessions. Only severely injured survivors were referred for long-term psychotherapy.

Play therapy

Play therapy is used for children at the Marcelino Children Centre in the Philippines (Protacio-Marcelino, 1989). Furthermore, art therapy is being developed as both an investigative and a treatment tool for children. Art therapy is also employed for adults when survivors are motivated and able to express themselves in this way.

Psycho-social treatment

The rehabilitation model of the RCT is based upon a biopsycho-social approach. Other centres have chosen to work within a frame of reference in which less emphasis is placed on the integration of the somatic and psychological aspects of the problem and more emphasis is given to psycho-social factors and support during the process of social reintegration. This model views the role of the professionals as only 'facilitators' of community activities and thus focuses on self-help and mutual help within the community. An attempt is made to provide a social-psychological explanation of the damage inflicted by the perpetrators and to explain the crises experienced by the survivors as part of a social process. Within this context, the survivors's dialogue with the community plays a central role for their re-integration process. The work does not end with remedying the harmful effects of torture and exile but involves the enhancement of public awareness of the conditions of political oppression. In this model the somatic problems and their treatment are not neglected but may be considered of secondary importance.

Spiritual dimensions in therapy

Religious issues may have to be dealt with at some stage during the therapy or sometimes from the outset. Many survivors are religious, and although religion may have a less prominent place in con-temporary thought in the westernized world than in other societies, it is nevertheless a reality for many survivors. Many survivors find solace in religious texts as such texts address general humanitarian issues and emotions. Survivors may wish to discuss 'eternal ques-tion' such as guilt, sin, and suicide as they relate to religion. In addition, they may search for basic ethical and moral values in religious texts in order to regain 'a basic belief in humanity' or to 'find faith again'.

Imagery

Relaxation therapy may be accompanied by imagery, even to the point of confronting the survivor with imaginal scenes of the torture chamber and thus releasing repressed emotions. A well-integrated personality is a prerequisite, and the therapist needs extensive experience before attempting such an approach. These treatment techniques are described in another chapter (see Başoğlu, this volume).

Testimony

The testimony method involves a contract between the therapist and the patient and the preparation of a document giving the details of the torture, including names, dates, and addresses. If this method is possible and if it is desired by the patient, the psychological reactions of the patient may be addressed through this process. In this respect, the testimony method is similar to insight therapy. Testimony therapy also attempts to restore the patient's political awareness since it is believed that the torture may have had an impact on the ideological beliefs of the survivor. It is argued that, if the patient has lost interest in devoting his/her life to a certain cause, the torturers have succeeded in achieving their goal (Cienfuegos & Monelli, 1983; Buus & Agger, 1988).

CONCLUSION

Torture induces predictable reactions of physical and psychological nature that disrupt the individual's ability to live a full life. Many psychotherapeutic techniques are now available, but their relative efficacy has not been scientifically assessed. We know that a large proportion of survivors undergoing therapy may experience significant improvement in their psychological functioning. Memories may persist but no longer affect daily life. We still lack, however, investigations focusing on the short- as well as long-term effects of treatment.

Important areas for future research include studies of the relationship between a) initial severity of symptomatology and treatment outcome, b) symptom profiles and treatment outcome, c) presenting symptoms and duration of treatment, and d) cultural background and outcome. Also needed are comparative studies of different models of rehabilitation.

REFERENCES

Bentsen, E-M, Hermansen, A., Knudsen, I. H. & Pentz-Moller, V. (1989). Interpretation in the rehabilitation of torture victims. *Transcultural Psychiatric Research Review*, **26**, 26–9.

Buus, S. & Agger, I. (1988). The testimony-method: The use of therapy as a psychotherapeutic tool in the treatment of traumatised refugees in Denmark. *Refugee Participation Network*, **3**, 14–18.

Cienfuegos, A. J. & Monelli, C. (1983). The testimony of political repression as a therapeutic instrument. *American Journal of Orthopsychiatry*, **53**, 43–51.

Danieli, Y. (1984). Psychotherapist's participation in the conspiracy of silence about the Holocaust. *Psychoanalytical Psychology*, **1**, 23–42.

Eitinger, L. (1969). Rehabilitation of concentration camp survivors (following concentration camp trauma). Proceedings of 7th International Congress of Psychotherapy, Wiesbaden 1967, part V rehabilitation. *Psychotherapy and Psychosomatics*, **17**, 42–9.

Foster, F. (1987). *Detention and Torture in South Africa*. Cape Town and Johannesburg: David Philip.

Grupo Colat (1982). *Psicopatologia de la tortura y el exilio*. Madrid: Editorial Fundamentos.

Gunderson, E. K. E. & Rahe, R. H. eds. (1974). *Life Stress and Illness*. Springfield, Illinois: Charles C. Thomas Publisher.

Kordon, D. R., Edelman, L. I., Lagos, D. M., Nicoletti, E. & Bozzolo, R. C. (1988). *Psychological Effects of Political Repression*. Buenos Aires: Sudamericana/Planeta.

Larsen, H. & Pagaduan-Lopez, J. (1987). Stress–tension reduction in the treatment of sexually tortured women: an exploratory study. *Journal of Sex and Marital Therapy*, **13**, 210–18.

Malt, U. F. & Weisæth, I. (1989). Traumatic stress: empirical studies from Norway. *Acta Psychiatrica*, **80 (suppl. 355)**, 7–137.

Melamed, B. G., Melamed, J. L. & Bouhoutsos, J. C. (1990). Psychological consequences of torture – a need to formulate new strategies for research. In P. Suedfeld, ed. *Psychology and Torture*. Hemisphere Publishing Corporation.

Ochberg, F. M. (1988). *Posttraumatic Therapy and Victims of Violence*. New York: Brunner Mazel.

Pagaduan-Lopez J. C. ed. (1987). *Torture Survivors, What Can We Do For Them?* Manila: Medical Action Group, Inc.

Protacio-Marcelino, E. (1989). Children of political detainees in the Philippines, sources of stress and coping patterns. *International Journal of Mental Health*, **18**, 71–86.

Somnier, F. & Genefke, I. K. (1986). Psychotherapy for victims of torture. *British Journal of Psychiatry*, **149**, 323–9.

17

CURRENT TRENDS IN THE TREATMENT OF POST-TRAUMATIC STRESS SYMPTOMS

Terence M. Keane, Anne Marie Albano and Dudley David Blake

With estimates of the prevalence of post-traumatic stress disorder (PTSD) ranging from 1–2% of the general population, it is not surprising that PTSD is a topic of rising concern for policy makers and clinicians alike (Davidson *et al.*, 1990; Helzer, Robins & McEvoy, 1987; Kulka *et al.*, 1988). The study of PTSD has consequently received increased attention from clinical researchers. Since inclusion of the disorder in the third edition of the *Diagnostic and Statistical Manual* (DSM–III) of the American Psychiatric Association (1980, 1987), there has been a proliferation of knowledge about the assessment, treatment, and prevalence of PTSD, as well as the biological and cognitive processes associated with it (Keane, 1989). The purpose of this chapter is to provide an overview of the advances made in the treatment of psychological trauma over the past decade.

While clearly the greatest advances in research on PTSD have stemmed from the study of combat-related PTSD, particularly in American survivors of Vietnam and Israeli survivors of the Yom Kippur and Lebanon Wars, many of the lessons learned from the study of these populations can be generalized readily to the study of survivors and victims of other life endangering experiences. Common themes appear to be associated with traumas of different origins and include conditions such as terror, helplessness, guilt over actions taken or avoided, fear of bodily injury, and consuming loss. Traumatic responses generally include common symptoms such as anxiety, depression, anger or rage, nightmares and concomitant sleep disorder, physiological hyperarousal and reactivity, and emotional numbing. Psychosocial problems also seem to occur and include alienation, substance abuse, vocational incapacity, and an impaired ability to form intimate attachments. With such extensive commonality in clinical phenomenology, the lessons learned from the study of combat trauma may provide a template for the development of assessment and treatment methods for other types of trauma.

The study of trauma secondary to torture can clearly benefit from an integration with the combat literature. With little extant empirical information on torture, it is relevant to consider the conditions of combatants and prisoners of war in trying to develop a comprehensive understanding of the clinical technology that might be of some assistance to the treatment of torture victims. While some of the sociopolitical issues surrounding torture may differ from those related to combat trauma, the issues of helplessness, terror, bodily injury, and guilt (or responsibility) over the experience seem especially common to both forms of trauma. This chapter, then, focuses on information currently available on the behavioral treatment of PTSD. When possible, an emphasis is placed on empirical studies so that the reader can benefit from the scientific knowledge accumulating in the study of PTSD.

A variety of treatments have been employed, separately and combined, to assist in the adjustment process of traumatized individuals. Exposure-based behavioral and cognitive-behavioral treatments have shown considerable promise in the amelioration of symptoms associated with post-traumatic stress disorder (PTSD) (Lyons & Keane, 1988; Fairbank & Brown, 1988; Keane *et al.*, 1989). Use of these treatments has been substantiated by empirical investigations that have demonstrated their efficacy. Moreover, therapy-process studies similarly have provided data that are consistent with predictions of the underlying theory (cf. Chemtob *et al.*, 1988; Foa, Steketee & Olasov Rothbaum, 1989; Keane, Zimering & Caddell, 1985; Levis & Hare, 1977). Findings on the biological substrates of PTSD (e.g. van der Kolk, 1983, 1987; Friedman, 1988; Krystal *et al.*, 1989) have also provided guidance for appropriate pharmacotherapeutic intervention. Similarly, other treatments such as group therapy (e.g. rap groups for combat veterans), skills training, and family therapy, have been used with notable success in treating traumatized individuals.

In the following sections, these main treatment approaches will be described, compared, and contrasted. Clearly, these treatments do not all provide the same therapeutic benefits to traumatized individuals. For example, cognitive treatments may minimize the catastrophic thinking and cognitive distortions that frequently are present in traumatized persons, while pharmacotherapy may serve to reduce physiological concomitants of the trauma response. Thus, it is important to view these treatments in light of their specific treatment effects. Given the multifaceted nature of post-traumatic stress, systematic observations of differential effects from treatment become crucial. Identifying the effects obtained from a given treatment will ensure an optimal patient-treatment match.

Each section below will include the following aspects: 1) the rationale/conceptual framework behind a treatment approach, 2) a review of pertinent treatment literature, 3) the differential symptom effects related to the described treatment, and 4) a summary and comments about the treatment.

While the focus of this book is torture and its effects, most of the work reviewed and discussed in this chapter relates to combat-related PTSD. As stated above, this was intentional since the war-related PTSD literature is substantial and exceeds that of the torture literature. It also contains several controlled studies of PTSD treatment. In addition, combat-related PTSD is phenomenologically similar to the traumatic stress of torture victims. Conceptually, both populations are similar also because the stress to which they are exposed is extreme and largely uncontrollable.

DIRECT THERAPEUTIC EXPOSURE

Direct therapeutic exposure (DTE) is widely regarded as a critical component of comprehensive treatment for intractable post-traumatic stress symptoms. DTE as a treatment approach can include desensitization, flooding, implosive therapy, and all other variants of *in vivo* and imaginal exposure. Exposure treatment studies with combat-related PTSD have generally involved desensitization and flooding or implosive therapy. These two groups of treatment procedures evolved from related but separate conceptual frameworks.

Rationale/conceptual framework

Imaginal, *in vivo*, and *in vitro* desensitization procedures stem from the pioneering work of Wolpe (1958), and are based on the principle of 'reciprocal inhibition', that is, certain behavioral responses take precedence over, and thus 'inhibit' the expression of others. One application of reciprocal inhibition is systematic desensitization which include three aspects: 1) establishing an alternative behavior that is incompatible with, or will inhibit, the undesired behavior (usually relaxation), 2) establishing a written hierarchy of feared stimuli scenes or images in which the individual can experience, in equal-interval steps, a gradient of increasing arousal until the final step, whereupon he or she is exposed to the full range of feared stimuli, and 3) exposing the individual to the feared stimuli in a titrated fashion while he or she engages in the inhibitory behavior (relaxation). Through this process, the individual receives increasing exposure to feared stimuli while fear responses are minimized, and eventually these fear responses are replaced by more adaptive ones.

Flooding and implosive therapy are based on early work by Stampfl & Levis (1967), and their use is linked conceptually with the work of Mowrer (1960; Levis & Hare, 1977; Keane *et al.*, 1985). Stampfl & Levis' (1967) model of psychopathology proposed the notion of 'serial conditioning' and the 'conservation of anxiety hypothesis' to explain why many trauma-induced symptoms, including those in torture victims, seem resistant to natural extinction effects. Extinction is the gradual weakening of the capacity of conditioned stimuli to evoke a conditioned response when the conditioned stimuli is presented without the unconditioned stimuli. Levis and Hare (1977) explain resistance to extinction by proposing that thoughts and feelings can become conditioned stimuli and they can 're-vitalize' other conditioned stimuli that have been extinguished or partially extinguished. In this way, trauma reactions become self-perpetuating (i.e. resistant to extinction) and the fear or anxiety is conserved. Also, more potent stimuli can condition less potent or non-trauma-related stimuli and the individual's anxiety/fear response can generalize beyond the originally present trauma cues. An example of this resistance to extinction can be seen in the (hypothetical) case of a torture victim who had been tied with rope and brutally assaulted. Presentation of a rope or any rope-like article could induce considerable arousal and anxiety. These fears could also generalize to any object that might be used to bind hands or feet (e.g. extension cords, shoe laces, etc).

The active elements of implosive or flooding therapy involve directing the victim to repeatedly and systematically imagine all aspects of the traumatic incident(s) in the context of a relationship with a knowledgeable and supportive professional. Typically this exposure occurs over many sessions and each memory is presented using imagery for a minimum of 100 minutes. In this approach, the individual is asked to vividly recall trauma stimuli using as many senses (sights, sounds, smells, tastes, tactile sensations) as possible. This comprehensive approach to cue presentation includes aspects of both stimulus and response propositions (Lang, 1977). Although there are variations of this approach (e.g. Farnsworth, Wood, & Ayers, 1975; Grigsby, 1987), the therapist typically serves as a facilitator, directing the individual to experience and reexperience a recollection of the traumatic event(s), reminding him or her to recall the event as if it were happening in that instant.

As opposed to systematic desensitization, the object of implosive therapy and flooding is to have the patient experience in the therapy session the arousal associated with the traumatic memories. This arousal is intentionally maintained until it is attenuated through extinction; within and across sessions the individual becomes less aroused to these trauma memories, and thus, symptomatology abates. The basic difference between implosive therapy and flooding is that while the latter entails having the individual image real or trauma-specific stimuli, implosive therapy also involves all possible conditioned stimuli, including hypothesized faulty beliefs and value systems (e.g. themes such as loss of control, eternal damnation, guilt, or humiliation and shame). The aim in implosive therapy is to address the anxiety and conflict associated with the many psychological issues related to the traumatic event, typically involving all stimuli hypothesized to be a part of the trauma response (e.g. thoughts and images directly and indirectly linked to the trauma stimuli).

PTSD and desensitization treatments

In an early report of the behavioral treatment of trauma, Kipper (1977) described *in vivo* desensitization treatment of four Israeli combat veterans of the Yom Kippur War who suffered from war-related fears (closed spaces, noises, bandages, and people and crowds). In short, these treatments were individualized and involved relaxation training followed by graduated and hierarchically sequenced exposure to circumstances, people, and materials, that were phobically avoided by or produced excessive physiological reactions from the respective veterans. Kipper reported the treated veterans to have attained success in mastering the phobic reactions (as shown by the veterans' ability to be exposed to greater steps in their hierarchies) and claimed that his findings support '... the inclusion of these modes of intervention in the list of treatments recommended for war neuroses ...' (p. 221).

Schindler (1980), also employing systematic desensitization, successfully treated a 29 year-old traumatized Vietnam combat veteran. Prior to treatment, the veteran reported nightly nightmares and anxiety about sleeping. After five 30-minute sessions the veteran reported experiencing no more nightmares. A seven-month follow-up revealed no reoccurrence of the disturbing nightmares.

Bowen and Lambert (1986) also reported on the successful use of systematic desensitization with combat traumatized veterans. These investigators treated eight Vietnam combat veterans, a World War II combat veteran/POW, and one veteran who witnessed a catastrophic airplane crash. All of the veterans were judged to have significant

Table 17.1. *Symptom changes in combat veterans undergoing deliberate therapeutic exposure*

Article	Treatment modality	Symptom changes from treatment
Black & Keane (1982)	Implosive therapy	Decreased anxiety
Boudewyns & Hyer (1990)	Implosive therapy	Decreased physiological responding (heart rate, forehead tension, skin conductance) when imaging trauma related scenes Improvements on measure of anxiety/depression, vigor, alienation, and confidence in skills
Bowen & Lambert (1986)	Systematic desensitization	Decreased heart rate and muscle tension (EMG) when exposed to trauma-related stimuli Decreased subjective stress
Cooper & Clum (1989)	Flooding therapy	Decreased state and trait anxiety Decreased sleep disturbance Decreased nightmares Decreased behavioral avoidance
Fairbank, Gross & Keane (1983)	Flooding therapy	Decreased motoric arousal when exposed to trauma cues Decreased depression ratings Decreased intrusive thoughts of trauma
Fairbank & Keane (1982)	Flooding therapy	Decreased daily anxiety Decreased anxiety related to traumatic cues Decreased intrusive thoughts of trauma Decreased heart rate and skin conductance when exposed to trauma-related stimuli
Grigsby (1987)	'Imagery' (flooding)	Decreased intrusive thoughts
Keane, Fairbank, Caddell & Zimmering (1989)	Implosive therapy	Decreased state anxiety Decreased reexperiencing symptoms Decreased startle Decreased depression Decreased self-reported fear Improvements in memory, concentration

Table 17.1. (*cont.*)

Article	Treatment modality	Symptom changes from treatment
Keane & Kaloupek (1982)	Implosive therapy	Decreased state anxiety Decreased anxiety ratings Increased sleep time Decreased nightmares Decreased flashbacks
Kipper (1977)	*In vivo* desensitization	Habituation to higher steps of hierarchies
Miller & DiPilato (1983)	Systematic desensitization	–
Mueser & Butler (1987)	Flooding therapy	Decreased auditory hallucinations
Saigh (1986)	*In vitro* flooding	Decreased anxiety Decreased behavioral avoidance Decreased depression Improved short-term memory, freedom from distraction, and concentration Decreased classroom hyperactivity
Saigh (1987a)	*In vitro* flooding	Decreased state and trait anxiety Decreased behavioral avoidance Decreased depression Increased self-report of assertiveness Improved short-term memory, freedom from distraction, and concentration
Saigh (1987b)	*In vitro* flooding	Decreased anxiety Decreased trauma-related thoughts Decreased behavioral avoidance Increased self-report of assertiveness Improved short-term memory, freedom from distraction, and concentration Decreased classroom hyperactivity Improved school grades
Schindler (1980)	Systematic desensitization	Remission of trauma nightmares

PTSD symptomatology and received several months of an outpatient treatment which included systematic desensitization; most of the veterans were also involved in group psychotherapy and received psychotropic medication. This treatment package was found to significantly reduce the veterans' physiological arousal and subjective stress when exposed to a series of combat verbally described scenes.

Collectively, the findings reported above indicate that systematic desensitization procedures are effective in reducing certain symptoms in traumatized individuals (Table 17.1). Given its efficacy with combat and other trauma populations (e.g. Williams, 1976; Wolff, 1977), the demonstration of systematic desensitization's efficacy with survivors of torture has promise and awaits empirical study.

PTSD and implosive therapy and flooding

Initially, evidence supporting the efficacy of implosive therapy and flooding with traumatized veterans came from case studies (Black & Keane, 1982; Fairbank, deGood & Jenkins, 1981; Fairbank, Gross & Keane, 1983; Fairbank & Keane, 1982; Keane & Kaloupek, 1982). More recently, randomized and controlled outcome studies have appeared that demonstrate clinical benefits from using this exposure-based procedure (Boudewyns & Hyer, 1990; Boudewyns *et al.*, in press; Cooper & Clum, 1989; Keane *et al.*, 1989).

Black and Keane (1982), used implosive therapy to treat a World War II Navy combat veteran with a 36-year history of combat-related fears. The investigators reported dramatic reductions in anxiety after three treatment sessions that led to lasting changes (18 months) in the individual's use of health care services. Fairbank and Keane (1982) used relaxation therapy and imaginal flooding to treat two Vietnam combat veterans with PTSD symptoms. Using a single case multiple-baseline methodology, these investigators found that treatment served to decrease psychological arousal to specific memories of combat experiences. This reduction in response to imagery of the events was documented using both subjective and psychophysiological measures (i.e. heart rate and skin conductance). Keane and Kaloupek (1982) also treated a Vietnam combat veteran using implosive therapy. In 19 sessions, the veteran's adjustment improved on measures of anxiety, nightmares, flashbacks, and increased sleep. This improvement was maintained at a 12-month follow-up.

Fairbank *et al.* (1983) treated a 32-year old Vietnam combat veteran with PTSD whose entire unit was decimated by an enemy assault wherein he eventually lost a leg from battle wounds. The patient had never previously discussed the incident with anyone, but experienced parts of intrusive memories of the assault in the form of recurrent, distressing nightmares and frightening flashbacks over an 11-year period. During exposure treatment the veteran reported considerable reductions in anxiety by the end of each session; by the end of treatment, he showed measurable decreases in motoric activity, depression ratings, and self-monitored intrusive memories of the event. A post-test probe assessment indicated that the patient could imagine the traumatic event with considerable reduced subjective and motoric arousal. At a 6-month follow-up, the veteran reported that he could more comfortably think about and discuss his trauma.

In a series of single-subject multiple baseline design treatments, Saigh (1986, 1987*a*, *b*) used flooding with traumatized child and adolescent bystanders of the Lebanon invasion and civil war. The trauma survivors evidenced anxiety, avoidance behavior, concentration problems, and depression. Flooding served to promote rapid positive changes in these children's affective, behavioral, and cognitive status.

In a randomized trial, Cooper and Clum (1989) compared a 'standard' individual and group PTSD treatment program with a standard program supplemented with flooding. Seven Vietnam combat veterans were assigned to each of the respective groups and the investigators found that only the flooding treatment group demonstrated significant symptom reduction. For the veterans receiving this treatment, improvements were shown in the form of decreased sleep disturbance, nightmares, subjective discomfort ratings during a behavioral avoidance task, and state anxiety. At three month follow-up, the flooding group continued to show decreases in sleep disturbance and psychotic-like symptoms.

In a controlled treatment outcome study of 24 Vietnam veterans with PTSD, Keane *et al.* (1989) provided 12 to 14 sessions of implosive therapy. The treatment focused on assisting the patients in exposure to traumatic events in imagery. This treatment was found to be superior to a no treatment (waiting list control) in effecting changes in the veterans' re-experiencing symptoms, anxiety, and depression, but did not appear to influence the affective numbing or social avoidance aspects of PTSD. These treatment gains were maintained at a six month follow-up.

Similarly, Boudewyns and Hyer (1990) compared direct therapeutic exposure (DTE; i.e. imaginal flooding) with conventional one-to-one counseling in the treatment of combat-related PTSD. Thirty-eight PTSD inpatients were randomly assigned to receive either 10–12

Table 17.2. *Positive and negative symptoms of post-traumatic stress disorder*

Positive symptoms	Negative symptoms
Recurrent and intrusive distressing recollections of the event	Efforts to avoid thoughts or feelings associated with the trauma
Recurrent distressing dreams of the event	Efforts to avoid activities or situations that arouse recollections of the trauma
Sudden acting or feeling as if the traumatic event were recurring	Inability to recall an important aspect of the trauma
Intense psychological distress at exposure to events that symbolize or resemble an aspect of the traumatic event	Markedly diminished interest in significant activities
Sense of a foreshortened future	Feeling of detachment or estrangement from others
Difficulty falling or staying asleep	Restricted range of affect
Irritability or outbursts of anger	
Difficulty concentrating	
Hypervigilance	
Exaggerated startle response	
Physiologic reactivity upon exposure to events that symbolize or resemble an aspect of the traumatic event	

sessions of DTE or counseling. Participants from neither group showed significant decreases in daily self-ratings of anxiety. However, the DTE group did show decreased arousal, especially heart rate, when exposed to slides of combat, and the individuals from this group showed significant improvements on components of a structured psychological assessment (in anxiety/depression, vigor, alienation, and confidence in skills).

Differential symptom effects

In reviewing the results of studies described above it is clear that exposure-based behavior therapy can significantly reduce the effects of traumatization. It is also clear that these treatments do not reduce all of the symptoms in the PTSD syndrome to an equal extent. Exposure appears to have the greatest impact on the more anxiety-based and observable, or 'positive' symptoms (e.g. startle, psychophysiological arousal, nightmares, irritability and anger), while negative ones (e.g. numbing, alienation, restricted affect) remaining relatively unchanged (Keane, 1989; Litz *et al.*, in press; see Table 17.2). For more uniform therapeutic benefit, additional or alternative treatments may be necessary. For example, Keane *et al.* (1985) recommended a stress management package that includes relaxation training, cognitive restructuring, and problem-solving skills training. Litz *et al.* (in press) suggest that clinicians might encourage their traumatized patients who show a preponderance of negative symptoms to increase interpersonal risk-taking and to arrange for success and mastery experiences via skills training and *in vivo* exercises. Alternately, Williams (1987) described a treatment program which addresses trauma survivors' experience of guilt. This program was designed to help veterans abreact, with the therapist playing an active role in probing and soliciting from the veteran a description of the traumatic incident(s). Other activities included in the guilt-reducing regiment are cognitive restructuring, the empty chair techniques (enabling the survivor express sentiments about those who did not survive or to explain behavior required for survival), and helping the veteran to give up sole responsibility for what happened, and to recognize his developmental level at the time of the incident(s).

Summary and comments

The differential effect on symptoms shown by the several DTE treatments suggests the need for treatment–patient matching at the treatment planning stage. Ascertaining whether an individual can possibly benefit from DTE is a primary consideration. With respect to this issue, Litz *et al.* (1990) have outlined decision rules for the proper use of DTE. The factors identified as important in determining the appropriateness of DTE treatment include an ability to provide a concise description of the traumatic event(s), no debilitating concurrent psychiatric or medical diagnosis, adequate motivation for change, and a demonstrated psychophysiological reactivity to traumatic memories. On the other hand, patients unsuited for DTE are those with characteristics that might interfere with the boundary conditions of DTE (e.g. poor ability to imagine, inability to tolerate intense arousal) or lead to unsatisfactory compliance or premature termination of treatment.

Exposure treatments may work best in combination with other treatments. For example, supportive therapy, cognitive therapy, anger or stress management, and social skills training are logical adjuncts to DTE. Pharmacotherapy may also be used to promote short term symptom relief. Combining therapies in a sensible way to maximize treatment success is a topic worthy of additional clinical and research exploration.

Due to the potential problems associated with the increase arousal and symptom escalation that accompanies implosive therapy (e.g. Giles, 1988; Kilpatrick & Best, 1984), stress management or desensitization approaches may be preferable. By virtue of how these 'milder' approaches are implemented, the individual never experiences high levels of arousal and consequently feels only manageable discomfort. However, other (e.g. Shipley & Boudewyns, 1980, 1988) have argued against implosive therapy's iatrogenic effects; these investigators argue that the published research data show implosive therapy to be as safe as, and in some ways safer than, traditional psychotherapeutic approaches. The patient who receives these mild treatments may also experience less extinction and consequently derive less benefit.

COGNITIVE BEHAVIORAL THERAPY

Recently, cognitive and information processing models for explaining post-trauma symptomatology have appeared in the literature (Chemtob *et al.*, 1988; Foa *et al.*, 1989; Jones & Barlow, 1990; Kreitler & Kreitler, 1988; Litz & Keane, 1989). Each of these theoretical formulations contains various common components that focus on cognitive processing, attentional processes, perception, and memory integration. A comparison of these various cognitive conceptualizations follows, with an emphasis on the unique elements of each.

Rationale/conceptual framework

Foa and Kozak (1986) proposed a fear memory network, for conceptualizing the anxiety disorders in accordance with the information processing model of fear outlined by Lang (1977, 1979). This network includes information: 1) about the feared stimulus, 2) about potential verbal, behavioral, and physiological responses, and 3) for assigning meaning to 1) and 2). This fear network is considered to be an executable program for escape and avoidance. Foa and Kozak argued that fear reduction occurs only when the fear network is activated and information is presented that is counter to and corrects the fear network, as is accomplished in the extinction based DTE treatments. This reconstituted fear network as a result contains weaker escape and avoidance behavior components. Foa *et al.* (1989) contend that the information-processing model of fear (Foa & Kozak, 1986) more adequately explains PTSD symptomatology than does conditioning theory. In their view, conditioning theory sufficiently accounts for those symptoms involving fear and behavioral avoidance but falls short in explaining other trauma symptoms, such as aggressive responses from victims, emotional numbness, and social withdrawal often seen with trauma survivors. Support for this model has also been articulated by other PTSD researchers (e.g. Litz & Keane, 1989).

Recently, Chemtob *et al.* (1988) described an encompassing cognitive action theory of PTSD that incorporates theoretical propositions introduced by Beck & Emery (1985), Foa and Kozak (1986), Lang (1977, 1979), and Horowitz (1976). This framework specifies that fear is conceptually organized as hierarchically arranged action structures involving cognitive schemata that range from abstract constructs to discrete responses. At each level of the action structure is associative information about stimuli and responses ('nodes'). Node activation is controlled by the combined effect of neural potentiation and inhibition received from other nodes or environmental stimuli (external and internal).

Chemtob *et al.* (1988) proposed that PTSD is distinguished from other anxiety disorders by three features: 1) a higher standard level of potentiation for threat arousal nodes, 2) greater susceptibility to and escalation in arousal and threat interpretation, and 3) higher limits on arousal magnitude. The investigators also proposed that trauma survivors are more apt to select information that confirms their expectations of the (threatening) world around them. From this theoretical framework, Chemtob *et al.* (1988) recommend exposure-based and stress management treatments in work with PTSD.

Horowitz (1978, 1986) presents a psychodynamic formulation of stress response that contains a cognitive conceptualization of trauma. Two themes, denial and the compulsive tendency to repeat some aspect of the trauma, play a central role in his formulation. In addition to the use of brief dynamic therapy, Horowitz advocates behavior therapy, including systematic desensitization and implosive therapy, as treatment variations in work with trauma survivors.

Other cognitive theories of PTSD have also appeared recently. Kreitler & Kreitler (1988) posited a cognitive approach to anxiety and to the 'complex of clinically significant long term responses [that are] characteristic of individuals who have been exposed to an unusually strong stressor' (p. 35). In describing why some individuals and not others develop long standing trauma responses, these investigators proposed that chronic anxiety originates in perceptual tendencies and is a reflection of a pattern of (maladaptive) meaning assignment. According to these investigators, meaning can be systematically analyzed along four sets of dimensions, including: 1) meaning dimensions (e.g. range of inclusion, consequences and results, temporal qualities, etc), 2) types of relation (e.g. attributive, comparative, etc), 3) forms of relation (e.g. positive, conjunctive, etc), and 4) shifts of referent (e.g. identical, associative, etc). In a systematic inquiry, these investigators found that higher anxiety individuals assign meaning to experiences in a unique way, including that they are

> ... highly sensitive to internal cues, bodily sensations, and pain; they are preoccupied with their body and incline toward hypochondriasis; emotionally they are excitable, tense, sensitive, and unstable; they tend toward worry, depression, and occasional hysteric swings; they tend to concentrate on fantasies, daydreams, and internal problems rather than on external reality; they tend to turn away from action and behave in a shy or withdrawn manner; they often adopt a critical judgmental-evaluative approach; they are concerned with moral standards, are highly conscientious, are stable in their attitudes and values, and take evaluations by others seriously; they tend to be guilt-prone and suffer from a sense of inadequacy; they are likely to delay gratifications; they tend to be introspective; they are often fast in reaction and may overestimate the duration of an event or action; they prefer the known and the familiar to the new and sensation-evoking; in the cognitive domain they tend toward rigidity, intolerance of ambiguity, and restriction in cognitive contents; in their approach to issues they tend to be subjectively biased, evaluative, and emotional rather than objective, factual, and analytic; they often deviate from presented situations to themes that are hardly, if at all, associated to the starting point; and they often perceive issues and solve problems in metaphoric-symbolic terms rather than rely on interpersonally shared considerations and common logical rules. (p. 46).

These investigators suggested that treatment for trauma victims should assist them in reassigning meaning, thereby cognitively altering their psychological condition.

PTSD and cognitive therapy

In a recent review of the trauma literature (Blake, Albano, & Keane, 1990), only one report was found evaluating the efficacy of cognitive therapy (McCormack, 1985). This report describes the use of a cognitively oriented counseling intervention with a Vietnam combat veteran which lead to successful progress on all treatment goals, including improved communication with the veteran's offspring. However, by virtue of relying on a case study design, the findings outlined in the report are subject to threats to both internal and external validity; controlled study is warranted in order to more fully evaluate the efficacy of cognitive therapy with PTSD patients. In addition to the paucity of articles on the cognitive treatment of PTSD, there were no studies directly testing the cognitive conceptual models described above. It is thus not possible to determine whether treatment focusing on changing cognitive schemas or belief systems will result in any lasting behavioral change or promote psychological adjustment. Given the importance of these approaches to treating trauma patients, clearly research is needed on the efficacy of cognitive therapies.

Summary and comments

The lack of published reports on cognitive therapy approaches to trauma raises several questions. First, how *do* these cognitive models translate to treatment? At present it appears that exposure-based, rather than cognitive, approaches are the treatments of choice. Foa and Kozak (1986) proposed that the changes resulting from exposure are a product of the emotional processing proposed by Rachman (1980), which incorporates altered cognitive processing. They proposed that four factors interfere with emotional processing: 1) cognitive avoidance, 2) absence of short-term habituation, 3) depression, and 4) overvalued ideation. In this view, the cognitive therapist's role might be to address and eliminate the barriers to optimal emotional processing, for example, by treating a coexisting depression or an excessively rigid cognitive style. However, research is needed to fully evaluate each of the four factors proposed by Foa and Kozak for their contribution to PTSD treatment.

Another question raised by the limited literature on cognitive factors associated with trauma involves the utility of currently available cognitive treatments. Applications to trauma can certainly be found in the cognitive behavior therapy of Beck (1976; Beck & Emery, 1987), the rationale emotive therapy of Ellis (Ellis & Grieger, 1986), the cognitive behavior modification of Meichenbaum (1974, 1977), and the self-efficacy theory of Bandura (1977, 1986). Most of these approaches involve changing cognitive patterns by modifying maladaptive cognitions, irrational beliefs, negative self-statements, or increasing self-efficacy and expectations. The degree to which these therapies are helpful in the treatment of PTSD awaits further empirical documentation.

PHARMACOTHERAPY

The literature on the pharmacotherapy of PTSD is largely composed of numerous preliminary and exploratory efforts. The application of pharmacotherapy in the treatment of post-traumatic stress has been addressed in detail elsewhere (i.e. Roth, 1988; Friedman, 1988), but descriptions of representative studies and accompanying theoretical bases are presented here.

Rationale/conceptual framework

Review of the literature reveals few controlled studies of pharmacotherapy in the treatment of traumatic stress. Friedman (1988) identified three main reasons for the limited pharmacological treatment research on trauma: 1) post-traumatic stress disorder is conceptualized largely by the 2-factor psychological-behavioral model (Mowrer, 1960) of conditioned emotional arousal and reinforced avoidance; 2) the reluctance, in some mental health and societal circles, to acknowledge the validity of posttraumatic stress as a diagnosis; and 3) the short span of time since the publication of DSM–III (American Psychiatric Association, 1980) limiting systematic psychopharmacological investigations.

Clearly, in the treatment of trauma medications are a viable treatment option when the intensity or duration of a symptom compromises an individual's ability to participate in psychological treatment. It is likely that pharmacotherapy in conjunction with psychotherapy may prove necessary for providing effective treatment to some severely traumatized individuals. While most experts agree that pharmacotherapy alone is not sufficient for providing complete remission of PTSD, it may enable traumatized patients to optimally benefit from psychotherapy (Friedman, 1988). While exposure to torture and atrocities may result in permanent alterations of an individual's biological and biochemical status, the mechanisms of action and biological markers of the disorder must first be identified and the medications systematically evaluated in controlled clinical trials in order to ascertain effective pharmacotherapy.

Decisions regarding whether to use a medication, or a combination of medications, should be based on sound biological models of trauma effects (cf. van der Kolk, 1987) and from idiographic assessment of identified symptoms. For example, van der Kolk's (1987) model of trauma includes viewing post-traumatic stress in part as a state of prolonged central nervous system (CNS) hyperreactivity and autonomic nervous system arousal. Accordingly, medications such as anxiolytic agents and beta-adrenergic blockers are often recommended. Therefore, the typical medication regime is a combination of drugs that focus on specific symptoms or symptom clusters. Medications that address specific symptom clusters (positive and negative) can be sensibly administered and monitored. Medications that have been utilized with trauma patients include mood stabilizers (antidepressants and lithium), beta-blockers, anti-convulsants, and minor tranquilizers. Research on the biological factors associated with PTSD is at a rudimentary level. As this research expands our base of knowledge on the biological changes of PTSD, we will be able to employ and develop medications that will assist these patients in their adjustment.

PTSD and pharmacotherapy

Several early preliminary studies suggested that the monoamine oxidase inhibitor (MAOI), phenelzine, is effective in the treatment of traumatized individuals (Hogben & Cornfield, 1981; Milanes *et al.*, 1984). The MAOI's are considered antipanic agents, antidepressants, and they inhibit REM sleep. Hogben and Cornfield (1981) reported the rapid remission of nightmares, flashbacks, startle response, panic and anxiety in five traumatized patients treated with phenelzine. It was also reported that these symptoms failed to remit when the patients had earlier received a regime including an antipsychotic and an antidepressant to reduce their symptoms. While Milanes *et al.* (1984) suggest phenelzine is effective in the treatment of nightmares, hyperalertness, irritability and anxiety, van der Kolk (1983) reported an increase in vividness, and hence *worsening*, of daytime traumatic memories in four of seven patients. Friedman (1988) cautions also that phenelzine may not be the best treatment option for PTSD patients with alcohol and substance abuse problems (due to increased risk for relapse via response generalization), and that its applicability may be limited to groups with low alcoholism rates.

Tricyclic antidepressants are used most often in treating PTSD. The use of tricyclics has been justified by the phenomenologic overlap between symptoms of PTSD and those disorders known to respond to antidepressants. van der Kolk *et al.* (1985) conceptualized post-traumatic stress as neurochemically-mediated autonomic hyperarousal and hyperreactivity in response to inescapable stress (i.e. 'trauma'), involving noradrenergic pathways and as a physiological state resembling dependence on high levels of stressor-activated endogenous opioids. Since tricyclics appear to enhance endogenous opioid release through potentiation of synergistic serotonergic mechanisms (Malseed & Goldstein, 1986), their utility in PTSD may be due to their modulating effect on this process. In addition, by their antipanic action, tricyclic antidepressants work to dampen hyperarousal, reduce intrusive memories, decrease flashbacks, and reduce traumatic nightmares, and appear to be especially efficacious with traumatized patients who also are clinically depressed. Antidepressant medications that affect serotonin release may also prove to be valuable treatment adjuncts for traumatized patients (e.g. fluoxetine).

Falcone, Ryan and Chamberlain (1985) reported improvements in retrospective data and clinician ratings of traumatized patients treated with tricyclics. These investigators compared the effects of amitriptyline, imipramine, desipramine, and doxepin with 17 combat veterans over a 6–8 week trial. Results suggest the most beneficial effects were evidenced with amitriptyline treatment, which led to reductions of nightmares, flashbacks, and panic symptoms. The investigators reported some improvement in all patients treated, and attributed a poor response to patients dually diagnosed with substance abuse problems. Burstein (1984) found a reduction of positive symptoms of PTSD in 10 patients treated with imipramine, but no change in or an exacerbation of avoidant symptoms. Most recently, Davidson *et al.* (1990) compared the use of amitriptyline with placebo regimens with 46 PTSD-diagnosed combat veterans (World War II, Korea, and Vietnam), and found that the tricyclic but not the placebo produced significant reductions in Hamilton Depression and Anxiety Interview scores, number and severity of PTSD symptoms, and Clinical Global Impression (for improvement). In a recent review, Ross, Ball, Sullivan & Caroff (1989) also indicated that tricyclics might be useful in treating the positive symptoms and sleep disturbance of PTSD. Moreover, when compared to the MAOIs, the tricyclics have less risk for patients with histories of alcohol or substance abuse (Friedman, 1988), common coexisting diagnoses of PTSD.

Consistent with the behavioral model of PTSD, Kolb and Mutalipassi

(1982) conceptualized the symptoms of PTSD as conditioned emotional responses to environmental stimuli that are reminiscent of the traumatic event; this conditioned response is thought to be related to excessive central and peripheral adrenergic sympathetic activation. Accordingly, trials of the antihypertensive, clonidine, and the beta adrenergic blocker, propranolol, were found to improve sleep and decreased hyperalertness. In a more recent study, patients who were treated with either clonidine or propranolol reported a decrease in startle responses, explosiveness, and intrusive reexperiencing, while those on both drugs concurrently reported decreased nightmares (Kolb, Burris & Griffiths, 1984). Follow-up at six months revealed continued symptom reduction for the majority of subjects (reduced explosiveness, decreased nightmares, improved sleep, decreased intrusive recollections, less startle, reduced hyperarousal).

Benzodiazepines have often been the drug of choice for many anxiety disorders. The anxiolytic effects of these drugs appear to be due to their effect on the CNS GABAergic system, which directly influences the symptoms of autonomic arousal and anxious mood by exerting an inhibitory effect in the central nervous system. While alprazolam has demonstrated antipanic and antidepressant properties, this drug causes concern due to its addiction potential and withdrawal effects (Friedman, 1988). Treatment with the benzodiazepines in patients with alcoholism, chemical abuse histories or dependence may also be problematic due to cross over tolerance effects. While this class of drugs improves sleep and decreases nightmares in some patients, their effects may increase the likelihood of abuse or overmedication (van der Kolk, 1987). Furthermore, recent findings with alprazolam suggest that minor tranquilizers may interfere with the long-term benefits derived from behavior therapy (Klosko et al., 1990).

Conceptualizing post-traumatic stress as a result of a neurobehavioral kindling process provides a rationale for trials of the anticonvulsant, carbamazepine. While one carbamazepine treatment study reported improvement in combat-related dreams, flashbacks and intrusive recollections (Lipper et al., 1986), another described reductions in violent behavior and angry outbursts (Wolfe, Alavi & Mosnaim, 1988). Lithium carbonate has also been used to treat the symptoms of loss of control and anger outbursts seen in trauma patients (van der Kolk, 1983). Of 22 patients treated with lithium, 14 reported gaining a subjective sense of control over their lives with a decrease in the hyperreactivity to stress and hyperarousal. The precise mechanism of action for these effects is debatable and the effects of the anticonvulsants on diversely different symptoms in the studies to date

Table 17.3. *Symptom changes in combat veterans receiving pharmacotherapy*

Article	Medication	Symptom changes from treatment
Burstein (1984)	Imipramine	Decreased positive symptoms
Davidson, Kudler, Smith, Mahorney, Lipper, Hammett, Saunder & Cavenar (1990)	Amitriptyline	Decreased depression Decreased anxiety Decreased PTSD score Increased clinical global impression (for improvement) score
Falcone, Ryan & Chamberlain (1985)	Amitriptyline Imipramine Desipramine Doxepin	Decreased nightmares Decreased flashbacks Decreased panic symptoms (effects most notable with Amitriptyline)
Hogben & Cornfield (1981)	Phenelzine	Decreased nightmares Decreased flashbacks Decreased startle response Decreased panic symptoms Decreased anxiety symptoms
Kolb, Burris & Griffiths (1984)	Clonidine Propranolol both drugs	Decreased startle response Decreased hyperalertness Decreased flashbacks Decreased nightmares
Kolb & Mutalipassi (1982)	Clonidine Propranolol	Improved sleep Decreased hyperalertness
Lipper, Davidson, Grady, Edinger & Cavenar (1986)	Carbamazepine	Decreased nightmares Decreased flashbacks Decreased intrusive thoughts
Milanes, Mack, Dennison & Slater (1984)	Phenelzine	Decreased nightmares Decreased hyperalertness Decreased irritability Decreased anxiety symptoms
van der Kolk (1983)	Phenelzine	*Increased* vividness of daytime traumatic memories
van der Kolk (1987)	Lithium	Decreased hyperreactivity Decreased hyperarousal Increase in subjective sense of control
Wolfe, Alavi & Mosnaim (1988)	Carbamazepine	Decreased violence Decreased anger outbursts

raises questions about the conceptual basis for these medications. Clearly, more research is needed to help us understand these effects.

Differential symptom effects

Review of the studies described above suggests pharmacotherapy may provide relief from the positive symptoms of PTSD, but is relatively ineffective in or has not been properly evaluated for ameliorating negative symptoms (see Table 17.3). Pharmacotherapy appears effective for reducing target symptoms of intrusive recollections, sympathetic arousal (startle, flashbacks, explosiveness) and disturbances of sleep (nightmares). Negative symptoms such as alienation, detachment, and psychic numbing have not been successfully treated with medication. The uneven effect found for pharmacotherapy may be due in part to the inconsistencies in the dependent variables employed.

The medications reviewed above were selected in part on the basis of their effectiveness for reducing symptoms shared by post-traumatic stress with other disorders, mainly panic and depression. Etiological differences between these disorders may account for the limited treatment effects described above. While post-traumatic stress and panic disorder share the features of heightened psychophysiological arousal, startle, and sleep disturbance, Friedman (1988) outlines several key differences. In panic disorder, attacks seem to be nonspecific and spontaneous, presumably involving a physiological basis; post-traumatic stress appears to be primarily psychological, tied to a clearly identifiable traumatic precipitant. Sleep is also different in both disorders, with stage 4 sleep reduced in PTSD but increased in panic disorder (Ross *et al.* 1989). Friedman also points out differences in shared symptoms of PTSD and depression, most notably in terms of amount of REM sleep and REM latency, sympathetic arousal levels, and differential response of the hypothalamic–pituitary–adrenocortical axis. Clearly, there is need for comparative studies evaluating specific symptomatology and drug response across disorders.

Summary and comments

The decision to use medication in the treatment of trauma may best be guided by a conceptual framework about traumatic stress. Such a framework would assist in decisions regarding which medication is appropriate for which patients showing which symptoms. Clearly, more biological modeling is needed in this process. Overall, however, the tricyclic antidepressants may be the best treatment option, in light of the potential for abuse and withdrawal and tolerance effects apparent with some medications, such as the benzodiazepines (Friedman, 1988), as well as the growing evidence that these medications may interfere with the therapeutic process of psychological treatment (specifically exposure based therapy; see Barlow, 1988, and Klosko *et al.*, 1990). Serotonergic medications such as fluoxetine, while only now being tested in clinical trials, also shows promise for the treatment of PTSD.

OTHER TREATMENTS

Skills training

Skills training with trauma populations involves the identification of behavioral excesses and deficits (symptoms) that cause significant psychological distress or impair an individual's ability to function. Skills training interventions can be employed in a prescriptive fashion to address a variety of symptoms. The efficacy of skills training has been demonstrated across a variety of target problems such as anger control (Novaco, 1975) and deficits in interpersonal skills (Kelly, 1982); problem solving skill (Nezu & Carnevale, 1987), and assertiveness (Rimm *et al.*, 1974). It has also been used with diverse populations.

Skills training may be especially useful in ameliorating the negative symptoms of PTSD (including avoidance, withdrawal and alienation), which can be considered as behavioral deficits (Keane *et al.*, 1989). Experience with trauma can disrupt previously learned behavior patterns in such a way that an individual previously described to be socially outgoing may become withdrawn and avoidant following the trauma. Skills training interventions typically involve promoting previously learned and new adaptive behaviors. Examples include social, job, and dating skills, assertiveness, and stress management. Similarly, for a behavioral excess such as recurrent anger outbursts, skill training in anger control would be one appropriate intervention. For example, McWhirter and Liebman (1988) describe a six-week group intervention program for anger management with Vietnam veterans. Cognitive restructuring, structured experiential activities, and assertiveness training are combined in this program, with a focus on reintegration into society.

Skills training interventions often involve training in identification of setting events. By definition, in PTSD the traumatic event (or series of events) is readily identified. Stimulus features of the event are then assessed and the individual is trained to recognize cues which elicit and reinforce the deficit/excess problem behavior. The intervention is then devoted to skill acquisition, using techniques such as role playing, cognitive restructuring, *in vivo* exposure exercises, and relaxation training. The consequences of adaptive and maladaptive behaviors, with a focus on reinforcement mechanisms, are elucidated. Throughout training, feedback is given to the individual through verbal instructions, participant modeling, and constructive criticisms.

The positive symptoms of PTSD may also be treated using a prescriptive intervention approach. For example, relaxation training, guided imagery, and stimulus control procedures may be utilized to treat the insomnia and sleep disturbance symptoms. The patient may be trained to utilize relaxation techniques to address initial insomnia, and utilize both relaxation and imagery for disrupted sleep. Symptoms of fear and heightened anxiety may be treated with cognitive restructuring and guided exposure to stress-provoking situations. Similarly, systematic desensitization has proven effectiveness and can be used to treat trauma-related fears and anxiety.

Family therapy

For the individual trauma survivor, stress is experienced acutely during and immediately after the traumatic incident(s), and again later when readjusting to family and the routines of life. Figley (1978) suggested that at times family interaction may exacerbate an individual's symptoms of PTSD. Several investigators have described the adverse effects on the families of trauma survivors (Figley, 1985; Masters, Friedman & Getzel, 1988).

Consistent with a family systems theory perspective, family interactions both affect and are affected by the victim's psychological distress. Accordingly, attention has been directed toward family interventions with individuals suffering from PTSD. Employing this approach, the therapist's goal is to assess the severity of the victim's disorder, and the impact of the disorder on family interactions. Interventions to address both the stress disorder and the related dysfunctions within the system (Stanton & Figley, 1978) are appropriate. Silver and Iacono (1986) evaluated family interactions *vis a vis* symptom patterns in combat veterans suffering PTSD. Results suggested that family therapy had a beneficial impact on both the veteran and the family system. Family interactions as a whole also appeared to be more important in the maintaining the disorder than were traumatized individual's responses, and positive changes in family functioning often predicted improvement in individual functioning. Improvements in family functioning also indirectly yielded improvement in such symptomatology as withdrawal and avoidant behaviors, which as earlier described, tend to be less responsive to other approaches.

Figley (1988) developed a five-phase family systems model to facilitate the individual's return to pre-trauma functioning within the family system. The therapeutic goals were to rebuild rapport and trust, promote self disclosure, and enable the family to handle future stressors. The intervention phases of the model involved: 1) gaining commitment to therapeutic objectives; 2) framing the problem through testimonials and resolving interpersonal animosity; 3) reframing the problem to help better equip the family for managing crises; 4) developing a 'Healing Theory', which describes descriptions of adaptive statements concerning the traumatic event, individual family members' responses, and a positive approach to solving future crises; and 5) closure and reinforcing the family's accomplishment. While this model offers promise as an addition to other therapeutic approaches, it also remains to be tested via controlled clinical research.

Group therapy

Group therapy has traditionally been viewed as a mechanism for providing therapeutic benefits separate from those gained through individual therapy (Yalom, 1975). In his classic work with groups, Yalom (1975) posited the many benefits derived from the group process and functions including: 1) instillation of hope, 2) universality, 3) imparting of information, 4) altruism, 5) the corrective recapitulation of the primary family group, 6) development of socializing techniques, 7) imitative behavior, 8) interpersonal learning, 9) group cohesiveness, 10) catharsis, and 12) existential factors. One might also add that the group environment also provides a forum for *exposure* to trauma-related stimuli, such as other victims, and in sharing experiences reactivating painful memories of traumatic incident(s). Thus, group therapy may provide a valuable forum for the treatment of torture victims.

Group treatment has been successful in the treatment of a number of traumatized populations, including Vietnam combatants (Ben-Yakar, Dasberg & Plotkin, 1978; Egendorf, 1975), and rape victims (Cryer & Beutler, 1980). Its use with survivors of torture would, with the appropriate structure, provide an important component to comprehensive treatment of PTSD.

PREVENTION OF POST-TRAUMATIC STRESS DISORDER SYMPTOMS

Several implications for the prevention of chronic symptoms of PTSD may be drawn from the research on assessment and treatment of victims of trauma. First, not all people who experience a traumatic event develop subsequent disabling psychological disorders. Brom and Kleber (1989) reported that approximately 80% of all people who are confronted with a trauma, utilize their own resources and social support to work through the after effects. Thus a minority of cases solicit professional assistance in coping with any adverse psychological sequelae. While not every victim needs intensive professional care, most would derive benefit from some form of support or crisis intervention. Timely access to services for the individual, group and family, may also be critical for preventing the development of persistent problems.

The following section reviews three factors to consider in efforts to prevent chronic PTSD: 1) the role of social support, 2) trauma debriefing, and 3) a cognitive behavioral treatment package which may preclude the progression of acute to chronic PTSD symptoms in trauma survivors.

SOCIAL SUPPORT

Social support has received considerable attention as a mediating variable between the experience of trauma or stress and development of related disorders (for an early review, see Leavy, 1983). Solomon (1986) outlined four components of social support: 1) emotional support, which may include providing information that one is loved, cared for, and respected; 2) reciprocity of obligation, in which the individual is a part of a support system of reciprocal help and mutual obligation; 3) task-oriented assistance, which involves the provision of direct aid (to the victim), and 4) provision of information relevant to coping, which may involve validating feelings and providing feedback about the appropriateness and impact of one's fears, beliefs and opinions.

Several studies have reported that the *absence* of social support in stressful situations acts to increase the likelihood of developing post-trauma difficulties (Cobb, 1976; Hobfoll & Walfish, 1984; Murphy, 1988; Solomon, Mikulincer & Avitzur, 1988). Murphy (1988) suggests that social support which is developed and maintained over time and exists prior to traumatic stress may protect individuals from the negative effects of trauma. She cites research evidence where the perception of spousal love and a stable network of supportive others predicted stress-related health consequences (Antonovsky, 1979; Burke & Weir, 1977; Miller, Ingram & Davidson, 1976).

While pre-trauma social support appears to moderate the negative effects of trauma, several investigations have studied the role of post-trauma support (Barrett & Mizes, 1988; Foy *et al.*, 1987; Kadushin, Boulanger & Martin, 1981; Keane *et al.*, 1985). In one study, combat veterans who had high social support after discharge reported significantly less psychological distress than those who reported low social support (Kadushin, Boulanger & Martin, 1981). Results indicated that positive emotional support from a spouse resulted in considerably less acute distress (one fourth the level seen without support) than in men with low spouse support. Furthermore, nearly half the married men in this study with acute post-trauma symptoms did not develop chronic distress as opposed to 71% of unmarried men who continued to experience chronic stress. Keane *et al.* (1985) compared a group of Vietnam veterans with PTSD with two groups of Vietnam era veterans without PTSD. The levels of social support prior to military service among the three groups were equivalent. However, the PTSD veterans reported a steady decline in social support since the time of their discharge from the military. Social support among the comparison groups was stable across the three time periods measured.

It has been suggested that American society as a rule rejects trauma survivors (Janoff-Bulman, 1982) and certainly the sociopolitical controversy surrounding America's involvement in Vietnam adversely affected the readjustment of many veterans. Laufer & Gallops (1982) explored the influences of society on the exacerbation of PTSD symptoms in Vietnam veterans. In this retrospective self-report study, the authors found a significant relationship between combat exposure and feelings of withdrawal and alienation upon return stateside. Further, the authors suggested this relationship applies only to combat veterans returning after the year 1967, a point of departure in Americas' support for the war and it's participants. Foy *et al.* (1987) reported similar results comparing PTSD to non-PTSD veterans in their perceived experience of cynicism, alienation, physical neglect and demeaning experiences upon their return from Vietnam.

Barrett and Mizes (1988) studied the influence of social support and exposure to combat in the development of PTSD in 52 Vietnam combat veterans. Results demonstrated that veterans who received high social support reported fewer symptoms of PTSD, depression, and other psychological disturbance than those receiving low social support.

However, the investigators correctly suggested that the display of PTSD symptoms may have decreased the social support the veterans received, rather than *vice versa*, i.e. traumatized individuals have an impaired capacity to access and utilize social support due to PTSD symptomatology. This contention is supported empirically by several studies which show that combat veterans with PTSD tend to have problems with intimacy and sociability (Roberts *et al.*, 1982) as well as problems with self disclosure, increased aggressiveness, and poor marital adjustment (Carroll *et al.*, 1985).

In a recent study, Solomon *et al.* (1988) examined the relationship between coping, locus of control, social support and combat-related PTSD in 262 Israeli soldiers who suffered combat stress reactions during the 1982 Lebanon War. Veterans were assessed two and three years after their tour of combat to evaluate the process of recovery. Results indicate that PTSD intensity declined between the two points in time, suggesting an ongoing recovery process. Further, veterans with an internal locus of control perceived greater social support. While the direction of causality was unclear, results suggest a significant link between post-traumatic stress intensity with personal and social resources. The investigators report that social withdrawal and emotion-focused coping led to increased PTSD intensity, whereas less introspective focusing and more social contacts lessened PTSD intensity. The avoidant symptoms of PTSD were viewed as a contributing factor in orienting a veteran's coping toward his internal state, and thus rendering him unable to access external support.

In sum, research with trauma victims and combat veterans with PTSD suggests that social support may provide important benefits to trauma survivors. Social support can be provided by positive emotional affiliation with and caring from significant others, and from the perception of respect and acceptance from the community. The individual's ability to access social support is related to the intensity of the avoidant and intrusive symptoms of PTSD, and thus while support may be available, the nature and extent of PTSD symptoms may prevent accessing such support or alienating potential support providers.

Provision of social support following a traumatic event can be a complicated matter. Social systems are complex and do not always have a beneficial impact on trauma survivors. For example, one study of disaster suggests that experience with established social support systems may in fact increase victims level of distress. For example, Hartsough (1985) described how the activities required of victims following a disaster in accessing temporary housing, and obtaining loans and grants to facilitate return to suitable housing compounded distress and delayed recovery. Additionally, the victim can be secondarily traumatized if he or she is in some fashion held responsible for the event, or is viewed to have been in collusion with the perpetrators (for a review, see Janoff-Bulman, 1982). Examples of such reasoning can be seen in perceiving a rape or incest victim as one who 'asked for it' and seduced the perpetrator, and in communities that view individuals who have been tortured as a result of their political beliefs and activities as having deserved punishment for unpatriotism or dissidence.

Relatedly, it is not certain whether trauma victims are more symptomatic without social support, or that trauma victims with greater symptomatology advertently or inadvertently reject support from those around them. In the former case, the remedy is to give the trauma victims support and resources as soon as possible. In the latter case, remedial efforts are not as clear cut. Certainly one might engage in efforts to decrease the post trauma symptomatology (relaxation training, group debriefing, exposure-based therapy, pharmacotherapy) or to train the victim in skills for appropriately soliciting help from their social support system.

TRAUMA DEBRIEFING

Immediately following trauma exposure, the treatment of choice is to permit survivors or victims to emotionally and cognitively process the incident(s), either with other survivors or professionals prepared to debrief them.

A critical aspect in treating trauma survivors and victims is the timing of the intervention. In general, interventions that are implemented soon after the trauma seem to produce the greatest benefit (Moses, 1977). It can be said that during this period the victim's disrupted cognitive, physiological, and behavioral patterns have not yet had time to become firmly established and attempts to mitigate chronic disorder will be maximally effective. Evidence for this contention can be found in the military psychiatry treatments on or near the battlefield in Vietnam (Bloch, 1969) and Israel (Jones & Johnson, 1975), and in rape crisis treatment (Haywood, 1975).

If treatment is best delivered immediately after traumatization, behavioral interventions can easily be modified to accommodate the more acute manifestations of the disorder. For example, re-exposure to the traumatic stimuli might take other forms, such as keeping traumatized combatants in safe quarters as near to the event as is reasonably possible so that conditioned responses to war related stimuli do not develop, or for the same purpose by encouraging torture victims to discuss their experiences and memories of the trauma.

During this acute-crisis period for treatment, overwhelming arousal, in the form of anxiety (Fairbank, Keane & Malloy, 1983) or mood disturbances (Helzer, Robins & Davis, 1976; Helzer *et al.*, 1979; Rickarby, 1977), can be treated in the short term with medication (e.g. anxiolytics or sedatives). This practice permits the delivery of primary therapeutic efforts in which control of overwhelming symptoms is achieved.

Evidence from other studies suggests that the best treatment strategy is to enhance the traumatized individual's sense of 'belongingness' (Dasberg, 1976). A key ingredient here may be the social support, seen lacking with some traumatized populations (Keane *et al.*, 1985).

Possibly the most important task to accomplish during a critical incident debriefing is to educate the victims and survivors about the psychological sequelae frequently experienced by all. This normalization of stress can reduce people's responses to the inevitable symptoms of stress, depression, guilt, sleep disturbance, and traumatic intrusions.

STRESS INOCULATION TRAINING

Experiencing traumatic stress can inculcate feelings of helplessness and despair, symptoms resulting in large part from a loss of control during the episode. Stress Inoculation Training (SIT; Meichenbaum, 1977; Meichenbaum & Turk, 1976) is a cognitive behavioral treatment package utilized by clinicians to ameliorate the psychological consequences of many forms of stress.

The concept of stress inoculation as an intervention and prevention measure has been represented in the early psychoanalytic and behavioral literature (for a review see Meichenbaum & Jaremko, 1983). Similar to the biological notion of immunization from disease, stress inoculation proposes that graded exposure to anxiety-provoking stimuli positively affects an individual's ability to tolerate anxiety, and thus inoculates the individual from higher intensities of stress. Through graded exposure, an individual also becomes aware of behavioral, subjective, and physiological signs of heightened anxiety while practising and mastering cognitive and behavioral coping skills. Janis (1983) proposed that stress inoculation training increased self confidence, hope, perceived control, and self-efficacy.

Stress Inoculation Training involves three phases. Phase 1, the *Education Phase*, introduces participants to information about stress, anxiety, and how they affect us. Participants are told that maladaptive emotions (anxiety, rage, avoidance) provide important cues and that these emotions contain a modifiable cognitive component. Cognitive self-statements are identified and monitored during this phase to help the participants assess their own anxiety experience, so that when confronting an anxiety provoking event (such as exposure to cues which remind the individual of the original trauma), they respond with effective coping statements and action.

In Phase 2, the *Skill Acquisition Phase*, participants are taught specific coping skills in four stage stages: 1) generation of positive self statements, which will assist the individual in preparing for a stressor, 2) confrontation of a stressor while practising positive self statements (usually through imagery), 3) rehearsal of self-statements aimed at coping with elements of a situation that may elicit a subjective feeling of being overwhelmed or panicked, and 4) instruction in verbal self-reinforcement for mastery of the stress. This skill acquisition phase is designed to help develop coping techniques that serve both to modify self-defeating cognitions to and control physiological arousal. A major focus is to teach constructive reactions to early signs of arousal and anxiety.

The final phase of SIT, the *Application Phase*, is introduced once the participants demonstrate mastery of relaxation and therapeutic self statements. In this phase, participants are exposed to imaginal and real stressors in a graded series of presentations. The purpose of this phase is to assist in the generalization of the skills learned in therapy to other spheres of their lives.

Research on the effectiveness of stress inoculation training has been demonstrated in patients with chronic pain (Wernick, 1983), victims of terrorism (Ayalon, 1983), military recruit training (Novaco, Cook & Sarason, 1983), and other stress provoking situations (for a review see Meichenbaum & Jaremko, 1983). While the package may be applied on an individual or group level, Meichenbaum and Jaremko (1983) stress the importance of tailoring the program to meet individual situational needs and to reflect the specific stressors and related stimuli for the particular trauma.

SUMMARY AND COMMENTS

Methods for preventing PTSD symptoms are reflected in stress inoculation training, trauma debriefing, and utilization of social support networks. Clearly, services to victims and survivors are most effective when they are multifaceted and available immediately. Intervention programs that are easily accessible and provide the needed education, social support, and peer exchange can effectively reduce long term psychological consequences of trauma. Programs specifically for family members and significant others that include education about stress and its consequences would also promote positive family adjustment. Resources for learning coping skills and stress management training are conceivably the most important techniques to be taught to survivors. Clearly some survivors have individual needs beyond critical incident debriefing and treatment needs to proceed according to these differences. Individual therapy might include education about stress, self monitoring, discussions on personal experiences and their cognitive appraisal, assertiveness skills and stress management training, expressive therapy, problem solving training, and methods to enhance social support.

FUTURE DIRECTIONS

Research on PTSD needs to proceed in a systematic fashion in order to evaluate fully treatment effectiveness. Studies that empirically evaluate components of treatment are clearly needed. With the advances that have been made in the assessment of PTSD, clinicians and researchers are in a unique position to determine precisely the effects of different treatments for trauma. Indeed, instruments are now available to assist researchers in understanding the differential effectiveness of treatment on the reliving/intrusive symptoms, the numbing/avoidance symptoms, and the arousal symptoms of trauma (Blake *et al.*, in press; Watson, 1991*a*; Watson *et al.*, 1991*b*). These advances in assessment will undoubtedly enhance our ability to determine which treatments are most effective with what types of patients and in what time periods following traumatic events.

Victims of torture and other forms of trauma are now benefiting from the advances made in the psychological sciences and the neurosciences as applied to PTSD. It is incumbent upon our society to continue to support such advances since trauma appears to be occurring with high frequency as our society becomes increasingly technological and the population of the world struggles to meet the accompanying economic and social challenges. The treatment of torture victims and their psychological trauma will continue to be a top priority in social policy for the foreseeable future.

P

REFERENCES

American Psychiatric Association (1980). *Diagnostic and Statistical Manual of Mental Disorders* (3rd edn.). Washington, DC: Author.

American Psychiatric Association (1987). *Diagnostic and Statistical Manual of Mental Disorders* (3rd ed.) – revised. Washington, DC: Author.

Antonovsky, A. (1979). *Health, Stress and Coping.* San Francisco: Jossey-Bass.

Ayalon, O. (1983). Coping with terrorism: The Israeli case. In D. Meichenbaum & M. E. Jaremko (eds), *Stress Reduction and Prevention.* pp. 293–340, New York: Plenum Press.

Bandura, A. (1977). Self-efficacy: toward a unifying theory of behavioral change. *Psychological Review,* **84,** 191–215.

Bandura, A. (1986). *Social Foundations of Thought and Action: A Social Cognitive Theory.* Engelwood Cliffs, NJ: Prentice Hall.

Barlow, D. H. (1988). *Anxiety and Its Disorders: The Nature and Treatment of Anxiety and Panic.* New York: Guilford Press.

Barrett, T. W. & Mizes, J. S. (1988). Combat level and social support in the development of posttraumatic stress disorder in Vietnam veterans. *Behavior Modification,* **12(1),** 100–15.

Beck, A. T. (1976). *Cognitive Therapy and Emotional Disorders.* New York: International University Press.

Beck, A. T. & Emery, G. (1985). *Anxiety Disorders and Phobias: A Cognitive Perspective.* New York: Basic Books.

Ben-Yakar, M., Dasberg, H. & Plotkin, I. (1978). The influence of various therapeutic milieus on the course of group treatment in two groups of soldiers with combat reaction. *Israel Annals of Psychiatry and Related Disciplines,* **16,** 183–95.

Black, J. L. & Keane, T. M. (1982). Implosive therapy in the treatment of combat related fears in a World War II veteran. *Journal of Behavior Therapy and Experimental Psychiatry,* **13,** 163–5.

Blake, D. D., Albano, A. M. & Keane, T. M. (October, 1990). *Trends in Trauma: Psychology Abstracts 1970 to 1990.* Paper presented at the annual meeting of the Society for Traumatic Stress Studies, New Orleans.

Blake, D. D., Weathers, F., Nagy, L. M., Kaloupek, D. G., Klauminzer, G., Charney, D. S. & Keane, T. M. (in press). A clinician rating scale for assessing current and lifetime PTSD: The CAPS-1. *The Behavior Therapist.*

Bloch, H. S. (1969). Army clinical psychiatry in the combat zone: 1967–1968. *American Journal of Psychiatry,* **126,** 289–98.

Boudewyns, P. A. & Hyer, L. (1990). Physiological response to combat veterans and preliminary treatment outcome in Vietnam veteran PTSD patients treated with direct therapeutic exposure. *Behavior Therapy,* **21,** 63–87.

Boudewyns, P. A., Hyer, L., Woods, M. G., Harrison, W. R. & McCranie, E. (in press). PTSD among Vietnam veterans: An early look at treatment outcome with direct therapeutic exposure. *Journal of Traumatic Stress.*

Bowen, G. R. & Lambert, J. A. (1986). Systematic desensitization therapy with post-traumatic stress disorder cases. In C. R. Figley, ed, *Trauma and its Wake* (Vol. II), pp. 281–291, New York: Brunner/Mazel.

Brom, D. & Kleber, R. J. (1989). Prevention of post-traumatic stress disorder. *Journal of Traumatic Stress*, **2**, 235–51.

Burke, R. & Weir, T. (1977). Marital helping relationships: moderators between stress and well being. *Journal of Psychology*, **95**, 121–30.

Burstein, A. (1984). Treatment of post-traumatic stress disorder with imipramine. *Psychosomatics*, **25**, 681–7.

Carroll, E. M., Rueger, D. B., Foy, D. W. & Donahoe, C. P. (1985). Vietnam combat veterans with post traumatic stress disorder: analysis of marital and cohabitating adjustment. *Journal of Abnormal Psychology*, **94**, 329–37.

Chemtob, C., Roiblat, H. L., Hamada, R. S., Carlson, J. G. & Twentyman, C. T. (1988). A cognitive action theory of Post-traumatic Stress Disorder. *Journal of Anxiety Disorders*, **2**, 253–75.

Cobb, J. (1976). Social support as a moderator of life stress. *Psychosomatic Medicine*, **38**, 300–14.

Cooper, N. A. & Clum, G. A. (1989). Imaginal flooding as a supplementary treatment for PTSD in combat veterans: a controlled study. *Behavior Therapy*, **20**, 381–91.

Cryer, L. & Beutler, L. (1980). Group therapy: an alternative approach for rape victims. *Journal of Sex and Marital Therapy*, **6**, 40–6.

Dasberg, H. (1976). Belongingness and loneliness in relation to mental breakdown in battle: with some remarks on treatment. *Israel Annals of Psychiatry and Related Disciplines*, **14**, 307–21.

Davidson, J., Kudler, H., Smith, R., Mahorney, S. L., Lipper, S., Hammett, E., Saunders, W. B. & Cavenar, J. O., Jr. (1990). Treatment of posttraumatic stress disorder with amitriptyline and placebo. *Archives of General Psychiatry*, **47**, 259–66.

Egendorf, A. (1975). Vietnam veteran rap groups and themes of postwar life. *Journal of Social issues*, **31**, 111–24.

Ellis, A. & Grieger, R. (1986). *Handbook of Rational Emotive Therapy* (Vol. 2). New York: Springer Publishing.

Fairbank, J. A. & Brown, T. A. (1987). Current behavioral approaches to the treatment of posttraumatic stress disorder. *The Behavior Therapist*, **10**, 57–64.

Fairbank, J. A., DeGood, D. E. & Jenkins, C. W. (1981). Behavioral treatment of a persistent posttraumatic startle response. *Journal of Behavior Therapy and Experimental Psychiatry*, **12**, 321–4.

Fairbank, J. A., Gross, R. T. & Keane, T. M. (1983). Treatment of posttraumatic stress disorder: evaluating outcome with a behavioral code. *Behavior Modification*, **7**, 557–68.

Fairbank, J. A. & Keane, T. M. (1982). Flooding for combat-related stress disorders: assessment of anxiety reduction across traumatic memories. *Behavior Therapy*, **13**, 499–510.

Fairbank, J. A., Keane, T. M. & Malloy, P. F. (1983). Some preliminary data on the psychological characteristics of Vietnam veterans with post-traumatic stress disorder. *Journal of Consulting and Clinical Psychology*, **51**, 912–19.

Falcone, S., Ryan, C. & Chamberlain, K. (1985). Tricyclics: possible treatment for posttraumatic stress disorder. *Journal of Clinical Psychiatry*, **46**, 385–9.

Farnsworth, B. K., Wood, E. H. & Ayers, E. G. (1975). Implosive psychodrama. *Psychotherapy: Theory, Research and Practice*, 12, 200–1.

Figley, C. R. (1988). A five-phase treatment of post traumatic stress disorder in families. *Journal of Traumatic Stress*, 1, 127–41.

Figley, C. R. (1985). The family as victim: mental health implications. *Psychiatry*, 6, 283–91.

Figley, C. R. (1978). Psychosocial adjustment among Vietnam veterans: an overview of the research. In C. R. Figley, ed, *Stress Disorders Among Vietnam Veterans: Theory, Research, and Treatment*, pp. 57–90, New York: Brunner/Mazel.

Figley, C. R. & Sprenkle, D. H. (1978). Delayed stress response syndrome: family therapy indications. *Journal of Marriage and Family Counseling*, 4, 53–6.

Foa, E. B. & Kozak, M. J. (1986). Emotional processing of fear: exposure to corrective information. *Psychological Bulletin*, 99, 20–35.

Foa, E. B., Steketee, G. & Olasov Rothbaum, B. (1989). Behavioral/cognitive conceptualizations of post-traumatic stress disorder. *Behavior Therapy*, 20, 155–76.

Foy, D. W., Resnick, H. S., Sipprelle, R. C. & Carroll, E. M. (1987). Premilitary, military, and postmilitary factors in the development of combat-related posttraumatic stress disorder. *The Behavior Therapist*, 10, 3–9.

Friedman, M. J. (1988). Toward a rational pharmacotherapy for posttraumatic stress disorder: an interim report. *The American Journal of Psychiatry*, 145, 281–5.

Giles, T. R. (1988). Phobia and suicide: an influence of treatment? *The Behavior Therapist*, 11, 26–42.

Grigbsy, J. P. (1987). The use of imagery in the treatment of Posttraumatic Stress Disorder. *Journal of Nervous and Mental Disease*, 175, 55–9.

Hartsough, D. M. (1985). Measurement of the psychological effects of disaster. In J. Laube & S. A. Murphy, eds, *Perspectives on Disaster Recovery*. East Norwalk, NJ: Appleton-Century-Crofts.

Haywood, C. H. (1975). Emergency, crisis and stress services for rape victims. *Crisis Intervention*, 6, 43–8.

Helzer, J. E., Robins, L. N. & Davis, D. H. (1976). Depressive disorders in Vietnam returnees. *Journal of Nervous and Mental Disease*, 163, 177–85.

Helzer, J. E., Robins, L. N. & McEvoy, L. (1987). Post-traumatic stress disorder in the general population. *The New England Journal of Medicine*, 317, 1630–4.

Helzer, J. E., Robins, L. N., Wish, E. & Hesselbrock, M. (1979). Depression in Vietnam veterans and civilian controls. *American Journal of Psychiatry*, 136, 526–9.

Hobfoll, S. E. & Walfish, L. (1984). Coping with a threat to life: a longitudinal study of self concept, social support and psychological distress. *American Journal of Community Psychology*, 12, 87–100.

Hogben, G. L. & Cornfield, R. B. (1981). Treatment of traumatic war neurosis with phenelzine. *Archives of General Psychiatry*, 38, 440–5.

Horowitz, M. J. (1976). *Stress Response Syndromes*. New York: Jason Aronson.

Horowitz, M. J. (1986). *Stress Response Syndromes* (2nd edition). New York: Jason Aronson.

Janis, I. L. (1983). Stress inoculation in health care: Theory and research. In D. Meichenbaum & M. E. Jaremko, eds, *Stress reduction and prevention,* pp. 67–100, New York: Plenum Press.

Janoff-Bulman, R. (1982). Esteem and control bases of blame: 'Adaptive' strategies for victims versus observers. *Journal of Personality,* **50,** 180–92.

Jones, J. C. & Barlow, D. H. (1990). The etiology of post-traumatic stress disorder. *Clinical Psychology Review.*

Jones, F. D. & Johnson, A. W. (1975). Medical and psychiatric treatment policy and practice in Vietnam. *Journal of Social Issues,* **31,** 49–65.

Kadushin, C., Boulanger, G. & Martin, J. (1981). Medical and psychiatric treatment policy and practice in Vietnam. *Journal of Social Issues,* **50,** 180–92.

Keane, T. M. (1989). Post-traumatic stress disorder: current status and future directions. *Behavior Therapy,* **20,** 149–53.

Keane, T. M., Fairbank, J. A., Caddell, J. M. & Zimering, R. T. (1989). Implosive (flooding) therapy reduces symptoms of PTSD in Vietnam combat veterans. *Behavior Therapy,* **20,** 245–60.

Keane, T. M., Fairbank, J. A., Caddell, J. M., Zimering, R. T. & Bender, M. E. (1985). A behavioral approach to the assessment and treatment of post-traumatic stress disorder in Vietnam veterans. In C. R. Figley, ed., *Trauma and its Wake: The Study and Treatment of Post-traumatic Stress Disorders,* pp. 257–294, New York: Brunner/Mazel.

Keane, T. M. & Kaloupek, D. G. (1982). Imaginal flooding in the treatment of a post-traumatic stress disorder. *Journal of Consulting and Clinical Psychology,* **50,** 138–40.

Keane, T. M., Scott, O. N., Chavoya, G. A., Lamparski, D. M. & Fairbank, J. A. (1985). Social support in Vietnam veterans with post-traumatic stress disorder: a comparative analysis. *Journal of Consulting and Clinical Psychology,* **53,** 95–102.

Keane, T. M., Zimering, R. T. & Caddell, J. M. (1985). A behavioral formulation of post-traumatic stress disorder in combat veterans. *The Behavior Therapist,* **8,** 9–12.

Kelly, J. A. (1982). *Social Skills Training: A Practical Guide to Interventions.* New York: Springer Publishing.

Kilpatrick, D. G. & Best, C. L. (1984). Some cautionary remarks on treating sexual assault victims with implosion. *Behavior Therapy,* **15,** 421–3.

Kipper, D. A. (1977). Behavior therapy for fears brought on by way of experiences. *Journal of Consulting and Clinical Psychology,* **45,** 216–221.

Klosko, J. S., Barlow, D. H., Tassinari, R. & Cerny, J. A. (1990). A comparison of alprazolam and behavior therapy in treatment of panic disorder. *Journal of Consulting and Clinical Psychology,* **58,** 77–84.

Kolb, L. C., Burris, B. C. & Griffiths, S. (1984). Propranalol and clonidine in the treatment of chronic post-traumatic stress disorders of war. In B. van der Kolk, ed., *Post-traumatic Stress Disorder: Psychological and Biological Sequelae.* Washington, DC: American Psychiatric Press.

Kolb, L. C. & Mutalipassi, L. R. (1982). The conditioned emotional response: a subclass of the chronic and delayed post-traumatic stress disorders. *Psychiatric Annals,* **12,** 979–87.

Kreitler, S. & Kreitler, J. (1988). Trauma and anxiety: the cognitive approach. *Journal of Traumatic Stress*, 1, 35–56.

Krystal, J. H., Kosten, T. R., Perry, B. D., Southwick, S., Mason, J. W. & Giller, E. L., Jr. (1989). Neurobiological aspects of PTSD: review of clinical and preclinical studies. *Behavior Therapy*, 20, 177–98.

Kuch, K. (1987). Treatment of PTSD following automobile accidents. *The Behavior Therapist*, 10, 224–42.

Kulka, R. A., Schlenger, W. E., Fairbank, J. A., Hough, R. L., Jordan, B. K., Marmar, C. R. & Weiss, D. S. (1988). *National Vietnam Veterans Readjustment Study Advance Data Report: Preliminary Findings From the National Survey of the Vietnam Generation.* Executive Summary. Washington, DC: Veterans Administration.

Lang, P. J. (1979). A bioinformational theory of emotional imagery. *Psychophysiology*, 16, 495–510.

Lang, P. J. (1977). Imagery in therapy: an information processing analysis of fear. *Behavior Therapy*, 8, 495–510.

Laufer, R. S. & Gallops, G. (1982). *A Modal of War Stress and Post-war Trauma: The Vietnam Experience.* Paper presented at the American Sociological Association convention, San Francisco, CA.

Leavy, R. L. (1983). Social support and psychological disorder: a review. *Journal of Community Psychology*, 11, 3–21.

Levis, D. J. & Hare, N. A. (1977). A review of the theoretical rationale and empirical support for the extinction approach of implosive (flooding) therapy. In M. Hersen, R. M. Eisler & P. M. Miller, eds, *Progress in behavior modification* (Vol. 4), pp. 299–374, New York: Academic Press.

Lipper, S., Davidson, J. R. T., Grady, T. A., Edinger, J. & Cavenar, J. O. (1986). Preliminary study of carbamazepine in post-traumatic stress disorder. *Psychosomatics*, 27, 849–54.

Litz, B. T., Penk, W. E., Gerardi, R. G. & Keane, T. M. (in press). The assessment of post-traumatic stress disorder. In P. Saigh, ed., *Post-traumatic Stress Disorder: A Behavioral Approach to Assessment and Treatment.* New York: Pergamon Press.

Litz, B. T., Blake, D. D., Gerardi, R. J. & Keane, T. M. (1990). Decision making guidelines for the use of direct therapeutic exposure in the treatment post-traumatic stress disorder. *The Behavior Therapist*, 13, 91–3.

Litz, B. T. & Keane, T. M. (1989). Information processing in anxiety disorders: application to the understanding of post-traumatic stress disorder. *Clinical Psychology Review*, 9, 243–57.

Lyons, J. A. & Keane, T. M. (1989). Implosive therapy for the treatment of combat-related PTSD. *Journal of Traumatic Stress*, 2, 137–52.

Malseed, R. T. & Goldstein, F. J. (1986). Enhancement of morphine analgesia by tricyclic antidepressants. *Neuropharmacology*, 18, 827–9.

Masters, R., Friedman, L. N. & Getzel, G. (1988). Helping families of homicide victims: a multidimensional approach. *Journal of Traumatic Stress*, 1, 109–25.

Meichenbaum, D. (1974). *Cognitive Behavior Modification.* Morristown, NJ: General Learning Press.

Meichenbaum, D. (1977). *Cognitive-Behavior Modification: An Integrative Approach*. New York: Plenum Press.

Meichenbaum, D. & Jaremko, M. E. (eds.) (1983). *Stress Reduction and Prevention*. New York: Plenum Press.

Meichenbaum, D. H. & Turk, D. C. (1976). The cognitive behavioral management of anxiety, anger, and pain. In P. O. Davidson, ed., *The Behavioral Management of Anxiety, Depression and Pain*. New York: Brunner/Mazel.

McCormack, N. A. (1985). Cognitive therapy of posttraumatic stress disorder: a case report. *American Mental Health Counselors Association Journal*, **7**, 151–5.

McWhirter, J. J. & Liebman, P. C. (1988). A description of anger-control therapy groups to help Vietnam veterans with PTSD. *Journal for Specialists in Group Work*, **13**, 9–16.

Milanes, F. J., Mack, C. N., Dennison, J. & Slater, V. L. (1984). Phenelzine treatment of post-Vietnam syndrome. *VA Practitioner*, **1**, 40–9.

Miller, W. R. & DiPilato, M. (1983). Treatment of nightmares via relaxation and desensitization: A controlled evaluation. *Journal of Consulting and Clinical Psychology*, **51(6)**, 870–7.

Miller, P., Ingram, J. & Davidson, S. (1976). Life events symptoms and social support. *Journal of Psychosomatic Research*, **20**, 515–22.

Moses, R. (1977). Community mental health services in times of an emergency. *Israel Annals of Psychiatry and Allied Disciplines*, **15**, 277–88.

Mowrer, O. H. (1960). *Learning Theory and Behavior*. New York: Wiley.

Mueser, K. T. & Butler, R. W. (1987). Auditory hallucinations in combat-related posttraumatic stress disorder. *American Journal of Psychiatry*, **144**, 299–302.

Murphy, S. A. (1988). Mediating effects of intrapersonal and social support on mental health 1 and 3 years after a natural disaster. *Journal of Traumatic Stress*, **1**, 155–72.

Nezu, A. M. & Carnevale, G. J. (1987). Interpersonal problem solving and coping reactions of Vietnam veterans with post-traumatic stress disorder. *Journal of Abnormal Psychology*, **96**, 155–7.

Novaco, R. W. (1975). *Anger Control: The Development and Evaluation of an Experimental Treatment*. Lexington, MA: D. C. Heath.

Novaco, R. W., Cook, T. M. & Sarason, I. G. (1983). In D. Meichenbaum & M. E. Jaremko, eds, *Stress Reduction and Prevention*, pp. 377–418, New York: Plenum Press.

Rachman, S. (1980). Emotional processing. *Behaviour Research and Therapy*, **18**, 51–60.

Rickarby, G. A. (1977). Four cases of mania associated with bereavement. *Journal of Nervous and Mental Disease*, **165**, 255–62.

Rimm, D. C., Hill, G. A., Brown, N. N. & Stuart, J. E. (1974). Group assertive training in the treatment of expression of inappropriate anger. *Psychological Reports*, **34**, 791–8.

Roberts, W. P., Penk, W. E., Gearing, M. L., Robinowitz, R., Dolan, M. & Patterson, E. (1982). Interpersonal problems of Vietnam combat veterans with PTSD. *Journal of Abnormal Psychology*, **91**, 444–50.

Ross, J. R., Ball, W. A., Sullivan, K. A. & Caroff, S. N. (1989). Sleep disturbance as the hallmark of posttraumatic stress disorder. *American Journal of Psychiatry*, **146**, 697–707.

Roth, W. T. (1988). The role of medication in post-traumatic therapy. In F. M. Ochberg, ed., *Post-traumatic Therapy and Victims of Violence*, pp. 39–56.

Saigh, P. A. (1986). *In vitro* flooding in the treatment of a 6-yr-old boy's posttraumatic stress disorder. *Behaviour, Research and Therapy*, **24**, 685–8.

Saigh, P. A. (1987a). *In vitro* flooding of childhood posttraumatic stress disorders: a systematic replication. *Professional School Psychology*, **2**, 135–46.

Saigh, P. A. (1987b). *In vitro* flooding of an adolescent's post-traumatic stress disorder. *Journal of Clinical Child Psychology*, **16**, 147–50.

Schindler, F. E. (1980). Treatment by systematic desensitization of a recurring nightmare of a real life trauma. *Journal of Behavior Therapy and Experimental Psychiatry*, **11**, 53–4.

Shipley, R. H. & Boudewyns, P. A. (1980). Flooding and implosive therapy: are they harmful? *Behavior Therapy*, **11**, 503–8.

Shipley, R. H. & Boudewyns, P. A. (1988). The mythical dangers of exposure therapy. *The Behavior Therapist*, **11**, 162–78.

Silver, S. M. & Iacono, C. (1986). Symptom groups and family patterns of Vietnam veterans with posttraumatic stress disorders. In C. R. Figley, ed., *Trauma and its Wake* (vol. 2), pp. 78–98, New York: Brunner/Mazel.

Solomon, S. (1986). Mobilizing social support networks in times of disaster. In C. R. Figley, ed., *Trauma and its wake* (vol. 2), pp. 232–263, New York: Brunner/Mazel.

Solomon, Z., Mikulincer, M. & Avitzur, E. (1988). Coping, locus of control, social support, and combatrelated posttraumatic stress disorder: a prospective study. *Journal of Personality and Social Psychology*, **35**, 279–85.

Stampfl, T. G. & Levis, D. J. (1967). Essentials of implosive therapy: a learning-theory-based psychodynamic behavioral therapy. *Journal of Abnormal Psychology*, **72**, 157–63.

Stanton, D., & Figley, C. R. (1978). Treating the Vietnam veteran within the family system. In C. R. Figley ed., *Stress Disorders Among Vietnam Veterans: Theory, Research, and Treatment*. New York: Brunner/Mazel.

Tsai, M. & Wagner, N. U. (1978). Therapy groups for women sexually molested as children. *Archives of Sexual Behavior*, **7**, 417–27.

van der Kolk & Bessel, A. (1987). *Psychological Trauma*. Washington DC, American Psychiatric Press, Inc.

van der Kolk, B. (1987). The drug treatment of post-traumatic stress disorder. *Journal of Affective Disorder*, **13**, 203–13.

van der Kolk, B. (1983). Psychopharmacological issues in post-traumatic stress disorder. *Hospital and Community Psychiatry*, **34**, 683–91.

van der Kolk, B., Greenberg, M., Boyd, H. *et al.* (1985). Inescapable shock, neurotransmitters, and addiction to trauma: Toward a psychobiology of posttraumatic stress. *Biological Psychiatry*, **20**, 314–25.

Watson, C. G. (1991a). Psychometric posttraumatic stress disorder measurement techniques: a review. *Psychological Assessment: A Journal of Clinical and Consulting Psychology*.

Watson, C. G., Juba, M. P., Manifold, V., Kucala, T. & Anderson, P. E. D. (1991*b*). The PTSD Interview: Rationale, description, reliability, and concurrent validity of a DSM–III-based technique. *Journal of Clinical Psychology*.

Wernick, R. L. (1983). Stress inoculation in the management of chronic pain: applications to burn pain. In D. Meichenbaum & M. E. Jaremko, eds, *Stress reduction and prevention*, pp. 191–218, New York: Plenum Press.

Williams, T. (1987). Diagnosis and treatment of survivor guilt. In T. Williams, ed., *Posttraumatic Stress Disorder: A Handbook for Clinicians*, pp. 75–92, Cincinnati, OH: Disabled American Veterans.

Williams, W. (1976). Acute traumatic neurosis treated by brief intensive behaviour therapy. *Journal of Behavior Therapy and Experimental Psychiatry*, **7**, 43–5.

Wolfe, M. E., Alavi, A. & Mosnaim, A. D. (1988). Posttraumatic stress disorder in Vietnam veterans: clinical and EEG findings; possible therapeutic effects of carbamazepine. *Biological Psychiatry*, **23**, 642–4.

Wolff, R. (1977). Systematic desensitization and negative practice to alter the aftereffects of a rape attempt. *Journal of Behavior Therapy and Experimental Psychiatry*, **8**, 423–5.

Wolpe, J. (1958). *Psychotherapy by Reciprocal Inhibition*. Stanford, CA: Stanford University Press.

Yalom, I. D. (1975). *The Theory and Practice of Group Psychotherapy*. New York: Basic Books.

18

BEHAVIOURAL AND COGNITIVE APPROACH IN THE TREATMENT OF TORTURE-RELATED PSYCHOLOGICAL PROBLEMS

Metin Başoğlu

INTRODUCTION

Today, a variety of psychotherapeutic approaches are being used in treating the psychological problems that arise after torture and other forms of organized violence. As most systematic treatment efforts are confined to small groups of mental health professionals or rehabilitation centres located in different parts of the world (van Willigen, this volume), the choice of psychologial treatment depends largely on the professional orientation of these workers. Among the most widely used approaches, psychodynamic psychotherapy appears to be the most popular, particularly in Latin American countries. This is understandable given the strong psychoanalytic tradition in Latin American psychiatry together with a long history of human rights abuses in those countries. However, part of this psychoanalytic tradition in treating torture survivors is probably a reflection of the experience with Holocaust survivors after World War II. Most Holocaust survivors who have come to the attention of mental health professionals, particularly those who have migrated to the United States, have been treated by psychodynamic methods. Judging by critical reviews of this experience, these methods, by and large, have not produced encouraging results in alleviating the suffering of Holocaust survivors (Solkoff, this volume).

There have been two systematic studies (Horowitz *et al.*, 1984; Lindy *et al.*, 1983) of the efficacy of psychodynamic psychotherapy in other stress response syndromes, both uncontrolled. In the Horowitz *et al.* (1984) study, although patients did show improvement over time, a meta-analysis of psychotherapy outcome (Nicholson & Berman, 1983) showed that this improvement did not differ from that of untreated controls (Fairbank & Nicholson, 1987). In the second study (Lindy *et al.*, 1983) only 10 of the 30 patients completed the study with some improvement.

Alternative methods in treating torture survivors include various other forms of individual and group psychotherapy, 'insight therapy' (Vesti *et al.*, this volume), and 'testimony' method (Cienfuegos & Monelli, 1983; Agger & Jensen, 1990). It is difficult to judge the efficacy of these treatments for several reasons. First, most reports of effective treatment do not provide a sufficiently detailed description of the method; many appear to be a mixture of various psychotherapeutic elements and not based on a consistent theory. Secondly, no controlled evaluation of treatment outcome has been undertaken. There is thus no way of estimating the role of non-specific factors and spontaneous recovery in positive outcome often attributed to treatment. Furthermore, most outcome evaluations are not based on careful measurement of problem areas. Although there are some recent efforts to standardize evaluation methods (van Willigen, personal communication), to date, very few standardized rating instruments exist. Finally, lack of follow-up assessments preclude any judgment on the long-term efficacy of these methods.

Psychological problems following severe trauma have been classified as Post-Traumatic Stress Disorder (PTSD) in the third edition of the diagnostic manual of the American Psychiatric Association. Torture is recognized as one of the aetiological factors for this condition. Despite the controversy surrounding the validity of this term as a diagnostic entity, it has aroused much interest and stimulated research in this area. In the last decade, promising advances have been made in treating this condition with the use of behavioural techniques (Keane, this volume). So far very little of this experience has been used in the treatment of torture survivors. The purpose of this chapter is to review the implications of the recent progress in treating PTSD and other anxiety disorders for work with torture survivors.

Although post-torture psychological problems show considerable variability from one individual to another, most commonly encountered symptoms are anxiety related. It is, in fact, this characteristic of the condition that has led to its classification as an anxiety disorder. It is therefore useful first to review briefly the recent advances in treating other anxiety disorders.

TREATMENT OF ANXIETY DISORDERS: A BRIEF REVIEW

There is now general agreement that behaviour therapy is the treatment of choice in anxiety disorders (for a review see Marks, 1987). Behaviour therapy is based on the exposure principle: prolonged exposure to a feared or anxiety-evoking situation diminishes anxiety (habituation) (Gelder, Marks & Wolff, 1967; Marks, 1985; Marks *et al.*,

1988). Exposure can be imaginal or can take place in a real life situation (*in vivo*).
In vivo exposure has been found to be particularly useful in anxiety disorders with
a strong behavioural avoidance component such as specific phobias, agoraphobia,
and obsessive–compulsive disorder (OCD) (Marks, 1987). Previous treatments
included various drugs of dubious therapeutic value, grossly invasive techniques such
as psychosurgery in OCD, or psychodynamic psychotherapy which took years to
complete. Today, these disorders can be treated in 10–15 sessions with lasting
improvement (O'Sullivan & Marks, 1990). Treatment is relatively easy to administer
and therapist training is much less arduous in comparison with other psychotherapies
such as psychodynamic psychotherapy. It is thus easier to disseminate the necessary
knowledge and skills to mental health professionals throughout the world.

Cognitive therapy (Beck *et al.*, 1979) is recognized as an effective way of treating
depression (Brewin, 1988, p. 183) although its role in anxiety disorders still remains
largely untested (Marks, 1987; Marks & Marks, 1990). Although its usefulness in
trauma-related anxiety problems remains yet to be confirmed (Keane *et al.*, this
volume) it may have an important place in treating depression that so often
accompanies PTSD.

Two groups of drugs have been used in anxiety disorders. Benzodiazepines provide
only transient relief from anxiety and carry the risk of undesirable side effects and
addiction. Relapse is common on discontinuation and withdrawal symptoms are a
major problem (O'Sullivan & Marks, 1990). Antidepressants can be useful when
depression complicates the picture but their effect on non-depressed anxiety patients
is still controversial. Their effect often vanishes after discontinuation and side effects
can be a problem (Marks, 1987).

BEHAVIOURAL TREATMENT OF PTSD

The effectiveness of behavioural treatments in anxiety disorders seem to have
implications for the treatment of trauma-induced stress symptoms. Certain post-trauma
symptoms do indeed respond to exposure treatment in the same way as the symptoms
of other anxiety disorders. The reader is referred to Keane *et al.* (this volume) for
a review of the conceptual framework for exposure treatments in PTSD and the
evidence for their effectiveness.

The similarity between PTSD and other anxiety disorders such as phobias in their
response to exposure treatment is perhaps not surpris-

ing in view of the other similarities between these conditions. Both conditions involve fear and avoidance reactions when confronted with certain situations. Compared with simple phobia, agoraphobia is closer to PTSD in that it involves fear of multiple situations and also generalized anxiety in the absence of phobic cues. There are, however, important differences between phobias and PTSD (Foa, Steketee & Rothbaum, 1989). While there is always a traumatic onset for PTSD, this may not be true for phobias. Furthermore, certain PTSD symptoms such as intrusive recollections, nightmares, flashbacks, startle reactions, cognitive impairment, emotional numbing and estrangement from others are not characteristic of phobias. Nevertheless, most positive symptoms of PTSD show the same response pattern (initial anxiety followed by habituation) to exposure treatment (Keane *et al.*, this volume).

COGNITIVE/BEHAVIOURAL TREATMENT OF POST-TRAUMATIC STRESS SYMPTOMS IN TORTURE SURVIVORS

So far, there have only been few attempts to study the efficacy of cognitive–behavioural treatment in torture survivors. The following discussion of the treatment method is therefore largely based on the author's own clinical experience. The various components of treatment are outlined below.

Initial interview
1 Identification of problem areas: presenting complaints, most distressing/disabling symptoms, impact of problems on social functioning
2 Assessment of suitability and motivation for treatment
3 Re-education concerning the nature of the symptoms
4 Discussion of treatment, its method, rationale and aims
5 Setting of treatment goals
Treatment phase
1 Implosive therapy (imaginal exposure to anxiety-evoking imagery and thoughts)
2 Exposure *in vivo*: behavioural exposure to anxiety-evoking/ avoided situations
3 Cognitive therapy

Initial interview

Identification of problem areas

A semi-structured interview is used to elicit the information necessary for the subsequent therapy sessions. The interview often starts with a discussion of the presenting complaints and reasons for referral. The major problem areas are then outlined in a hierarchical fashion from the most to the least distressing and/or disabling in order to determine treatment priorities. Setting treatment priorities correctly is crucial for providing rapid relief from the most distressing symptoms and thereby enhancing the client's motivation for treatment. The hierarchy is based mainly on two criteria: subjective distress associated with the symptom and the impact of the symptom on social functioning. For example, extensive avoidance of various situations for an unrealistic fear of re-arrest, torture, or of being killed is both a distressing and a socially incapacitating symptom and thus could be assigned a higher priority. As part of the assessment of social impairment, the impact of symptoms on the client's ability to fulfil political commitments should also be taken into account, particularly in individuals for whom political functioning is central to their lives.

Assessment of suitability and motivation for treatment

Various personality characteristics that make individuals better candidates for psychotherapy in general also apply to torture survivors and will not be discussed in detail here. The socio-cultural background of the survivor may be an important consideration in the screening process. Some survivors may be from certain cultures or from certain parts of a particular country where psychotherapy is not recognized as a form of treatment. In such cases an offer of psychotherapy may be rejected by the client, or even when accepted, premature termination of treatment is always a serious possibility.

History of a past psychotic episode is not in itself an exclusion criterion. Transient psychotic reactions to extreme stress are not uncommon in torture survivors and sometimes are followed by typical post-traumatic stress symptoms which are often amenable to behavioural treatment. On the other hand, a full-blown current psychosis, particularly of the paranoid type, is an exclusion factor. In other cases where there is a likelihood of psychotic reactions during treatment, therapy is best undertaken under controlled conditions, preferably on an inpatient basis.

As implosive therapy requires a certain level of arousal in response to mental images of past traumatic experience for habituation to occur, those individuals who are capable of evoking more vivid mental imagery seem to do better in treatment. The client's capacity to evoke mental imagery often becomes evident during the process of eliciting information about past traumatic experiences.

Assessment of motivation for psychological treatment is crucial since many survivors present with psychosomatic symptoms and request traditional medical care. Those survivors who are aware of the connection between their symptoms and their past traumatic experience appear to be more motivated for psychological treatment. Sometimes there may be a realistic reason for their request for physical treatment such as medication. Certain symptoms such as severe sleep disturbance, incapacitating somatic anxiety symptoms as part of an underlying depression or other depressive symptoms may require rapid relief. In such cases, antidepressants are often useful in providing this relief, which in turn makes the client more motivated for and amenable to psychotherapy.

Re-education

Re-educating the client about the nature of the symptoms not only enhances motivation for treatment but is also therapeutic in itself. This is particularly important for those who tend to somatize their anxiety and believe that the symptoms are a result of an internal physical damage caused by torture. Such survivors often insist on having some form of physical treatment and tend to discontinue contact with the therapist if their demands are not met. A careful explanation of how such symptoms can be brought about by severe psychic trauma may help the client develop insight into his/her problems. Some cognitive restructuring may be required at this stage aimed at irrational beliefs underlying their refusal to acknowledge the psychological nature of symptoms. One such belief is to view psychological problems as a sign of a 'weak character'. These beliefs may need to be tactfully challenged and replaced by the understanding that theirs has only been a normal response to an extremely traumatic situation. More will be said about the cognitive restructuring process later in the chapter.

Once a common understanding of the nature of the problems is established between the therapist and the client, the next step is to clarify for the client how his/her symptoms affect social functioning. For example, irritability and outbursts of anger and hostility might disrupt relationships and enhance social isolation. Concentration and memory difficulties might impair performance at work or school. Depressive symptoms might alter realistic perceptions of life and inhibit the will and the energy to continue with much valued social and political activities. Fear and avoidance of various situations might preclude social activities and so on. Once this process of mapping-out of symptoms onto their social consequences is completed, the client is ready for a discussion of treatment prospects.

Discussion of treatment method, rationale and aims

The rationale for behavioural treatment needs to be carefully explained to the client. The client needs to understand fully that the reason behind confronting anxiety-evoking situations (e.g. painful memories) is to allow anxiety and other painful emotions to habituate so that the memory of the trauma no longer evokes them. Avoidance of painful thoughts and situations that remind the client of past trauma only serve to sustain the symptoms. If confronted for sufficiently long without avoidance, anxiety evoked by these situations does not last forever and eventually subsides. This understanding is vital since much of the treatment outside therapy sessions will need to be undertaken by the client himself/herself in the form of homework sessions.

Alleviating symptomatic distress is not the sole aim of the treatment. The ultimate objective is to facilitate return to normal and productive social functioning by removing the disabling symptoms. For many survivors, inability to pursue political activities as a result of debilitating symptoms is a major problem in itself which may compound feelings of defeat, helplessness, hopelessness and ultimately depression.

Informing the client of the possibility of an initial worsening of symptoms may help prevent a premature termination of treatment later. An increased arousal and exacerbation of symptoms during the early stages of treatment is often due to recollection of painful memories. An increase in irritability, generalized anxiety, sleep disturbance, outbursts of hostility and aggressive behaviour, and depressed mood may be observed. Similar changes have also been observed in phobic patients (Giles, 1988) and sexual assault survivors (Kilpatrick & Best, 1984) treated by implosive therapy. Agoraphobics treated by exposure often experience an initial increase in their panics which is then followed by lasting improvement (Marks et al., in preparation). Such effects of implosive therapy are not harmful (Shipley & Boudewyns, 1980, 1988; Keane et al., this volume); they are often transient and subside with continuation of treatment.

Setting of treatment goals

As noted earlier, the most distressing and disabling problems are given priority in treatment. These are often positive symptoms such as intrusive recollection of traumatic events, re-experiencing of the trauma through flashbacks and nightmares, severe sleep disturbance, fear and avoidance of situations which resemble the torture setting or which evoke an unrealistic fear of re-arrest, further torture or of being killed, and depression with or without suicidal ideation.

Even without a suicide risk, depression needs priority attention since it often undermines motivation for and compliance with treatment. Further, experience with other anxiety disorders has shown that depression impedes information processing and habituation to anxiety-evoking stimuli (Foa & Kozak, 1986; Başoğlu *et al.*, 1988). Anti-depressants, particularly those with sedative properties such as amitriptyline, are often useful in providing rapid relief from the most disabling anxiety and depressive symptoms (Falcon, Ryan & Chamberlain, 1985; Davidson *et al.*, 1990; Başoğlu, Marks & Sengün 1992). Once depression has lifted, therapy can commence.

Treatment priorities are fully discussed with the client and a consensus achieved. Rather than imposing tasks on the client, his/her active participation in the decision-making process is encouraged. This is important since the client will need to adopt a problem-solving approach and show initiative in dealing with numerous problem situations as they arise in daily life. Active participation in goal-setting also implies a commitment to therapy which in turn enhances treatment compliance.

Treatment phase

Implosive therapy

Therapy sessions are initially carried out at least twice, preferably three times, a week. Sessions usually last 1 ½ to 2 hours or sometimes longer depending on the amount of material covered and the speed with which the desired outcome is achieved. The total number of sessions may vary from 10 to 20.

The session The session begins with the therapist asking the survivor to relate his/her story starting from the events that lead up to arrest, detention and torture. A chronological account of events is desirable since it allows a gradual build-up to the most distressing memories and also helps the therapist to detect possible gaps in memory as well as suppressed events and associated painful emotions. For effective guidance through the session, the therapist needs to have elicited sufficient information during the initial interview about the most traumatic events for the survivor. Critical information, however, may also emerge during the session through verbal and non-verbal behaviour of the survivor.

When most distressing aspects of past traumatic events are reached, the survivor is asked to imagine repeatedly the traumatic situation, retain the anxiogenic imagery in his/her mind as vividly and as long as possible and go through the disturbing thoughts over and over again. At this stage, the survivor relates the events in the present tense, as if they were happening at that moment. The therapist intentionally helps sustain the state of arousal by having the client recall various aspects of the torture situation such as sounds, sights, smells and tactile sensations (e.g. 'You are waiting in the dark, tell me what you hear. Do you hear the footsteps?', 'They put you in a filthy room. What did it smell like?', 'They brought your friend from the torture chamber. What was his condition like?'). This is continued until a clear reduction in anxiety becomes evident either through verbal and non-verbal behaviour or direct feedback from the survivor who may rate his/her anxiety as a 0–10 scale.

There are two types of stimuli that can be presented during the session: trauma-specific stimuli and conditioned stimuli (Keane *et al.*, this volume). Trauma-specific stimuli involve the real aspects of the trauma situation such as the torture setting itself, the methods used and the physical and psychological pain suffered during torture. Conditioned stimuli concern the individual's cognitive and emotional responses to the traumatic events such as fear, guilt, self-blame, humiliation, shame and loss of control. Such stimuli are particularly important in torture survivors since the very act of torture is designed to produce such emotions. Feelings of guilt and self-blame may concern past behaviour seen as giving in to the torturers, causing harm to friends, comrades, relatives or to the political cause, or 'undignified' behaviour (e.g. pleas for mercy) displayed in order to avoid further torture. Loss of control during torture may result in disorganized behaviour, later remembered with regret, shame and humiliation. The conflict imposed upon the survivor by forced 'impossible choices' during torture may be sustained long after the incident.

The therapist's role is to guide the survivor through a series of painful memories and facilitate vivid recall and free emotional expression against the background of a safe environment. A non-judgmental, caring and supportive attitude on the part of the therapist is essential. The therapist would need to take care, however, to preserve a certain degree of detachment from the emotional impact of the often extremely disturbing material uncovered during the session in order to maintain an objective view and control of the session.

Another word of caution concerns the amount of material covered in one session. Although there is no hard and fast rule in this respect, care is taken not to drive the client to a point of physical and emotional exhaustion. Such a state may impede emotional processing and can also be confused with anxiety extinction. An exhausted client would still perceive and report the presented stimuli as distressing but would be unable to emotionally respond to them. The presentation of stimuli is thus terminated after anxiety subsides and before exhaustion sets in.

Some time is set aside at the end of the session for a discussion of the material covered. A cognitive reappraisal of session material is often useful in resolving emotional conflicts that may be left relatively untouched by the extinction process. In the author's experience, trauma-specific emotional responses are more easily accessed and extinguished than conditioned responses such as guilt, shame, humiliation and other emotional conflicts. Such residual problems, when present, can be further reduced by cognitive interventions. It should be noted, though, that a general decrease in emotional arousability is often accompanied by a significant reduction in the intensity of conditioned responses, thereby making them more amenable to cognitive intervention. It is thus advisable to wait until the extinction process is completed before attempting any cognitive restructuring.

Not uncommonly, extinction of anxiety alone achieves cognitive change without any therapist intervention. Once the emotional upheaval has subsided, the survivor might spontaneously say, for instance, in reference to a 'double-bind' situation imposed by the torturers 'There is no point in blaming myself, is there? I was left with no choice'. Any cognitive change is reinforced by the therapist. In situations where there is a need for a lengthy discussion of the session material but not enough time left for it, the next session might be used for this purpose before moving on to other trauma themes.

Setting homework tasks

Self-administered exposure outside therapy sessions is a critical ingredient of behavioural treatment programmes in anxiety disorders (Marks, 1987; Marks *et al.*, 1988; Al-Kubaisy *et al.*, 1988). Setting homework exposure tasks is straightforward in cases where there are identifiable external anxiety cues and overt behavioural avoidance such as in agoraphobia or OCD. In cases where anxiety cues are internal (e.g. thoughts, images, conditioned emotional and autonomic responses) and avoidance is cognitive (e.g. suppression of painful thoughts, distraction), setting implosive therapy tasks is more difficult. In situations where the primary problem is anxiety-evoking thoughts (e.g. catastrophic thoughts in panic disorder or pure obsessions), repeated listening to tape-recorded sessions of imaginal flooding has been found useful as a homework exercise (Richards & Rose, 1991; Başoğlu & Noshirvani, unpublished case studies).

In cases where this technique is feasible, homework tasks consist of daily sessions of listening to the taped material until extinction occurs. Alternatively, the client may set aside time every day to go through the session material along the lines practised during the session.

Factors determining treatment success

As in most psychotherapies, success in therapy largely depends on the client's motivation for, and compliance with, treatment. There are a number of other factors, however, that may determine therapy outcome. Incomplete exposure to trauma-related (conditioned) stimuli is suggested as a factor that may impede extinction (Keane, Zimmerling & Caddell, 1985). This theory may explain why spontaneous exposures to stimuli through re-experiencing of the trauma (e.g. flashbacks, intrusive recollection of trauma) do not lead to extinction (Keane *et al.*, 1985). In view of the evidence that prolonged exposure is more effective than short exposure (Stern & Marks, 1973; Chaplin & Levine, 1980; Rabavilas, Boulougouris & Stefanis, 1976; Marshall, 1985; Matthews, Gelder & Johnston, 1981; for a review see also Marks, 1987), an alternative explanation is the brief duration of spontaneous exposures (Foa, Steketee & Rothbaum, 1989). Thus, if the latter theory is correct, incomplete extinction during the therapy session may be due to insufficient duration of exposure.

Another factor concerns memory gaps or suppression of painful memories and associated emotions, a common feature of post-trauma symptomatology. This is said to be due to a discrepancy between the emotional state at the time of the trauma (high arousal) and that which is present at the time of recall (low or no arousal) (Keane *et al.*, 1985). That such discrepancy impedes recall has indeed been demonstrated in an experiment (Bower, 1981). Thus, an increased arousal level at the time of recall provides a better match for the emotional state that was present during the trauma, which, in turn, facilitates recall of details of the event (Foa *et al.*, 1989). Cognitive avoidance of anxiety-evoking stimuli (e.g. by distraction or dissociation) or inability to recall vivid imagery relating to the trauma during the therapy session may result in low arousal and thus impede extinction. Such avoidance strategies should be blocked to facilitate arousal. There is evidence to suggest that the individual has to experience anxiety during exposure for a successful outcome (Borkovec & Sides, 1979; Kozak, Foa & Steketee, 1988; Lang, Melamed & Hart, 1970).

Current theories of aetiology in PTSD explain the long-term persistence of PTSD symptoms and their resistance to natural extinction effects by the concept of 'serial conditioning' and the 'conservation of anxiety hypothesis' (Keane *et al.*, this volume). In other words, once the trauma (unconditioned stimulus-UCS) has occurred, external and internal cues can become conditioned stimuli (CS) and generalize to a wide variety of situations. While this may, in part, explain the chronic nature of symptoms in some torture survivors, it does not take account of the additional factor of repeated traumas (multiple UCSs) experienced by many survivors. Survivors often confront a series of traumatic situations or may live under serious threat over a long period of time (e.g. continual persecution and harassment by the authorities, threat of further detention and torture or of being killed, having to go into hiding, witnessing violence due to civil strife or death of loved ones). This is, in fact, why some have challenged the validity of the term post-traumatic stress disorder for torture survivors (van Willigen, this volume). In such cases anticipation of a real threat (UCS) may play a more important role in 'conservation of anxiety' than do the CS. This may indeed pose problems in therapy. For instance, in treating a survivor who is still at serious risk of further arrest and torture, presentation of CS may have the effect of UCS and increase anxiety rather than extinguish it. In such cases it may be better to defer behavioural treatment until the real or perceived threat has abated.

Exposure *in vivo*

Behavioural exposure is often useful in treating fear and avoidance of various situations – a problem which may be extremely distressing and socially incapacitating. Panics and an agoraphobia-like condition with extensive avoidance or even house-bondage may occur. Torture survivors often show fear and avoidance of various situations that resemble certain aspects of the torture experience (Bøjholm & Vesti, this volume). Survivors subjected to electrical torture, for instance, may

avoid electrical appliances or medical procedures involving electrodes
such as EEG or ECG. Those who have been sexually tortured may
avoid gynaecological examination or sexual relationships. Solitary
confinement in small cells may lead to a fear of closed spaces. Being
awakened and dragged away for torture in the middle of sleep may
result in fear of sleeping at night. An interview with an authority
figure may evoke panic when it bears a slight resemblance to previous
interrogation experience. People in uniform, police stations, government offices or hospitals may be feared and avoided. In brief, fear can
be generalized to any aspect of the environment that evokes memories
of torture. These cues can also trigger flashbacks and sudden re-
experiencing of the torture trauma.

Preparation for exposure treatment is along the same lines as for
implosive therapy. After a detailed explanation of the rationale and
aims of treatment, targets are defined in consensus with the client.
Sessions are conducted once or twice weekly. The treatment principle
is the same: graded exposure to fear-evoking situations until anxiety
subsides. The therapist may need to accompany the client during the
initial sessions to provide encouragement and support and to monitor
progress. The speed of exposure and the level of anxiety that can be
tolerated at any one time depends on the individual. Clients who
respond to fear stimuli with extreme fear or terror may require a more
gradual exposure so as to keep anxiety within tolerable levels at each
step. Some survivors may readily lapse into flashbacks or re-
experience the trauma even at relatively low levels of anxiety. This
may pose a problem in treatment since such episodes, if too frequent
or prolonged, may preclude habituation by disengaging the client
from the stimulus situation. For habituation to occur, emotional information must access and activate central representation of fear (Borkovec, 1982; Foa & Kozak, 1986; Lang, 1979). In such cases, exposure
may need to be carried out at a slower pace, increasing the dose
gradually as habituation occurs at each step.

The therapist encourages self-exposure when the client is ready to
engage in further exposure tasks on his/her own. At the end of each
session progress is reviewed and targets for the next session are
discussed. The client is given strong emotional support, encouragement and verbal praise for any progress made.

As noted earlier, exposure homework is crucial in bolstering the
gains achieved during the sessions. The client is thus asked to practice
on tasks tackled during the session as well as on new ones. The client
also keeps a homework diary so that progress can be reviewed and
difficulties resolved at the next session.

Cognitive therapy

The effectiveness of cognitive therapy in PTSD (Keane *et al.*, this volume) or in other anxiety disorders (Emmelkamp and Mersch, 1982; Williams & Rappoport, 1983; Michelson, Mavissakalian & Marchione, 1985) is not yet established. Although some treatments with cognitive elements are said to be effective in torture survivors (Somnier & Genefke, 1986), there are no systematic controlled studies to verify the validity of these impressionistic observations.

The potential usefulness of cognitive interventions in torture survivors, however, cannot be dismissed in view of the common occurrence of depression in torture-induced PTSD (Allodi & Cowgill, 1982; Petersen *et al.*, 1985; Hougen *et al.*, 1988; Mollica, Wyshak & Lavelle, 1987; Mollica *et al.*, 1990) and the aetiological theories of symptom formation in trauma sufferers. If, as evidence suggests, loss of control under traumatic stress plays a role in anxiety, learned helplessness and depression (for a review see Başoğlu and Mineka, this volume), then treatments which help reverse this process by restoring sense of control in the individual may be effective in torture survivors.

Attributional style has been proposed as a factor which may account for low self-esteem and self-blame associated with helplessness (Abramson, Seligman & Teasdale, 1978). Three types of attributions have been pointed out: internal vs external, global vs specific, and stable *v*. unstable. Trauma victims who attribute the cause of uncontrollable events to themselves (internal), generalize them across situations (global), and perceive them to be chronic (stable) are more likely to have more and more severe behavioural deficits. Others have argued that the threat value of the uncontrollable event (e.g. perceived threat to life) better accounts for subsequent stress symptoms (Foa *et al.*, 1989).

These theories may have important implications in cognitive therapy with torture survivors. Individuals who perceive themselves as having failed to cope with torture or shown 'undignified' coping behaviours to prevent further torture may see their failure as a sign of an inherent 'weakness' in their personality or lack of firmness in their belief system – an attribution often reinforced by the normative culture of their political group. These attributions may cause considerable guilt, shame and social withdrawal. In such cases, survivors are encouraged to think that what they did under torture was a normal human response necessary for survival, that they were subjected to an extreme stress designed to break down their defence, that they have been confronted with an 'impossible choice' situation, that breaking under severe stress is not a sign of weakness and so on.

Self-blame may also concern behaviours that have led to friends or relatives being arrested, tortured or killed. For instance, the survivor, unaware of being kept under surveillance by the authorities, may have led the police to his/her comrades in hiding and caused their torture or perhaps even death. Or he/she may have been caught carrying a piece of paper with the names and addresses of comrades sought by the authorities. In such cases the circumstances which led to these mistakes should be explored and self-blame for any action should be directed away from the survivor's character to his/her behaviour (e.g. from 'I am worthless, untrustworthy, unreliable' to 'I made a mistake. This was because of my inexperience. I will be very careful next time').

Humiliation and degradation suffered during torture may result in low self-esteem, shame and guilt. The ensuing emotions are particularly intense if the survivor has been forced to violate religious and moral values, sexual taboos, and political/ideological beliefs. These emotions, though at times very slow to emerge, often surface during implosive therapy and can be dealt with as described earlier. Self-blame for the actions committed under torture are directed externally, i.e. to the torturers. Several propositions may be used in shifting the focus of blame: 1) an individual cannot be held responsible for an involuntary act committed under such extreme coercion, 2) it is the torturers who are to blame for having committed such atrocities, 3) such treatment was a deliberate attempt designed to undermine the survivor's self-respect and dignity. Therefore blaming one's self for what happened is an admission of defeat and of the torturers' victory, 4) the survivor is not unique in his/her experience; degrading treatment is a common form of torture.

The therapist often has to deal with moral, philosophical and political issues that emerge during therapy. This is a potentially problematic stage of therapy, particularly when the survivor's views on these issues are different from those of the therapist. How much agreement does there have to be on these issues for effective treatment to take place? There are conflicting views in this regard. Some have adopted a 'humanitarian' approach which presumably allows for some differences in views while others stress the importance of 'solidarity' with their clients (van Willegen, this volume). Although there is as yet no evidence to support either position, one might argue that gross differences in thinking is likely to undermine the therapeutic alliance. Therapist–client dissimilarity has been pointed out as one of the reasons for dropout in psychotherapy in general (Baeckeland & Lundwall, 1975).

An important issue that may need attention during therapy is the question of how someone can inflict so much pain and suffering on a fellow human being. This is, indeed, a relevant question given the abhorrent nature of the acts perpetrated during torture. Some survivors' inability to give a meaning to their experience seems to stem from a basic assumption that the world is just ('just-world hypothesis', Staub, 1990) and that human beings are not capable of inflicting pain on each other on a scale that was experienced during torture. This is consistent with the safety-signal theory (Seligman & Binik, 1977) and the proposition that individuals are more likely to develop PTSD if the trauma has violated formerly held basic concepts of safety (Foa *et al.*, 1989). This theory would predict that individuals who have been victims of state terror and who previously maintained uncritical faith in a 'just and benevolent' state and its institutions are more likely to suffer from the trauma. It would also predict that chronic fear induced by torture would be more generalized than that caused by other traumas of human design such as rape. The pervasive suspiciousness and generalised distrust of others commonly observed in torture survivors might perhaps be explained by the loss of the most fundamental safety signal: basic trust in others.

Most psychotherapies of torture survivors (e.g. Somnier & Genefke, 1986; Agger & Jensen, 1990; Agger, 1989; Allodi, 1986; Reid & Strong, 1988; Vesti *et al.*, this volume), implicitly or explicitly, aim to reverse such effects of torture. This aim is explicit in cognitive therapy. A discussion of the methods and aims of torture with reference to the survivor's own experience can help the survivor achieve an objective appraisal of the events during torture and his/her reactions to them. A global view of the function torture serves as an instrument of political repression against dissent can help place the traumatic experience in a political perspective and thereby 'de-personalize' it. Helping the survivor channel the pain and suffering caused by torture into useful action such as taking active stance against human rights violations may provide a meaning for the trauma and dispel feelings of helplessness. This is consistent with the 'constructive survival' hypothesis used in explaining the successful coping strategies of concentration camp survivors after their camp experience (Baker, this volume).

Some individuals are drawn into political activity without any clear understanding of the implications of engaging in a political movement against an oppressive regime. In contrast to those who were aware of the dangers involved and prepared to assume responsibility for their actions, these individuals seem to be more prone to traumatization. In therapy, they are encouraged to assume full responsibility for their own actions and regard their experience as a price one should be prepared to pay in the struggle for a better world.

Some survivors may have come out of prison to find that the political opposition in their country totally crushed, their political groups disbanded, friends and comrades killed, imprisoned or forced into exile. Their feelings of helplessness may thus be compounded by a sense of defeat. Furthermore, they may have to face public disgrace and blame for being 'troublemakers', 'criminals' or 'terrorists.' Far from receiving public sympathy for their inhumane treatment, they may be blamed for having brought it all upon themselves. Such examples of unsympathetic 'by-stander psychology' (Staub, 1985, 1989, 1990) may make cognitive appraisal of the trauma in a meaningful way considerably more difficult. In such cases, two questions that often arise in therapy are 'Given the extent of defeat suffered, is the cause lost? and 'Was what I went through all in vain?' Individuals who hold unrealistic expectations about the speed with which social and political change can be brought about in a society seem to have greater difficulty in resolving these issues. An appraisal of just how unrealistic such expectations are would obviously depend on the socio-political circumstances in any particular country. However, given the tremendous political and military pressures in the world against radical political change or even moderate demands for socio-economic reforms in Third World countries, it would be only fair to say that socio-political change is on the whole a painfully slow process involving considerable human misery and suffering. History is indeed replete with examples of positive social change being arrested, even thrown back at times, but in the longterm the world has witnessed a steady, albeit slow, progress forward. Individuals do have a personal responsibility in supporting this progress but need to be realistic about the timescale of change which may well exceed one's lifetime and avoid setting unattainable goals likely to lead to frustration and quick disillusionment. A discussion along these lines may help the survivor to review past mistakes, individual as well as ideological, and realistically appraise his or her own role in the process of social change.

It should be stressed here that a definition of the therapist's role as such does not necessarily imply an assumption of moral, ideological, or intellectual superiority over or a patronizing attitude towards the client. The therapist needs to take great care not to give the impression that he/she has all the answers to difficult questions and that his/her view of the world is closer to the truth than that of the survivor. It is all too easy for a naive cognitive therapist to slip into a 'know-all' role, only to realize later that this achieves nothing other than to drive the survivor into a defensive and possibly antagonistic position.

COGNITIVE-BEHAVIOURAL TREATMENT AND OTHER PSYCHOTHERAPIES: A BRIEF REVIEW OF COMMON ELEMENTS

The psychotherapy methods used in treating torture survivors, some of which are reviewed in this volume, have one important element in common: getting the survivor to talk about his/her traumatic experiences and encourage free emotional expression in a therapeutic context (Somnier & Genefke, 1986; Garcia-Peltoniemi & Jaranson, 1989; Agger, 1989; Ortmann et al., 1987; Roth et al., 1987; Allodi, 1986; Vesti et al., this volume). In psychodynamic psychotherapy, whatever psychodynamic formulation is used in explaining trauma-induced symptoms, the primary goal of treatment is integration of the traumatic experience by means of a therapeutic reliving of the trauma (Horowitz, 1973, 1974; Horowitz and Kaltreider, 1980; Horowitz et al., 1984; Brende, 1981; Brende & McCann, 1984; Blackburn, O'Connell & Richman, 1984; Crump, 1984). This goal is shared by behavioural procedures involving imaginal exposure to the trauma (e.g. Fairbank, Gross & Keane, 1983; Fairbank & Keane, 1982; Keane & Kaloupek, 1982; Schindler, 1980; see also Keane et al., this volume). It is thus conceivable that a therapeutic ingredient common to all these therapies may be extinction of anxiety through exposure to painful memories, followed (or accompanied) by cognitive change which ultimately enables integration of the traumatic experience.

Indeed, striking parallels can be observed between the cognitive-behavioural approach described in this chapter and the 'testimony method' (Agger & Jensen, 1990) developed in Chile in the 1970s (Cienfuegos & Monelli, 1983). This method involves the following procedures (Agger & Jensen, 1990) (possible common elements with behavioural treatment indicated in brackets): The therapist first informs the survivor about the procedures and 'reframes the situation and the symptoms and introduces the testimony method as a meaningful way of working with symptoms' [educating the client about the nature of symptoms and presenting the rationale of treatment]. The client's consent is obtained. Therapy starts with the client relating his/her story from the very beginning [imaginal exposure]. The testimony covers background (demographic) information about the client, events leading up to the traumatic event, the trauma story in details including dates, hours, and places, 'description of torture methods' [exposure to real or trauma-specific stimuli] and 'the reaction to them' [exposure to conditioned stimuli], and examples of daily life in prison. 'This can be complemented with drawings of places and situations' [thereby achieving more vivid imagery, facilitating recall of events and ensuring prolonged retention of painful imagery in mind]. The therapist may intervene 'by asking questions about emotional reactions then and now, or about situations which need clarification' [further exposure to conditioned stimuli]. Further painful memories uncovered in the process include flight from country of origin, 'why and how did the client escape', life in exile and 'dreams and hopes for the future and realistic possibilities'. The session is either tape recorded or written out by hand by the therapist [tape recording of sessions during implosive therapy for further practice at home]. 'Each session starts with a recapitulation of the last sentences from the former session' [thereby avoiding gaps in the account, enabling detection of memory deficits related to various traumatic events, facilitating recall of these events and ultimately ensuring complete exposure]. Therapy usually takes 12–20 weekly sessions [similar duration for behavioural treatment]. After the testimony is completed, 'Errors are corrected, situations are described more precisely. More therapeutic work on the emotional level is maybe done. The final document is written out' [further imaginal exposure outside sessions to reinforce gains]. The document may then be signed and read aloud by the client, with the therapist and the interpreter present as witnesses. The client keeps the document and can use it for private purposes (e.g. as evidence in asylum procedures or 'as a highly motivating text in language school'). The testimony can also be used for political purposes by sending it to international organizations, exile groups, or various professionals as documentation.

The bearing of testimony is seen as a cathartic healing process during which the traumatic experience is 'reframed' (Figley, 1988) or given a new meaning (Lindy, 1986). These procedures thus seem to share the same therapeutic ingredient with cognitive restructuring described earlier. Use of the testimony by the client for political purposes can also be viewed as a means of regaining control over events and dispelling feelings of helplessness. Perhaps the new meaning which emerges during either treatment is closely related to the process of regaining control and abandoning the victim role.

The current debate on cognitive versus behaviour therapy is also relevant here. What is the critical therapeutic ingredient in cognitive–behavioural treatment or testimony method in torture survivors:

cognitive restructuring or exposure? It is possible that cognitive intervention procedures, even when they do not involve live exposure, have an effect via imaginal exposure. It is thus difficult to disentangle the relative contribution of each component to the therapeutic process. Although no attempt has so far been made to investigate the effect of one component controlling for the other, controlled studies in anxiety disorders comparing cognitive–behavioural treatment with exposure alone have not found significant differences in outcome (Emmelkamp *et al.*, 1978; Emmelkamp & Mersch, 1982; Emmelkamp *et al.*, 1985; Mavissakalian, Michelson & Dealy, 1983; Williams & Rappoport, 1983). That significant improvement can be achieved by behavioural treatments without any cognitive intervention in combat survivors (Keane *et al.*, this volume) as well as in other anxiety disordered patients (Williams & Rappoport, 1983) is suggestive of an important role for exposure (see also Barlow, 1988, p. 425, for a review of the contribution of cognitive therapy to exposure treatment). Whether cognitive reattribution (e.g. giving a meaning to torture experience) alone achieves any improvement or enhances the effects of exposure when combined with it in torture survivors remains to be demonstrated.

Implications for treatment of torture survivors

The study of the therapeutic ingredients in the treatment programmes for torture survivors reviewed here and elsewhere in this volume has important treatment implications. If, as the evidence so far suggests, exposure is the critical ingredient in any treatment that involves a reconstruction of trauma memories, then care has to be taken that exposure is complete and sufficiently long to enable habituation to all aspects of the traumatic experience. Partial and brief exposures are usually ineffective, as noted earlier. This implies that conventional treatments without due emphasis on complete and prolonged exposure may be less than effective. Incomplete exposure may also explain the worsening of symptoms observed in some survivors (Mollica & Lavelle, 1988, cited in Agger, 1989) following a review of the trauma story. Lack of treatment response in such cases may be due to inadequate exposure rather than to a lack of 'reframing' of the trauma experience, as some have suggested (e.g. Agger, 1989).

This issue also concerns certain treatment policies adopted by rehabilitation centres for torture survivors. For instance, it is suggested that great care should be taken not to remind the survivors of their past experience while they undergo a rehabilitation programme (e.g.

Bøjholm & Vesti, this volume). There is no doubt this policy reflects a humanitarian concern to avoid causing further suffering for already severely traumatized individuals. Given the evidence supporting the efficacy of exposure-based treatments, such an avoidance approach might be potentially anti-therapeutic. This is not to say that the rehabilitation programme described by the above-mentioned authors is ineffective. On the contrary, their programme appears potentially effective since, judging by their description, it seems to contain intensive exposure to trauma cues, despite the 'anti-exposure' policy adopted by the staff. There are a number of points in their description to support this point. First, this intentional anti-exposure policy seems limited to staff-patient interactions during medical examinations and treatments; psychotherapy sessions seem to involve a fair amount of imaginal exposure during the review of the trauma story (Vesti et al., this volume; Somnier & Genefke, 1986).

Secondly, great emphasis is placed on physiotherapy during the rehabilitation programme and special importance is paid to administering physiotherapy and psychotherapy concurrently. It is conceivable that the setting and procedures involved in physiotherapy (e.g. a closed space, various instruments applied to the body, water, nakedness, close physical proximity of strangers, bodily contacts, authority figures, etc), by way of their association with the torture experience, act as conditioned stimuli and thus provide an opportunity for prolonged exposure and ultimately habituation to take place. Indeed, the survivors are said to show strong emotional reactions (e.g. fear) to these procedures. The fact that concurrent psychotherapy sessions are viewed as essential is probably another indication of the intensity of emotional arousal during physiotherapy.

Thirdly, the rehabilitation programme involves a fair amount of medical investigations ranging from simple physical examinations, blood tests, EEG, ECG to more complex procedures such as gastroscopy, rectoscopy, dental treatment, and surgery. The associations between these procedures and torture methods are obvious and indeed they evoke the same fear reactions observed during physiotherapy (Bøjholm & Vesti, this volume).

In brief, this rehabilitation programme appears to provide ample opportunity for both imaginal and behavioural exposure to generalized fear/anxiety cues. When the programme is taken in its entirety, its parallels with the principles of cognitive–behavioural treatment described in this chapter are striking. The efficacy of this programme might perhaps be further increased if the staff adopted an exposure rather than anti-exposure approach. There is evidence to show that reinforcing anxious patients' tendency to avoid feared situations is not only anti-therapeutic (Greist *et al.*, 1980; Telch *et al.*, 1985; Marks *et al.*, 1988) but can also wipe out gains from other treatments such as anti-depressant medication (Marks *et al.*, 1988).

The cognitive–behavioural paradigm can easily be implemented in multidisciplinary rehabilitation programmes with torture survivors. It can be used on an individual basis or in a group context. At an appropriate stage the patients might be told that some of the procedures they will be going through are likely to be emotionally disturbing but that this is not entirely undesirable since it will help them to overcome their generalized anxiety and fears. In other words, the patients might be prepared for the rehabilitation programme along very much the same lines as those described for behavioural treatment. The programme might be tailored according to the needs of each individual so that the survivor has an opportunity to deal with as many anxiety-evoking situations as possible to avoid incomplete exposure. The exposure programme can be extended to cover other anxiety-evoking situations outside the rehabilitation setting. Exposure can be gradual, if necessary, to keep levels of anxiety within tolerable limits. It need not be administered indiscriminately, e.g. to unwilling, unmotivated individuals, but patients can be selected on the basis of their clear understanding of the rationale, motivation and other suitability criteria. Clearly, cognitive–behavioural treatment is not an alternative to existing rehabilitation programmes; it can be integrated into 'comprehensive' treatment approaches to enhance their effectiveness.

Exposing a tortured individual to torture-related cues might at first seem a somewhat disturbing idea. It should be clear, however, from the discussion so far that the principle underlying behavioural approach, i.e. exposure, is probably common to most psychotherapies used with torture survivors, whichever conceptual formulations are used to define them. Perhaps the distinction between these therapies is one of style in administering a particular therapeutic intervention rather than theoretical. Given the plethora of evidence on the efficacy of behaviour therapy in treating anxiety, its use for torture survivors seem certainly to be in their own interest.

To summarize, the aims of cognitive–behavioural treatment are not incompatible with those of currently established treatments for torture survivors. It may also share important therapeutic elements with the latter. Obviously, it has its limitations, like any other treatment, but these limitations do not necessarily arise from its clear goal-oriented approach per se, as has been suggested by some authors (Turner & Gorst-Unsworth, 1990). As discussed earlier, its goals concern most problem areas deemed important in torture survivors. Furthermore, there is abundant evidence to show that the improvement achieved by cognitive–behavioural treatment in physiological, behavioural and cognitive problem areas often generalizes to social, family, marital and work problems. Its reliance on careful assessment, made possible by clear definition of goals, allows testability of hypotheses concerning its efficacy – a basic requirement of any scientific endeavour.

Excessive concerns about 'medicalizing' the consequences of torture may carry the risk of overlooking severely disabling psychological problems and thus not be in the interest of torture survivors. Social support may be helpful but only to the extent that the survivor is able to access and utilize it. Traumatic stress symptoms can impede the individual's capacity to utilize social support (Barrett & Mizes, 1988; Solomon, Mikulincer & Avitzur, 1988; Roberts *et al.*, 1982; Carroll *et al.*, 1985). Furthermore, social support may not always have the desired effect (Keane *et al.*, this volume).

CONCLUSION

We do not yet have any firm evidence in support of any therapeutic method in the treatment of torture survivors. Most treatments that are said to be helpful involve a reconstruction of the traumatic experiences in a therapy context. The critical components of these treatments have not yet been verified. Although recent advances in behavioural sciences have provided valuable insights into anxiety disorders and their treatment, this knowledge is not fully exploited in the search for effective treatments for torture survivors. Clearly, much research needs to be done before we can draw conclusions about the efficacy of existing treatments.

REFERENCES

Abramson, L. Y., Seligman, M. E. P. & Teasdale, J. D. (1978). Learned helplessness in humans: Critique and reformulation. *Journal of Abnormal Psychology*, 87, 49–94.

Agger, I. (1989). Sexual torture of political prisoners: an overview. *Journal of Traumatic Stress*, 2, 305–18.

Agger, I. & Jensen, S. B. (1990). Testimony as ritual and evidence in psychotherapy for political refugees. *Journal of Traumatic Stress*, 3(1), 115–30.

Al-Kubaisy, T., Marks, I. M., Sungur, M., Logsdail, S., Marks, M., & Headland, K. (1988). The role of self-exposure and therapist-aided exposure in phobia reduction: a controlled study. Paper presented at World Congress of Behaviour Therapy, Edinburgh, Scotland.

Allodi, F. (1986). Psychotherapy of post-traumatic stress disorders: a multicultural model. Workshop on Mass Violence and Post-traumatic Stress Disorders. Rockville, Md. April 14–15.

Allodi, F. & Cowgill, G. (1982). Ethical and psychiatric aspects of torture: a Canadian study. *Canadian Journal of Psychiatry*, **27**, 98–102.

Baeckeland, F. & Lundwall, L. (1975). Dropping out of treatment: a critical review. *Psychological Bulletin*, **82**, 738–83.

Barlow, D. H. (1988). *Anxiety and Its Disorders*. New York: The Guilford Press.

Barrett, T. W. & Mizes, J. S. (1988). Combat level and social support in the development of posttraumatic stress disorder in Vietnam veterans. *Behaviour Modification*, **12(1)**, 100–15.

Başoğlu, M., Lax, T., Kasvikis, Y. & Marks, I. M. (1988). Predictors of improvement in obsessive–compulsive disorder. *Journal of Anxiety Disorders*, **2**, 299–317.

Başoğlu, M., Marks, I. M. & Şengün, S. (1992). Amitriptyline for PTSD in a torture survivor: a case study. *Journal of Traumatic Stress*, **5(1)**, 77–83.

Beck, A., Rush, J., Shaw, B. & Emery, G. (1979). *Cognitive Therapy of Depression*. New York: Guilford Press.

Blackburn, A. B., O'Connell, W. E. & Richman, B. W. (1984). PTSD, the Vietnam veteran, and Adlerian natural high therapy. Individual psychology. *Journal of Adlerian Theory, Research and Practice*, **40**, 317–32.

Borkovec, T. D. & Sides, J. (1979). The contribution of relaxation and expectance to fear reduction via graded imaginal exposure to feared stimuli. *Behaviour Research and Therapy*, **17**, 529–40.

Borkovec, T. (1982). Functional CS exposure in the treatment of phobias. In Y. Boulougouris, ed. *Learning Theory Approaches to Psychiatry*, New York: Wiley.

Bower, G. H. (1981). Mood and memory. *American Psychologist*, **36**, 129–48.

Brende, J. O. (1981). Combined individual and group therapy for Vietnam veterans. *International Journal of Group Psychotherapy*, **31**, 367–78.

Brende, J. O. & McCann, I. L. (1984). Regressive experiences in Vietnam veterans: their relationship to war, posttraumatic symptoms and recovery. *Journal of Contemporary Psychotherapy*, **14**, 57–75.

Brewin, C. R. (1988). *Cognitive Foundations of Clinical Psychology*. Lawrence Erlbaum Associates, Publishers: Hove and London.

Carroll, E. M., Rueger, D. B., Foy, D. W. & Donahoe, C. P. (1985). Vietnam combat veterans with posttraumatic stress disorder: Analysis of marital and cohabiting adjustment. *Journal of Abnormal Psychology*, **94**, 329–37.

Chaplin, E. W. & Levine, B. A. (1980). The effects of total exposure duration and interrupted versus continuous exposure or flooding. *Behavior Therapy*, **12**, 360–8.

Cienfuegos, J. & Monelli, C. (1983). The testimony of political repression as a therapeutic instrument. *American Journal of Orthopsychiatry*, **53**, 43–51.

Crump, L. E. (1984). Gestalt therapy in the treatment of Vietnam veterans experiencing PTSD symptomatology. *Journal of Contemporary Psychotherapy*, **14**, 90–8.

Q

Davidson, J. Kudler, H., Mahorney, S. L., Lipper, S., Hammett, E., Saunders, W. B. & Cavenar, J. O., Jr. (1990). Treatment of posttraumatic stress disorder with amitriptyline and placebo. *Archives of General Psychiatry*, **47**, 259–66.

Emmelkamp, P. M. G., Kuipers, A. C. M. & Eggeraat, J. B. (1978). Cognitive modification versus prolonged exposure *in vivo*: A comparison with agoraphobics as subjects. *Behaviour Research and Therapy*, **16**, 33–41.

Emmelkamp, P. M. G. & Mersch, P. P. (1982). Cognition and exposure in vivo in agoraphobia: short term and delayed effects. *Cognitive Therapy and Research*, **6**, 77–88.

Emmelkamp, P. M. G., Brilman, E., Kurper, H. & Mersch, P. P. (1985). The treatment of agoraphobia: a comparison of self-instruction, rational-emotive therapy and exposure *in vivo*. *Behavior Modification*, **10**, 37–53.

Fairbank, J. A. & Keane, T. M. (1982). Flooding for combat-related stress disorders: assessment of anxiety reduction across traumatic memories. *Behavior Therapy*, **13**, 449–510.

Fairbank, J. A., Gross, R. T. & Keane, T. M. (1983). Treatment of posttraumatic stress disorder: evaluating outcome with a behavioral code. *Behavior Modification*, **7**, 557–68.

Fairbank, J. A. & Nicholson, R. A. (1987). Theoretical and empirical issues in the treatment of post-traumatic stress disorder in Vietnam veterans. *Journal of Clinical Psychology*, **43**, 44–55.

Falcon, S., Ryan, C. & Chamberlain, K. (1985). Tricyclics: possible treatment for posttraumatic stress disorder. *Journal of Clinical Psychiatry*, **46**, 385–9.

Figley, C. R. (1988). Post-traumatic family therapy. In F. M. Ochberg, ed., *Post-Traumatic Therapy and Victims of Violence*, pp. 83–109, New York: Brunner/Mazel.

Foa, E. B. & Kozak, M. J. (1986). Emotional processing of fear: Exposure to corrective information. *Psychological Bulletin*, **99**, 20–35.

Foa, E. B., Steketee, G. & Rothbaum, B. O. (1989). Behavioral/cognitive conceptualizations of post-traumatic stress disorder. *Behavior Therapy*, **20**, 155–76.

Garcia-Peltoniemi, R. E. & Jaranson, J. (1989). A multidisciplinary approach to the treatment of torture victims. Paper presented at the Second International Conference of Centres, Institutions and Individuals Concerned with the Care of Victims of Organised Violence. San Jose, Costa Rica, Nov. 27–Dec. 2.

Gelder, M. G., Marks, I. M. & Wolff, H. H. (1967). Desensitization and psychotherapy in the treatment of phobic states. *British Journal of Psychiatry*, **113**, 53–73.

Giles, T. R. (1988). Phobia and suicide: an influence of treatment? *The Behavior Therapist*, **11**, 26–42.

Greist, J. H., Marks, I. M., Berlin, F., Gourney, K. & Noshirvani, H. (1980). Avoidance versus confrontation of fear. *Behavior Therapy*, **11**, 1–14.

Horowitz, M. J. (1973). Phase oriented treatment of stress response syndromes. *American Journal of Psychotherapy*, **27**, 506–15.

Horowitz, M. J. (1974). Stress response syndromes, character style, and dynamic psychotherapy. *Archives of General Psychiatry*, **31**, 768–81.

Horowitz, M. J. & Kaltreider, N. B. (1980). Brief psychotherapy of stress response syndromes. In T. B. Karasu and L. Bellak, eds., *Specialized techniques in individual psychotherapy*. New York: Brunner/Mazel

Horowitz, M. J., Marmar, C., Weiss, D. S., Devitt, K. N. & Rosenbaum, R. (1984). Brief psychotherapy of bereavement reactions: the relationship of process to outcome. *Archives of General Psychiatry*, **41**, 438–48.

Hougen, H. P., Kelstrup, J., Petersen, H. D. & Rasmussen, O. V. (1988). Sequelae to torture. A controlled study of torture victims living in exile. *Forensic Science International*, **36**, 153–60.

Keane, T. M. & Kaloupek, D. G. (1982). Imaginal flooding in the treatment of posttraumatic stress disorder. *Journal of Consulting and Clinical Psychology*, **50**, 138–40.

Keane, T. M., Zimmerling, R. T. & Caddell, J. M. (1985). A behavioral formulation of post-traumatic stress disorder in Vietnam veterans. *The Behavior Therapist*, **8**, 9–12.

Kilpatrick, D. G. & Best, C. L. (1984). Some cautionary remarks on treating sexual assault victims with implosion. *Behavior Therapy*, **15**, 421–3.

Kozak, M. J., Foa, E. B. & Steketee, G. (1988). Process and outcome of exposure treatment with obsessive–compulsives: psychophysiological indicators of emotional processing. *Behavior Therapy*, **19**, 157–70.

Lang, P. J., Melamed, B. G. & Hart, J. (1970). A psychophysiological analysis of fear modification using an automated desensitization procedure. *Journal of Abnormal Psychology*, **76**, 220–34.

Lang, P. (1979). A bioinformational theory of emotional imagery. *Psychophysiology*, **16**, 495–512.

Lindy, J. D., Green, B. L., Grace, M. & Titchener, J. (1983). Psychotherapy with survivors of the Beverly Hills Supper Club fire. *American Journal of Psychotherapy*, **37**, 593–610.

Lindy, J. D. (1986). An outline for the psychoanalytic psychotherapy of post-traumatic stress disorder. In C. R. Figley, ed., *Trauma and Its Wake: Traumatic Stress Theory, Research and Intervention*, vol. II, pp. 195–212, New York: Brunner/Mazel.

Marks, I. M. (1985). *Psychiatric nurse therapists in primary care*. Research series, Royal College of Nursing, London.

Marks, I. M. (1987). *Fears, Phobias and Rituals*. Oxford: Oxford University Press.

Marks, I. M., Lelliott, P., Başoğlu, M., Noshirvani, H., Monteiro, W. & Kasvikis, Y. (1988). Clomipramine and exposure for obsessive–compulsive disorder. *British Journal of Psychiatry*, **152**, 234–8.

Marks, I. M. and Marks, M. (1990). Exposure treatment of agoraphobia/panic. In R. Noyes, Jr., M. Roth and G. D. Burrows, eds. *Handbook of Anxiety, The Treatment of Anxiety*, vol. 4, Elsevier Science Publishers B.V.

Marshall, W. L. (1985). The effects of variable exposure in flooding therapy. *Behavior Therapy*, **16**, 117–35.

Matthews, A. M., Gelder, M. G. & Johnston, D. W. (1981). *Agoraphobia: Nature and Treatment*. New York: Guilford Press.

Mavissakalian, M., Michelson, L. & Dealy, R. S. (1983). Pharmacological treatment of agoraphobia: imipramine versus imipramine with programmed practice. *British Journal of Psychiatry*, **143**, 348–55.

Michelson, L., Mavissakalian, M. & Marchione, K. (1985). Cognitive and behavioral treatments of agoraphobia: clinical, behavioral and psychophysiological outcomes. *Journal of Consulting and Clinical Psychology*, **53**, 913–25.

Mollica, R. F. & Lavelle, J. P. (1988). Southeast Asian refugees. In L. Comas-Diaz and E. E. H. Griffith, eds. *Clinical Guidelines in Cross-Cultural Mental Health*, New York: Wiley.

Mollica, R. F., Wyshak, G. & Lavelle, J. (1987). The psychosocial impact of war trauma and torture on Southeast Asian refugees. *American Journal of Psychiatry*, **144**, 1567–1572.

Mollica, R. F., Wyshak, G., Lavelle, J., Truong, T., Tor, S. & Yang, T. (1990). Assessing symptom change in Southeast Asian refugee survivors of mass violence and torture. *American Journal of Psychiatry*, **147**, 83–88.

Nicholson, R. A. & Berman, J. S. (1983). Is follow-up necessary in evaluating psychotherapy? *Psychological Bulletin*, **93**, 261–278.

Ortmann, J., Genefke, I. K., Jakobsen, L. & Lunde, I. (1987). Rehabilitation of torture victims: An interdisciplinary treatment model. *American Journal of Social Psychiatry*, **4**, 161–167.

O'Sullivan, G. & Marks, I. M. (1990). Longterm outcome of phobic and obsessive-compulsive disorders after treatment. In Noyes *et al.*, eds. *Handbook of Anxiety Disorders*, Vol. 4. Amsterdam: Elsevier.

Petersen, H. D., Abildgaard, U., Daugaard, G. *et al.* (1985). Psychological and physical long-term effects of torture. A follow-up examination of 22 Greek persons exposed to torture 1967–1974. *Scandinavian Journal of Social Medicine*, **13**, 89–93.

Rabavilas, A. D., Boulougouris, J. C. & Stefanis, C. (1976). Duration of flooding sessions in the treatment of obsessive–compulsive patients. *Behaviour Research and Therapy*, **14**, 349–55.

Reid, J. C. & Strong, T. (1988). Rehabilitation of refugee victims of torture and trauma: principles and service provision in New South Wales. *The Medical Journal of Australia*, **148**, 340–6.

Richards, D. A. & Rose, J. S. (1991). Exposure therapy for post-traumatic stress disorder: four case studies. *British Journal of Psychiatry*, **158**, 836–40.

Roberts, W. P., Penk, W. E., Gearing, M. L., Robinowitz, R., Dolan, M. & Patterson, E. (1982). Interpersonal problems of Vietnam combat veterans with PTSD. *Journal of Abnormal Psychology*, **91**, 444–50.

Roth, E. F., Lunde, I., Boysen, G. & Genefke, I. K. (1987). Torture and its treatment. *American Journal of Public Health*, **77**, 1404–6.

Schindler, F. E. (1980). Treatment by systematic desensitization of a recurring nightmare of a real life trauma. *Journal of Behavior Therapy and Experimental Psychiatry*, **11**, 53–4.

Seligman, M. E. P. & Binik, Y. M. (1977). The safety signal hypothesis. In H. Davis and H. M. B. Hurwitz, eds. *Operant–Pavlovian Interactions*. Hillsdale, NJ: Lawrence Erlbaum Associates.

Shipley, R. H. & Boudewyns, P. A. (1980). Flooding and implosive therapy: Are they harmful? *Behavior Therapy*, 11, 503–8.

Shipley, R. H. & Boudewyns, P. A. (1988). The mythical dangers of exposure therapy. *The Behavior Therapist*, 11, 162–78.

Solomon, Z., Mikulincer, M. & Avitzur, E. (1988). Coping, locus of control, social support, and combat-related posttraumatic stress disorder: a prospective study. *Journal of Personality and Social Psychology*, 35, 279–85.

Somnier, F. E. & Genefke, I. K. (1986). Psychotherapy for victims of torture. *British Journal of Psychiatry*, 149, 323–9.

Staub, E. (1985). The psychology of perpetrators and bystanders. *Political Psychology*, 6, 61–85.

Staub, E. (1989). The evolution of bystanders, German psychoanalysts, and lessons for today. *Political Psychology*, 10, 39–52.

Staub, E. (1990). The psychology and culture of torture and torturers. In P. Suedfeld, ed. *Torture and Psychology*. New York: Hemisphere Publishing Corporation.

Stern, R. S. & Marks, I. M. (1973). Brief and prolonged flooding: A comparison in agoraphobic patients. *Archives of General Psychiatry*, 28, 270–6.

Telch, M. J., Agras, W. S., Taylor, C. B., Roth, W. T. & Gallen, C. (1985). Combined pharmacological and behavioural treatment for agoraphobia. *Behaviour Research and Therapy*, 23, 325–35.

Turner, S. & Gorst-Unsworth, C. (1990). Psychological sequelae of torture: a descriptive model. *British Journal of Psychiatry*, 157, 475–80.

Williams, S. L. & Rappoport, A. (1983). Cognitive treatment in the natural environment for agoraphobics. *Behavior Therapy*, 12, 299–313.

Part VI

TORTURE IN PARTICULAR COUNTRIES:
EXPERIENCE WITH SURVIVORS OF
TORTURE IN THEIR HOME COUNTRY

19

TORTURE IN ARGENTINA
Diana Kordon, Lucila Edelman, Dario Lagos,
Elena Nicoletti, Daniel Kersner, Mirta Groshaus

HISTORICAL BACKGROUND

On May 19, 1813, three years after Argentina broke away from Spain, the nation's general assembly drew up its first package of laws, which included the prohibition of 'the heinous use of torments that were part of a legislation of tyranny'.

The Argentine Constitution, adopted in 1852 and in force today, ratified that prohibition: 'Abolished forever are the death penalty in political cases, as well as all forms of torture and beating. The jails of the nation will be safe and clean, to secure and not to punish the prisoners whom they hold.'

Even though the principal legal instruments of Argentina banned torture, it never ceased to be a part of the political landscape. Its forms have changed, but not its essence. Its use, even when secret, spread until it became a routine procedure used against political prisoners and even those accused of common crimes.

But beginning with the *coup d'état* of 1976, which brought to power a dictatorship that would last until 1983, there was a qualititative change in the forms of political repression. The forced disappearance of persons was the main manifestation of this new era in the use of violence to silence political expression.

FORCED DISAPPEARANCE OF PERSONS

Without explanation, thousands of people were kidnapped from their places of work, their homes or public places. No clue was ever given as to their fate. The justice system and the military government denied having information about the missing people. Relatives, friends and colleagues visited hospitals, police stations, jails, military barracks and morgues. But all attempts to find the missing persons were futile. They, literally, had disappeared.

The Inter-American Human Rights Commission (CIDH), part of the

Organization of American States, as a result of a visit to Argentina in 1979, gave a detailed description of this form of repression (CIDH, 1980). In its reports on the Human Rights situation in Argentina, the CIDH said:

> In relation to the respect for human rights, the Commission deems it to be of vital importance to present in this chapter an analysis of this phenomena, whose moral, social, domestic and legal implications are deeply affecting Argentine society.
>
> There are many cases, in a variety of nations, in which governments deny systematically detaining people, despite convincing evidence by those who seek to prove their claim that the missing people have been deprived of their liberty by the police or military authorities and, in some cases, that they are or have been held in specific places of detention.
>
> This practice is cruel and inhuman. As experience shows, 'disappearance' is not only an arbitrary detention, but it also seriously endangers personal integrity, security and the lives of the victims. It is, additionally, a true form of torture for the families and friends of the victims, due to the manifest uncertainty they sense regarding the fate of the missing people and the impotence they experience in efforts to give legal, moral and material assistance to the victims.
>
> The practice of forcing people to disappear appears to be an easy way of avoiding those legal dispositions upholding individual liberty, physical integrity, human dignity and the right to life. This practice nullifies the legal norms approved in recent years in some nations to prevent illegal detentions and the use of physical and psychological force against prisoners.
>
> It could be important to point out what might be the appropriate definition of the disappeared person. In a writ of *habeas corpus* presented to the Supreme Court, 1221 people petitioning on behalf of missing people described the situation in the following way:
>
> 'The people mentioned have been apprehended from their homes, from their places of work and from public places depending on the case, by armed men who are *prima facie*, and always claiming to be acting in the name of some manner of public authority. The fore-mentioned operations were carried out openly, with the deployment of large numbers of men – sometimes in uniform – arms and vehicles, and they generally had a duration and were so detailed in nature as to ratify the presump-

tion that those who intervened were backed by operational resources that are characteristic of the use of public force.

After being apprehended in the fore-mentioned fashion, the people in whose favor the undersigned petition was presented have disappeared without trace. All writs of *habeas corpus*, reports to police, criminal complaints and administrative actions have failed. The authorities approached in each case have invariably said that there was nothing indicating that the missing person has been detained.

Other complaints received by the CIDH have said that the armed men who carry out operations in the homes of the victims, apprehend the victim as well as that person's spouse and sometimes their children. They also rapidly search the residence, ransacking personal belongings and almost invariably covering all members of the family with a hood before taking them away.

The persons affected by these operations, and whose names are found in the lists in the power of the CIDH, are for the most part men and women between 20 and 30 years of age, although people both younger and older have also disappeared. Some children, who were kidnapped with their parents, have been freed, handed over to relatives or left abandoned in public places. Other children, nevertheless, are still missing.

According to information available to the Commission that phenomena of the missing people affects professionals, students, labor leaders, employees of different firms, journalists, religious leaders, draftees, businessmen: in other words, the better part of the many segments of Argentine society.

The immunity of the repressive forces

Security forces acted without any limits, working in broad daylight against defenceless people. The CIDH said:

The operations, for the most part similar in nature, were carried out by groups of between six and 26 people who showed up at the home or place of work of the victim, in several cars without any markings and with radios. In some cases the men were accompanied by additional forces supported by trucks, which after each mission were filled with the belongings of the victims.

The men participating in the missions dressed in civilian clothes and carried short and long arms, which they used to intimidate the victims and witnesses. If the mission was carried out in the victim's place of work or in a public place it generally was brief; but if it occurred at the victim's home it often would last several hours, particularly when the security forces had to wait for the victim to show up at home.

Claims also have been made that when the relatives, witnesses or doormen at apartment buildings reported what was happening to the local police, they almost always confirmed the operation and at the same time warned that they were not authorized to intervene. In the few cases that policemen appeared at the scene, they left shortly after talking with those people directly involved with the mission. This type of situation has been called the 'free zone', one favoring the force in action.

The existence of clandestine jails

Those few people who were freed after being abducted, were the first to report the existence of clandestine jails. Information provided by the former detainees, and other clues, led to the discovery of the jails and helped reveal the military jurisdiction to which they belonged.

Now, there is clear proof that 340 clandestine detention centres were in operation under military rule. Just one example is Tucuman province, where there were 11 detention centres.

Under military rule, the authorities denied operating any clandestine detention centres as well as any information relating to them.

The indiscriminate and massive nature of repression

Terror was widespread. It touched everybody – labour leaders, students, professionals, and political activists – sparing no one regardless of age or sex. Several of the thousands of missing people were pregnant women, young children and even newly born babies.

Relatives and neighbours who refused to help security forces were subject to the same danger. All who dissented were candidates to become missing people. People became regarded as guilty just by being detained. Judicial norms were inverted: everybody was guilty until the opposite could be proved. Many relatives of those sought by security forces were kidnapped and tortured for information, or to be used as hostages.

The complicity of the justice system

Writs of *habeas corpus* were useless. Courts rejected attempts to free the missing people, claiming that they had no information regarding the cases or that there were no legal grounds for action.

From 1976–1978, the mere act of presenting a writ of *habeas corpus* in favour of a missing person was an act of high risk for the petitioners, who in many cases also were abducted, disappearing without trace. Many others were detained or held under special powers of the National Executive Power (PEN). A total of 129 lawyers have been reported missing over the years.

The cover-up

The news media did not report what was occurring. In many cases there were express orders against doing so and in others journalists carried out auto-censorship, believing that they had to remain silent in order to survive or not endanger the lives of missing people. This idea was spread by government officials and by people linked to the government. Nevertheless, information regarding missing people spread in hushed conversations. There were signs, suggestive reports, telephone calls, etc, but there were never certainties about the fate of those who had been abducted.

The mandate of silence also affected relatives, friends and colleagues, who knew that any mention of the subject was implicitly or explicitly prohibited.

THE SYSTEMATIC USE OF TORTURE

Everybody who was detained knew that he or she would be tortured, and that is what happened. People were tortured either to extract information, which their jailers invariably sought to characterize as self-incriminating, or simply as punishment. There was no limit to how long one might be tortured. It could be longer or shorter, crueller or more gentle, but it was almost always unavoidable.

Most of the people who suffered systematic torture never resurfaced; they are still missing people. As a result, they have not been able to report the details of the physical and mental abuse they suffered. Their story, however, has been told by those who shared the horror of clandestine detention, who, for one reason or another, were freed, transferred to a public jail or managed to escape from detention.

The CIDH, in its report, gave the following description of torture in Argentina:

> The physical beatings and torture are believed to have been carried out mainly during the stage of questioning ... Many are the means by which illegal beatings were administered. The same is true in the cases of mental, psychological and moral torture. These are believed to have been carried out in special places of

detention where the people were taken for questioning. These places are known as 'chupaderos' (a place into which one is sucked), or also, in some cases, have been the nation's legal detention centres.

Among the modalities analyzed and chosen by the Commission from the abundant testimony that it has received, are the following:

a) Brutal beatings of the detainees which in many cases have caused broken bones and left people at least partially disabled; which, in pregnant women, have caused abortion and which in some other cases have helped death. These kinds of beatings have been inflicted with different kinds of weapons. People have been punched or kicked or struck with different instruments, either metallic, rubber, wooden or of other characteristics. There are reports referring to cases in which the victim's urinary bladder has burst, in which the sternum or ribs have been crushed and in which the victim suffered serious internal injuries.

b) For trivial reasons, the missing people suffered confinement in punishment cells for many weeks. They were left in conditions of desperate isolation and were subjected to baths of cold water.

c) The detained people often had their hands tied with chains, attached to the headboards of beds, or to the seats of airplanes or vehicles in which they were transported from one place to another. In these conditions, they were the victims of beatings and other abuse.

d) Simulated executions, using firearms, or in some cases the execution of detainees in the presence of other prisoners, including relatives, as has happened in places including but not limited to Cordoba, Salta, and in the Pavilion of Death in La Plata.

e) A form of simulated drowning called the 'Submarine', in which the victim's head – covered with a hood – was repeatedly ducked under water, causing asphyxia with the aim of forcing the person to talk.

f) The use of the electric prod, which was widespread. The victims were frequently tied to the metallic parts of a bed in order that they might receive high voltage shocks to areas including the head, the temples, the mouth, the hands, the legs, the breasts and the genital organs. In order to improve the electrical shocks, the victims were often soaked with water. According to reports, in some cases in which the electric prod was used a doctor was present to control the situation due to the 'shocks' that occur during the torture session.

g) The use of cigarettes to burn the victims. The cigarettes were applied to different parts of the body, frequently leaving areas of ulcerous sores.

h) The insertion of razor blades or other sharp instruments under the finger or toe nails.

i) The threat of rape of both men and women. Rape.

j) Surrounding prisoners with ferocious dogs, which were trained to threaten but stop short of attacking the prisoners.

k) Forcing the detainees to wear a hood for several weeks. They were also beaten while lying down with their feet and hands tied.

l) The hanging of the detainees, handcuffed or fastened to metal or wooden bars that hung from the ceiling, in such a fashion as to leave their feet just inches above the ground, which was covered with broken glass. There also were cases in which the victims were hung by their hands or by their feet, fracturing their hip bones or other parts of the body.

m) Forcing detainees to remain standing for long periods of time.

n) Administering drugs or injections to prisoners as a result of prolonged torture in which they passed out.

o) The detailed search of prisoners, abusing all parts of the body with the resulting humiliation.

p) The use of the so-called cube, consisting of a prolonged submersion of the detainee's feet in cold and then in hot water.

THE AIMS OF TORTURE

The above described conditions, which were common during military rule, made it difficult for the victims of abuse to receive immediate medical and psychological attention. That only became possible long after the abuse occurred.

Physical injuries were cared for with a great deal of negligence by personnel of the repressive forces. In other cases the assistance was given by the cell mates, always in very precarious conditions.

Many people developed psychological conditions following torture. They did not receive any type of medical attention or merely received sedatives from prison service doctors. Reports were received regarding the cases of various political prisoners who, having been tortured, committed suicide in jail without receiving any kind of medical attention.

Our experience is based on:

1 direct contact with victims of military repression, both during
   the years of the dictatorship and during the period of constitutional rule that followed,
2 an investigation carried out in 1983 by anonymous interviews
   of people who had been tortured, and
3 the treatment of people who had been tortured.

The aim of torture is to do away with the resistance of the subject.
The beatings and the abuse inflicted by sophisticated instruments both
aim at causing increasing levels of pain and testing the victim's limits
of resistance. All forms of psychological torture have a similar goal, i.e.
breaking the resistance of the victim. The torturer does this to obtain
information, to transform the victim into an informant and, in the most
extreme instance, to force the victim to abandon his/her stance as an
activist or a political dissident. The death of a prisoner during torture is
generally accidental. It is usually not one of the goals of torture.

Most of the information provided by survivors of torture suggests
that there is a clear difference between the torturers and those who
were in charge of killing the victims. This explains the presence of
doctors in the torture sessions. The doctor's function is to keep the
victim of torture alive as long as that person might be of some use and
until the torturer manages to break the victim's resistance.

The reports almost always describe another division of labour
among the torturers: those who inflict physical pain ('the bad ones')
and those who persuade and menace ('the good ones'). Both forms of
torture are aspects of the same system and have a common objective:
to break down the prisoner.

DISAPPEARANCE AND PSYCHOLOGICAL TORTURE

The torture that takes place during forced disappearance has certain
characteristics. Apart from the physical pain involved, it is a situation
of extreme uncertainty about the future which may bring total disappearance from the world, in life and in death. The outcome may
therefore be more than just a death caused by an 'excess of torture'.

Survivors of torture have told us that their captors said 'We can do
anything we want with you – Nobody knows you are here'. The
captors often even denied their prisoners the fantasy of escape by
death by saying 'We are not going to let you die – We are like God, we
control your life and death'.

Considering the fact that being in touch with and recognized by
other people is extremely important for one's mental health, isolating
the victim from the symbolic world constitutes a form of psychological

torture. This is highlighted by the experience of a survivor who was kidnapped and taken to an unknown place. After three days of physical torture with an electric prod, he was left on a patio, seated, handcuffed, blindfolded, and unable to talk. He had no idea what was going to happen to him but had a strong feeling that he was going to be killed. Under these circumstances he suffered an anxiety attack with feelings of depersonalization – something he had not experienced when he was being tortured the previous days. The anxiety attack lasted until he was recognized by other detainees who called him by his name; this produced an immediate relief.

Other aspects of psychological torture during forced disappearance include threats of torture and death to the victim and to his/her family, the torture of family members in the presence of the victim (typically occurring at the time of the kidnapping and in the home of the victim), repeated sham executions, and verbal insults and assaults on the individual's personality.

Although torture is a form of political repression that cannot be formulated only in psychological terminology, it nevertheless involves certain psychological processes which will be described below. In our clinical experience, each person is affected by and responds to torture in a unique fashion. This response is determined by the individual's personal history and the situation he/she is going through. Phrases like 'one responds with what one has' and 'one discovers one's true self' suggest that the individual discovers during torture previously unknown aspects of his/her character and, once this occurs, he/she is never the same as before. We will examine three aspects of torture: its effect on the individual's identity, self-esteem and the relationship between the body and pain.

Effects on the individual's identity

In addition to extracting information from the victim, torture targets the individual's identity which may be broadly defined as a complex of representations of self and value systems that produces the feeling of oneness and allows one to maintain internal coherence in time. Physical and psychological aggression during torture aims to generate a situation whereby the victims 'feel at the mercy' of others and experience depersonalization, fear of annihilation, and the destruction of their body image.

The torturers have a special interest in having the victim 'see' the physical consequences of torture, not only on one's body, but also on loved ones and others, in order to generate feelings of desperation and vicarious suffering. The victims are thus often told 'That's how you are going to end up' or 'That's what you look like'. In interviews, survivors often give accounts of having felt deeply concerned about their physical state (often described as 'a sack of potatoes') or that of others following torture.

Some of the procedures that are used from the moment of detention of kidnapping are similar to those employed in asylums for the mentally ill. These include removal of all personal items and clothes which are replaced by flimsy uniforms, banning of all visits from outside resulting in isolation from the family or other loved ones, denying the victims any information concerning the reasons for, and the duration of, detention, calling them by numbers rather than by their names, and keeping them in suspense about the possible outcome of the situation.

Feelings of depersonalization are further aggravated by sensory deprivation and immobilization of the body. Hands are often tied, eyes covered, and talking and moving prohibited. The sanitary and nutritional conditions during detention are subhuman. The victims are often deprived of any contact with the outside world and left without any idea where they are, although sometimes this may be figured out. They know that nobody outside knows where they are and they feel extremely uncertain about their future. Feelings of isolation are reinforced by comments such as 'nobody knows you are here. You have disappeared. You don't exist. You are not with the living and you are not with the dead'.

The prisoners who were held in official institutions were frequently transferred from one place to another, being blindfolded and beaten *en route*. The possibility of 'disappearing' or of being tortured outside the jail or in a torture chamber was always present.

Certain behaviours during detention, such as giving too much importance to a relatively trivial aspect of the experience, can be seen as an attempt to preserve one's identity. For example, a kidnapped woman, on being informed that she would be freed, insisted on having her identity documents and purse returned. Another woman, on being released, demanded a telephone token to make a phone call to her family who lived very near where she was held.

Effect on self-esteem

Self-esteem is a fundamental aspect of an individual's identity. It can be broadly defined as one's inner sense of value or self-worth. From a psychoanalytical perspective it is the relationship between the self and the self ideal which is shaped by certain values that the individual hopes to live up to.

Torture often poses a conflict between one's self-image and the behaviour that is deemed necessary for survival. The behavioural responses to torture are often diverse, being determined by individual personality characteristics and group processes. Torture is an experience that mobilizes all personality resources and the coping capabilities of the individual. Those people who have refused to respond to demands for information by the torturers have managed to maintain their self-esteem. They have also been better able to resume social and political connections without having to isolate themselves or to change their group of friends, colleagues or comrades. Refusing to comply with the torturers' demands may even reinforce the survivor's self-esteem since such behaviour is often consonant with his/her self-ideal.

In some cases the self-ideal does not have a direct relationship with certain moral values. Consequently, self-esteem is not directly affected by the behaviour displayed under torture. Sometimes a person could feel that s/he has not lived up to his/her own expectations, despite not having talked under torture ('I was a little lamb' 'I shouldn't have accepted the cookie'). Others, despite having revealed information, may have preserved their self-esteem by stressing certain aspects of their coping behaviour such as not having cried in front of the torturers.

In those people whose self-esteem is affected, there may be narcissistic collapses, with diverse clinical manifestations. These include mainly depression, loss of self-confidence, anxiety and even suicide attempts. In certain cases, as part of a process of adaptation, the self-ideal may be re-defined and goals set for oneself altered. One of the procedures frequently used by the torturers is to induce in the prisoner an intense sense of loss of values and self-denigration. For example, the most traumatic experience for a young woman who was detained and tortured in a variety of ways was being accused of being a lesbian by her guards after she refused to sign a statement renouncing her political ideology. These feelings induced by the torturers may later be reinforced by the survivor's reference group who may suspect him/her of having betrayed them.

The body and pain

The experience of torture puts one in contact with the body ravaged to its limits and subjected to intense humiliation. According to Anzieu (1987), an intense and lasting pain threatens the integrity of the psychic structure or leaves the psychic apparatus disorganised and affects the capacity to want and to think. Pain is not shared. Each person is alone in its experience. It engulfs everything and one no longer exists as one's self. What exists is pain. These experiences of pain are difficult, and sometimes impossible, to describe or to comprehend.

Other psychological effects

Although the psychological impact of torture on the individual is determined by his/her personality and personal history, in most cases the survivor undergoes irrevocable change. Torture often unleashes a traumatic neurosis with symptoms of recurrent dreams of the traumatic event, anxiety, fear, crying, panic and feelings of helplessness. The traumatic experiences may be relived when the survivor hears loud noises such as sirens, horns or shouting, etc. One woman said that she got extremely upset every time she heard footsteps near her apartment, thinking they were coming to get her. Another survivor told of how a chance encounter in public with a torturer produced paralysing anxiety. Some symptoms relate directly to the type of torture experienced and do not need a stimulus to be activated. Example include sexual dysfunctions following rape, such as frigidity and amenorrhea in women or impotence or lack of sexual drive in men. Some survivors may experience paranoid symptoms, having difficulty in distinguishing between real situations of danger and an internal feeling of persecution.

Psychological defences

Among the psychological mechanisms deployed in response to torture are intellectual understanding and the mind–body dissociation.

Intellectual understanding

An intellectual understanding of what is happening acts as a defence in its broadest sense – a defence that protects the self. But it should not be confused with a defence mechanism. 'The intellectual defence, by way of understanding, is the most effective assurance that one is not totally defenceless, and that one could even protect one's personality when faced with an extreme threat' (Bettelheim, 1973). This defence puts into play various forms of self-assertion, such as that of synthesis, of anticipation, of discrimination, all liked to the universe of symbols.

Intellectual understanding includes the plane of the ideological position and of the related general values. It substantially improves one's chances of resisting the demands of torturers. As noted by one survivor of torture, 'The problem is whether you believe in your own explanation or that which they give you.' Furthermore, intellectual understanding helps one to tolerate long periods of detention.

Linked with the defensive attitude is the recognition of one's role in the situation of torture. This recognition involves an understanding that the act of torture is a product of a social situation and that the roles of torturer and victim are determined by one's place in the social system and, in the case of the torturer, not by individual traits of sadism. Examples of such thinking are 'One is free to choose', 'My being tortured did not have anything specific to do with me', and 'The torturer does not use this method for any reason you might believe but because he happens to be there, in that place, in that situation.'

The dissociation between mind and body

One of the defence mechanisms used in the service of self-preservation during torture is the dissociation between the mind and the body: 'I knew that they were destroying my body but they did not get me.' Sometimes the survivors speak in an impersonal fashion when they are referring to their body: 'They were destroying my body, but my mind kept working and even though they did not know it, I was thinking. I was intent on keeping quiet ... no matter what they did.'

THE PSYCHOLOGICAL EFFECTS OF SOCIOPOLITICAL FACTORS FOLLOWING THE TRAUMA

The effects of the torture perpetrated by the dictatorship have only been evaluated over a short and medium term; the long-term effects still remain to be seen. Some of the after-effects are directly related to the impact of the trauma while others can be determined by the social circumstances in which the trauma took place.

After the constitutional government took power, people demanded and hoped for justice. Calls were made for the punishment of those responsible for kidnapping, torturing and killing people during the years of dictatorship, and for the fate of the missing people to be determined. But after seven years of constitutional government, no answer has been given regarding what happened to the 30 000 missing people. Apart from a handful of military officers who headed the armed forces during the military dictatorship and were tried and found guilty of having committed 'excesses', those responsible for the genocide are still at liberty.

The approval of laws bringing to an end the prosecution of members of the military for crimes committed during military rule (known as 'The Punto Final') as well as the law of 'due obedience' (exemption of lower ranking members of the armed forces from prosecution on grounds that they were just following orders), provided a legal situation of virtual immunity from prosecution. Those crimes already proved in court were prescribed. Those members of the armed forces who had tortured, kidnapped and assassinated people were let off the hook as they were considered to have been following orders. Finally, pardons granted by the present constitutional government further reduced the number of those punished, even though found guilty of committing crimes against humanity.

Thus the social context was marked by the fact that those people who had carried out the military repression were at large in society. There were widespread reports about the barbaric acts that occurred under military rule but there was no intention of punishing those responsible for these crimes. This left the survivors fearful and inhibited in their thought and actions. They feel the freedom of the repressors is a real threat to all the people.

TREATMENT

Our experience with tortured people is consistent with that of other workers, whether dealing with Holocaust survivors or the victims of state terror in Southern Latin America. The majority of survivors, once freed, describe a variety of feelings in relation to the horror they have suffered. These include bashfulness, regret, rage, confusion, and hate. They cannot, however, communicate their experience; they keep quiet. The most common reasons for seeking help are problems with interpersonal relationships, symptoms arising from the traumatic experience, and depression.

Treatment of torture survivors require an effective therapeutic alliance between the survivor and the therapist. A prerequisite for therapeutic alliance is the survivor's confidence in the therapist. The survivors need to know that they can share with the therapist opinions and value judgments concerning their traumatic experience. They also need to know that the person with whom they share their most intimate secrets is aware of the social and political dimensions of the trauma they suffered. Everything they say in the session must be guided by their free will and not by the impositions or demands of 'treatment'. The therapy setting must be protective and respectful.

The fact that the perpetrators of torture and other repressive acts have not been penalized generates a climate of distrust among the survivors which in turn undermines the development of therapeutic alliance with care providers. Consequently, the survivors often tend to seek help from institutions or therapists who are known for their stance against the abuse of human rights.

It should also be borne in mind that confidence in the therapist can impede progress in therapy to the extent that it is transformed into an unconscious pact of complicity which serves as a refuge for pathological defences. This issue needs attention and interpretation during treatment.

Two case vignettes may be useful in highlighting the importance of confidence in the therapist.

Case vignette I

A young human rights activist, who had been detained for several years and tortured, sought help with the Psychological Assistance Team of the Mothers of the Plaza de Mayo due to problems in his relationship with his partner. The team decided to send him to a hospital, deeming it appropriate for him to establish outside relationships given his tendency to act freely only in those groups with which he strongly identified himself. He embraced these groups as sources of protection but this made it difficult for him actively to adapt to reality.

On appearing at the hospital, he was seen by a doctor who took notes during the interview. He asked the doctor not to take notes. The doctor pointed out that taking notes on clinical history was a normal procedure at the hospital. The patient then returned to see the team of the Mothers of Plaza de Mayo and reported that, although he felt positively towards the doctor, he could not accept his words being taken down by the doctor because this made him feel intensely insecure and concerned about the future. These concerns were solidly founded since the patient had personal knowledge of raids on health centres and confiscation of medical records. Thus, although a potential for a therapeutic relationship between the survivor and the doctor existed, the prevailing atmosphere of mistrust caused by impunity granted to the perpetrators of torture in Argentina undermined the patient's confidence in health care institutions.

Case vignette II

A woman who had been raped during detention refused any psychological treatment despite the distressing psychological problems that followed the incident. Her husband had also been detained in the same establishment during the same period. After their release from prison, they were unable to share their traumatic experiences with each other in any meaningful way because of mutual accusations regarding who was to blame for their detention.

Even though she reported having normal sexual relations, she showed signs of panic at any suggestion of gynaecological examination. When asked about the reasons for her resistance to psychological treatment, she related an experience she had with a psychologist whom she saw shortly after being released. At the first interview the psychologist had suggested to her that her commitment to a political ideology could have reflected a suicidal tendency which might finally have led to her detention. This interpretation left her with an intense feeling of hostility to the therapist while also evoking feelings of guilt and responsibility for being detained. She realized that she needed a therapist who shared her views about the political repression in Argentina during the military dictatorship.

During the course of the treatment it became evident that the patient had a narcissistic problem in granting her partner a respected role in the family both as a husband and a father. She became the central point of reference in the family while placing him into the role of a child and encouraging the children to treat their father as an older brother. He nevertheless managed to establish an adequate relationship with his children.

When these events were interpreted to the patient, she rejected the interpretation and insisted that the therapist acknowledge her indispensable role as a human rights activist which she thought inevitably led her to assume an excessively dominant position in the family.

The therapeutic atmosphere and a trusting relationship facilitate the expression of the traumatic experiences. As we have noted in an earlier investigation (Kordon *et al.*, 1986) carried out under military rule, 'The majority of those people interviewed said that it was the first time they had talked about the subject. They said the experience of torture is so personal that they could not talk about it in their everyday life, especially when dealing with those people closest to them. In treating people who had been detained and tortured at the same time and in the same place, we discovered that they had not been able to talk among themselves about the experience' (patient described in Case vignette II).

We have formulated a hypothesis to explain the survivors' reluctance to talk about their traumatic experiences. This hypothesis is by no means complete and needs further investigation. Four possible mechanisms seem to deserve attention:

1 Intense and prolonged pain during torture induces a neuro-genic shock characterized by varying degrees of impairment in consciousness, ranging from mild clouding to stupor or a state of inertia, emptiness and total suspension of psychic activity. This affects memory retention during the trauma and sub-sequent recall of events. The resulting lacunal amnesia may last a long time and even forever.

2 The attack against the body affects the basic nucleus of the identity which is the corporal self. The person finds him/herself in an extreme state of defencelessness which is akin to primitive states of helplessness and forlornness. The ensuing narcissistic regression is so extreme that the events can no longer be described in psychological terms.

3 A 'schizophrenic', defensive dissociation occurs. Dissociation is a defence characteristic of the most primitive mental levels. It occurs in response to a fear of annihilation induced by torture. The body image is detached from and projected outside one's self, a phenomenon often described by the survivors as 'The body did not belong to me'. During this process, certain aspects of one's identity may be lost, leading to irrevocable changes in the personality of which the individual may not always be aware.

4 Feelings of shame, which make it difficult to relate the trau-matic experience, are associated with certain 'intimate' experi-ences during torture that are at variance with one's self-image or ego ideals prior to the trauma. The narcissistic disillusion-ment resulting from this conflict may not necessarily concern the survivor's fundamental behavioural responses to torture. It may also be related to apparently trivial details of the survivor's behaviour which may assume great importance when perceived as resisting or surrendering to the will of the torturer.

An important requirement for successful psychotherapy of torture survivors is due attention to the survivor's isolation from the outside world, at times for quite long periods, and its likely impact on the family. The space that had been occupied by the survivor in the family often becomes a nominal space and the family adapts itself to the absence of the survivor. The survivor's subsequent return to the family may disturb this adaptation and lead to serious interpersonal difficul-ties arising from a sense of exclusion on the part of the survivor, the perceived role of the family in actively bringing about this exclusion in its adaptation process, and feelings of resentment and guilt associated with this situation. It is therefore necessary to take the whole family unit into account in psychotherapy and even consider concurrent family therapy.

Another important issue in psychotherapy is an adequate understanding of the problems the survivor is likely to experience in his/her return to normal life in society. These problems do not only concern the social stigma attached to being arrested and detained but also the difficulties in adapting to conditions that have changed in the survivor's absence. The survivors also often have to face more concrete obstacles in their readaptation process such as getting a job. Such problems can be particularly serious in Third World countries such as Argentina. One also needs to bear in mind the ways in which a repressive state adversely affects the patient and his/her chances of successful re-integration into society.

An important problem that may arise during therapy is countertransference reactions between the patient and the therapist. Effective dealing with this problem requires regular team discussions about therapy process. The therapist's position regarding torture can be questioned during therapy. What may also come up is the therapist's own ideals and values and the patient's expectation that the therapist will act on them. Attention should be given to the different feelings (e.g. disillusionment, rejection, etc) the therapist might have regarding the conduct of the patient which may not coincide with his/her own values.

Physiotherapy may sometimes be of great help. It not only helps heal the physical sequelae of torture but also complements psychotherapy. Physiotherapy and the associated sense of protection, care and pleasure help restore the body image and bodily functions that may have been distorted or damaged during torture by the primitive process of mind-body dissociation discussed earlier. The physiotherapist may speed up recovery by setting examples of a healthy relationship with one's body and its functions.

CONCLUDING REMARKS

In concluding the chapter we would like to stress certain points we consider important in working with survivors of torture. Although many tortured individuals have symptoms similar to those described in the post-traumatic stress syndrome, we nevertheless refrain from defining a specific post-torture syndrome for several reasons. First, torture is a repressive act of a political and not of a psychological nature. Any nosologic categorization that would place the problem in the domain of psychiatry and reduce it to merely psychopathology cannot be acceptable. Secondly, psychiatric labelling is stigmatizing and any process of stigmatization in survivors seeking help should be avoided. Finally, in our experience with survivors of torture, we have not observed a complex symptom constellation that is unique and always present. Each person reacts to the trauma of torture in a unique way in accordance with his/her personality characteristics and personal history, the particular circumstances of torture, and the extent to which the social environment affords opportunities for recovery. It is important therefore that the therapy focuses on the subjective meaning of the trauma and of its short- and long-term effects.

REFERENCES

Anzieu, D. (1987). *El Yo Piel.* Editorial Biblioteca Nueva. Madrid.

Bettleheim, B. (1973). *El corazon bien informado.* Fondo de Cultura Economica. Mejico.

Comision InterAmericana de Derechos Humanos (1980). Report on the Human Rights situation in Argentina.

Kordon, D., Edelman, L., Lagos, D., Nicoletti, E., Bozzola, R., Siaky, D., L'Hoste, M. & Kersner, D. (1986). *Efectos Psicologicos de la Repression Politica.* Editorial Sudamericana Planeta, Buenos Aires.

20
TORTURE AND THE HELPING
PROFESSIONS IN SOUTH AFRICA
Terence Dowdall

Abuse and torture at the hands of the state became increasingly commonplace in South Africa in the decades following the 1950s. As human-rights activist David Webster wrote, a short while before his assassination:

> During this period South Africa earned its place in the rogues' gallery of repression. While regimes in countries like Argentina and Chile went in for spectacular abuses of human rights, they lacked the stamina and steady concentration of South Africa's security police. Webster, 1987

This chapter outlines the context in which repression and torture arose, and the kinds of abuses that have been seen. It also looks at the challenges which civil rights abuses – and in particular, torture – have posed for medicine and social services in this country, and how the professions have coped with these challenges.

THE DEVELOPMENT AND OPERATION OF THE APARTHEID SYSTEM

Torture is an instrument of power. It cannot be usefully understood separately from the historical, political and economic context of power relations in any country. To make sense of why and how torture became established in South Africa in the latter part of this century we need to consider briefly the history of power relations between black and white people in this country, and the implications of the ruthless social engineering experiment known as apartheid. These implications have been discussed elsewhere in detail (e.g. Wilson & Ramphele, 1987; De Beer, 1984; Steere, 1984; Seedat, 1984) and will be summarized briefly here.

Apartheid is in a sense the crystallization of the colonialism of previous centuries in South Africa. Originally inhabited sparsely by the KhoiKhoi, the country was settled from the north by Bantu-speaking peoples since around the first millennium, and from the south by Holland and Britain from the mid-seventeenth century. Wars of subjugation were waged against the black peoples of South Africa until the end of the nineteenth century, after which coercive economic measures were used to bring blacks to work as cheap labour in agriculture, mining and developing industries. In 1910, when the four colonies of South Africa were united in the Union of South Africa, racial segregation and discrimination were among the foundation stones of the Union. Opposed to this dispensation was the African National Congress, formed in 1923 from a group which arose shortly after Union to press black rights.

The South African political system has always practised discrimination in a free-wheeling way, but when the Afrikaner Nationalist Party came to power in 1948, this became institutionalized policy, prosecuted with ruthless attention to detail. In January 1963, Premier H. F. Verwoerd, the major architect of the policy, said in the House of Assembly:

> Reduced to its simplest form the problem is nothing else than this: we want to keep South Africa white. Keeping it white can only mean one thing, namely white domination. Not leadership, not guidance, but control, supremacy.

This policy was articulated under the name of apartheid, and was concerned with the entrenchment of white – particularly Afrikaner – power and economic advancement, and the removal of blacks from any position in which they might compete. To this end, a 'tribal homelands' policy was pursued, in which some three-and-a-half million blacks were forcibly uprooted and relocated to barren, overcrowded 'homelands' with minimal industrial infrastructure. Those blacks living in 'white' South Africa were increasingly hedged in by intrusive and demoralizing legislation which governed every aspect of their lives. It is not possible to convey the crushing burden of this legislation here; but some well-documented aspects of the structural violence of apartheid include:

1 Hunger, malnutrition and the disease of poverty, which cause stunting in about one-third of black children and result in an infant mortality rate some 15 times higher than in white children.
2 Calculated inferior education designed to condition black people to acceptance of roles of servitude. It is characterized by overcrowded, poorly equipped classrooms staffed by

underqualified and commonly authoritarian teachers. It was resentment and rejection of this 'gutter education' that precipitated the Soweto revolt of 1976. Inferior education plays an important role in sustaining the economic disadvantage which apartheid builds in for blacks.

3 The Group Areas Act forces black families who are legally permitted to reside outside the 'homelands' to live in cramped, depressing townships, usually far from the workplace. On township peripheries, huge numbers of people live in shacks built of whatever materials can be found. Townships and shanty towns are dangerous, violent and crime-ridden. Alcoholism and family violence are common. The quality of family life is severely eroded. The position for squatters is worse, in that their shacks may be bulldozed at any time. For those confined to the homelands, the lack of jobs forces them to become migrant workers, often in the mines. This means that they are away from their families (who are not allowed to accompany them) for up to a year at a time.

4 One of the most damaging aspects of apartheid is that it erodes not only family life but the self-concepts and self-confidence of great numbers of black people. Writing in the early 1970s, Steve Biko vividly depicts the way in which the ideology of racial superiority may come to be accepted by those classified as culturally and psychologically inferior.

But the type of black man we have today has lost his manhood. Reduced to an obliging shell he looks with awe at the white power structure and accepts what he regards as the 'inevitable position'. Deep inside his anger mounts at the accumulating insult, but he vents it in the wrong direction – on his fellow man in the township.... In the privacy of the toilet his face twists in silent condemnation of white society, but brightens up in sheepish obedience as he comes out hurrying to his master's impatient call.... His heart yearns for the comfort of white society and makes him blame himself for not having been 'educated' enough to warrant such luxury.... All in all the black man has become a shell, a shadow of a man, completely defeated, drowning in his own misery, a slave, an ox bearing the yoke of oppression with sheepish timidity. Biko, 1978, pp. 28–29

Apartheid ideology and its constructs seep into the self-concepts of blacks, and this is one of its most pernicious aspects. But, rejection of this intolerable vision of their parents and of their own prospective situation was also one of the driving forces of the Soweto revolt of 1976 and the civil conflict of the 1980s, which precipitated the present dismantling of apartheid.

RESISTANCE AND REPRESSION

As the Nationalist government began to enforce its apartheid policies in the 1950s, the African National Congress reorganized and rallied public protest. This evoked only police retaliation and, after a long period of debate, the ANC decided to resort to armed resistance. Major state repression followed and black leaders were imprisoned or fled into exile. In the years that followed, an increasingly powerful security police apparatus was built up and, simultaneously, legislation was passed and repeatedly refined which closed down all normal channels of protest, and provided the umbrella of unaccountability under which torture could flourish.

Formal repression has taken many shapes in South Africa (e.g. Human Rights Commission, 1989). It has been enabled by legislation which allows people to be detained without trial, banned or 'restricted' (which effectively removes people from political life under very onerous conditions). Criminalization of political activity permits the state to remove opponents from public life through political trials which may drag on for years. People may be 'listed' (banned from being quoted), their passports withdrawn, or they may be banished to a remote area. In addition, organizations may be banned or restricted or have foreign funding stopped; gatherings, meetings, demonstrations or even public funerals may be banned; publications are censored in large numbers, newspapers may be closed down or suspended, and, under the State of Emergency regulations, actions of the security forces or the treatment of detainees may not be reported on. Political actions such as boycotts or work stayaways are also forbidden under these regulations.

Outside of legislated provisions for repression is a shadowy and vicious set of 'informal' repressive forces, including police-based 'hit squads' which have, according to evidence, carried out assassinations and harassment of political figures; and vigilantes – apartheid-linked black groups which have acted with extreme violence and brutality. The central point to be made here is that, within the South African situation, detention and torture is only one of the elements – albeit a particularly visible element – in a wide spectrum of repression and oppression.

We are, however, concerned here particularly with legislation which has fostered the conditions in which torture can flourish. These are the provisions which allow political opponents of the state to be detained in conditions of secrecy, without recourse to the law or contact with the outside world; and legislation which indemnifies members of the security forces for abuses committed 'in good faith'. In South Africa this legislation falls under two broad headings: State of Emergency legislation (under the Public Safety Act of 1953); and the various provisions of the Internal Security Act of 1982. The latter Act represents the streamlining of a series of legislative steps, going back to the 90-day detention provisions of the General Laws Amendment Act of 1963, where, for the first time, provisions which had operated only under the extreme circumstances of a State of Emergency became part of the permanent law and everyday life of the country. Opening a legal conference in South Africa in 1982, Chaskalson summed up the position when he said

> The legislature has ... over the past thirty years made clear through its legislature and its actions that it is determined to suppress certain political and social views in conflict with its own, and that in the process of doing so it is willing to abrogate freedom and to rule by force. By curtailing the powers of the Courts it has made sure that its design is not frustrated by the antiquated principles of freedom and justice which sometimes find favour with judges. Chaskalson, 1985, p. 2

The different sections of the Internal Security Act provide for witness detention, preventive detention (where the Minister believes that person is likely to commit a security offence) and, under the notorious Section 29, detention for interrogation. Under Section 29 the detainee can be held indefinitely – until the police are satisfied that 'all questions are satisfactorily answered', or 'no useful purpose will be served by further detention'. The detainee has no access to anyone other than police, magistrate or district surgeon, and the courts have no jurisdiction over such detention.

In the early days of the 1950s and 1960s, whilst some individuals from the English language universities pointed out the need for the legal profession to oppose repressive apartheid legislation, the profession was, by and large, unresponsive. Scrutiny of South Africa's law journals during this period shows, with few notable exceptions, concern with expositions of rules and laws, rather than criticism or a moral stand. Court rulings have tended to ignore evidence of torture, (e.g. Tucker, 1985) or to exonerate police charged with abuses (e.g.

Foster & Luyt, 1986). In the circumstances, given a blank cheque, it was unlikely that the security police would show restraint in their treatment of detainees.

Under the various legal provisions, some 75,000 people have been detained without trial – the vast majority under State of Emergency regulations (Human Rights Commission, 1989b). From 1985 to 1989, some 24 000 children were detained amongst these – some as young as 12 – often in appalling conditions (Human Rights Commission, 1990a). Only 25% of people detained were charged, and only 3% actually convicted, giving credence to the claims that detention and abuse was primarily aimed at intimidation of activists, organisations and indeed the population at large.

THE EMERGENCE OF TORTURE AND ABUSE

Early criticism from legal and psychological quarters of Section 29 detentions (e.g. Mathews & Albino, 1966) referred to sensory deprivation studies and pointed out that prolonged detention in solitary confinement was likely to be harmful, and that evidence so obtained was questionable. But accumulating allegations from ex-detainees painted a grimmer picture of widespread physical and mental abuses inflicted upon people in detention by the security police. The courts tended to be sceptical of detainee allegations of torture made in their trials, were reluctant to reject confessions obtained in the circumstances of Section 29 detention (e.g. Dugard, 1985), and even where it seemed incontrovertible that witnesses had been assaulted, frequently failed to condemn or even rebuke these abuses (Tucker, 1985; Mathews, 1990). Dugard (1985) also pointed out that a restricted range of by and large conservative judges tended to be allocated to security trials, and suggested that their 'judicial discretion' was more likely to be exercised in favour of the state – as was the discretion of magistrates. Mathews (1990) excoriates these officials for contributing towards a climate in which abuses could flourish:

> Is it not both shameful and incredible that the judges, on proper occasions, have not denounced this practice in moral tones that reverberate right into the offices of the highest functionaries of government? Take the case of Mogale in which the Appellate Division, whilst recording evidence of a torture session in which the police broke the victim's teeth whilst attempting to extract them with a pair of pliers, uttered no words of condemnation or even disapproval (p. 1) Judges have not hesitated to condemn

other forms of uncivilised violence. Torture, like these other
forms of violence, is unlawful, and even the security forces
renounce it, nominally, at least. . . . Its moral repugnance is due in
large measure to the absolute vulnerability of the persons on
whom it is practiced and to the fact that it is a gruesome violation
of the law by the very persons whose duty it is to uphold
it. Mathews, 1990, p. 2

It is difficult to differ from Tucker when he concludes that

there is very little in the system which provides any degree of
protection for the detainee. Tucker, 1985, p. 41

This conclusion was steadily borne out during the late sixties into
the mid–1970s, as allegations of torture accumulated. By 1990, 73
political prisoners had died in detention (Human Rights Commisson,
1990b). The South African government has repeatedly denied allegations of abuse and torture of political prisoners, arguing that these are
merely propaganda intended to discredit the police and the state.
Like many authoritarian governments, they are also manifestly sensitive to being unmasked. For these reasons the five investigations into
torture in this country which will be cited, were important. Together
with the legal exposure of the Biko case and the Orr injunction, they
constituted a weight of evidence that could not be brushed aside, and
exposed the State to the full censure of the international community.
    An investigation by Amnesty International led them to report in
1978 that 'All the evidence indicates that torture is extensively inflicted
on political detainees, and that the government sanctions its use'
(Amnesty International, 1978 p. 56). Tortures identified as common by
the Amnesty report included beating and physical assault, electrical
shock applied to different parts of the body, prolonged standing or
forced exercise; and psychological abuse, including death threats,
threats to the safety of one's family and extended sleep deprivation.
    In 1982, The Detainees' Parents Support Committee brought out a
report based on interviews with over 70 ex-detainees. Torturers listed
included physical assaults – often extremely brutal – as the most
frequent (over 70%). These included punching, slapping, kicking,
assault with objects, crushing toes with chairs or bricks, heads banged
against walls or tables, etc. The next most common torture was
enforced standing or exhausting physical exercises (about 50%). Sleep
deprivation and prolonged interrogation was experienced by about
30% of this group, as was being kept naked for long periods, and
exposed to cold. About 35% of the people interviewed had suffered

'hooding' where a plastic or canvas bag is placed over the head and the detainee is partially suffocated or strangled. Electric shock torture to various parts of the body, including the genitals, was also common. This report also made mention of the 'helicopter' – a suspension technique where the victim is handcuffed at wrists and ankles and suspended on a pole, causing severe pain. Frequent psychological tortures included death threats, threats to loved ones and humiliation of various kinds.

The need was felt, however, by DPSC for a more scientifically devised assessment of torture in South Africa, and this was set in motion via the Institute of Criminology at the University of Cape Town (Foster & Sandler, 1985). This retrospective study assessed 176 cases of detention via a partially structured, partially open-ended interview schedule. As far as possible, the ratios (male/female, black/white, etc) matched current detention ratios. Some 83% of ex-detainees reported some form of physical torture whilst detained under Section 29. Of detainees, 75% reported beatings and assaults, with the next most frequent types of torture including forced standing and various other forms of exhausting physical exercise. Hooding was described by 25%, with a similar figure for electric shocks. Strangulation occurred in 18% of allegations with some form of suspension torture occurring in some 14% of reports. Major psychological tortures included false accusations (83%), solitary confinement (79%), verbal abuse (64%), alternating good/bad interrogators (57%), witnessing or knowing of the torture of others (45%), execution threats levelled against self or family members (41%), being forced to undress (27%), and prolonged interrogation (23%). The differences between black and white prisoners' experiences were not unexpected in the South African context: generally, the younger and the blacker the detainee, the greater the physical and verbal abuse.

The results of this study do not depart in any radical way from the less formal picture gained in early data collection. Officials of the SA Government were, expectedly, incensed and embarrassed, and berated the study as biased and unscientific, though the criticisms themselves were characterized as emotional and inept (Foster, Davis & Sandler, 1987). The study is, of course, open to the charge that ex-detainees are likely to have an axe to grind, and there seemed to be no way of telling whether, either consciously or unconsciously, they may have been exaggerating or fabricating in a retrospective interview. This is why two studies that followed were important in lending validation to Foster and Sandler's findings.

Wendy Orr was a courageous young district surgeon whose duties included working with State of Emergency detainees at St Alban's Prison in Port Elizabeth, subsequent to sessions they had spent with the security police. Appalled at the 'unrestrained abuses' which she saw being inflicted daily, and fobbed off when she complained to her superiors, she systematically collected data on her medical examinations and made an appeal to the Supreme Court to prevent the police from further assaulting the detainees at the prison.

Figures from Orr's first affidavit, which dealt only with physical injuries, showed that 153 detainees sustained injuries unlikely to have been caused by resisting arrest or during the dispersal of a riotous assembly. They included 50 cases of facial injuries, 8 perforated eardrums, 26 cases of injuries on unusual parts of the body, such as palms of hands, 7 cases of injuries of an unusual nature, consistent with assault on a restricted victim, and 48 cases of such a multiplicity of injuries that they could not have been sustained in the manner described by the police.

A second set of figures (Orr, 1990) concerned the approximately 1500 State of Emergency detainees held in St Alban's prison between 20 July and 24th September 1985:

- 706 men complained of assault or had injuries consistent with assault, or both (46%).
- 434 detainees were recorded as having lodged complaints, with 406 of these identifying the police as perpetrators of the assault.
- 296 of the detainees who alleged assault by the SAP had injuries recorded that were consistent with their allegations.
- 4 allegations of assault were investigated by the SA police.

None of these cases ever came to court.

These figures, together with Dr Orr's daily first-hand experience in contact with detainees, constitute a compelling naturalistic study with substantial medical validation of allegations. A second more formal study was carried out by Browde (1988), who analysed the data obtained by a group of National Medical and Dental Association (NAMDA) doctors in medical and psychological examination of all 131 detainees referred to the Detainee Clinic in Johannesburg from December 1985 to June 1986. The majority were examined within 19 days of their release.

In this sample, 92 (72%) claimed to have been physically assaulted, with 89% of this group reporting physical beating with fists, hands, kicking, beating with sjambok or baton, or hit against other objects. 25% alleged suffocation; 15% reported being forced into postures or physical exercises; 14% reported being given electrical shock. Of the 92 who alleged assault, 23 did not show physical evidence of assault. Of individuals 69 who alleged physical assault and on whom evidence of assault was found were evaluated for signs of physical injury consistent with the alleged assault. In 97% of cases, the examining doctor reported findings on physical examination that were consistent with the alleged assault.

This latter observation, together with Orr's data, lends weight to the likelihood that when ex-detainees describe assaults and abuses, they are accurately relating what really happened. This is, of course, a matter of common cause amongst all who have had any contact with the detention system; but detention and torture are political issues extending far beyond individuals involved; and international conviction was crucial to increase pressures on the South African regime.

PSYCHOLOGICAL SEQUELAE OF TORTURE

Ex-detainees in the Institute for Criminology study reported sleeping problems (60%), headaches (53%), excessive recourse to fantasy (45%), appetite loss (44%), concentration difficulties (44%) and nightmares (41%) as common psychological reactions during detention. A variety of other anxiety- and depression-related symptoms were also reported. Subsequent to release the most common reported sequelae included tiredness (42%), problems relating to friends (39%) and family (35%), sleep difficulties and nightmares (around 34%), and a wide range of psychosomatic problems, and anxiety- and depression-linked symptoms. On average, ex-detainees experienced around four problem areas on release. Further analysis suggested, as could be expected, that longer periods of detention and solitary confinement were associated with increased numbers of problems (Foster *et al.*, 1987).

Browde's (1987) report noted that in a group of 83 ex-detainees showing psychological symptoms, 33% were diagnosed as suffering from post-traumatic stress disorder, 19% from depression and 11% from anxiety reactions. At the stage at which they visited the Detainee Clinic the most common symptoms were sleep disturbances (68%), impaired memory and concentration (65%), recurrent and intrusive recollections (43%), recurrent nightmares (30%, and symptoms of anxiety or depression (18%).

Friedlander (1986) examined 28 ex-detainees – mostly State of Emergency detainees, the majority of whom were seen within a month of release. The most common symptoms reported were concentration problems (96%), disturbed sleep (88%), intrusive, fearful thoughts about the future (73%), depression (69%), irritability (65%) and tension headaches (62%). Friedlander diagnosed over half of his sample as having a major depressive disorder or post-traumatic stress disorder, and noted that stress does not end with release, given the stressful and dangerous environment into which the detainees were released.

By and large, the results of these three studies show a similar picture, although the first study relies on self-report inventories and essentially lay interview, whilst the second two lean towards formal psychiatric diagnosis.

Aside from these more statistical studies, clinical studies have presented aspects of this work in more depth. Solomons (1989) has explicated, from a psychodynamic point of view, the dynamics of post-traumatic stress disorder with ex-detainees. The concept of PTSD has received some critical attention in the South African context, notably by Straker (1987), and has been further discussed in clinical context (e.g. Friedman, 1987; Dowdall, 1990*a*). The circumstances prevailing within a country where repression and civil conflict is endemic do not fit the picture of a discrete traumatic event, followed by a 'post-trauma' disorder. Detainees in South Africa are likely to have lived in stressful circumstances long before their detention, and after release into black townships are commonly subjected to ongoing traumatic stress. Continuing and unpredictable harassment and danger is common. Police may burst in at any time of the day or night, and may question, threaten or redetain people. In many parts of the country, an even grimmer threat exists, where groups of black vigilantes may arrive and threaten, harm or kill the ex-detainee or members of the family. Members of rival anti-apartheid groups may pose similar dangers. In these circumstances some South African psychologists now speak rather of a continuous traumatic stress syndrome (CTSS). The detention/torture survivor is in a position where vigilance and defences must be sustained, where life remains deeply unsettled and he or she may be for long periods 'on the run'. In this ongoing picture, chronic suspiciousness, deep feelings of anger or hatred and severe depressions are common.

The impression should not, however, be created that everyone who has been detained and abused emerges psychologically impaired. Despite residual stress effects, large numbers of activists emerge with resolve and commitment strengthened – although at the other end of the spectrum are severely damaged individuals. Obviously, the psychological stability of individuals before detention will have bearing on their level of resilience, as will the duration and severity of abuse. Availability of supportive relationships after release is important, and so, in our experience, is the construction which the detainee is able to put on the experience. Where the detainee has a coherent ideological way of making sense of the experience, this often acts as an important resilience factor, minimizing the confusion and profound demoralization often felt by relatively apolitical detainees who were tortured. Accounts of political imprisonment over the ages have emphasized the importance of active strategies engaged in by prisoners to retain areas of control in their lives and to resist; and these contribute to the resilience which detainees manifest. Activists connecting to progressive helping services in South Africa have always stressed the importance of professionals bringing a 'good attitude' to therapeutic work, i.e. a positive attitude which affirms strengths and political commitment, and does not subtly undermine the struggle by focusing only on damage and 'sympathy', conceiving of the ex-detainee as a 'victim' of unassailable forces, and thus generating pessimism and despondency. Health workers in turn have repeatedly cautioned resistance organizations against the unreflective macho stance of the township activists – that to admit to any stress reactions is weak, and that weakness is unacceptable. The dialogue has been mutually constructive, and has contributed to the transformation of counselling services on the one hand, and has raised mental health on the agendas of resistance organizations on the other.

The conceptualization of detention and torture and their sequelae have tended to reflect the orientation and involvement of the writers. Practising clinicians involved directly with the treatment of survivors are concerned with the picture which they see on a daily basis and are concerned to ameliorate. Many of these lean towards a PTSD/CTSS model with its natural linkage to the body of literature on dynamics and treatment (e.g. Solomons, 1989; Friedman, 1987; Straker, 1987). Social psychologists have tended to opt for social psychological models such as Tajfel's work, which allows a primary emphasis on social and political identity (e.g. Foster, 1989). Theories and models are, of course, constrained by their range of intent and by their levels of analysis, and neither of these approaches is able to satisfactorily encompass the other; but useful cross-fertilization is possible. Both share fundamental assumptions about the inseparability of political identity from detention, torture and the interpersonal transactions of the treatment process. The sociopsychological approach has its contribution to make in underlining the broader context within which torture takes place, and that torture constitutes not only an arena for medical and psychological support, but also a 'site of struggle' in broader sociopolitical terms. Perhaps the most useful current models are those that recognize that different levels of analysis, which may interact but cannot be conflated, are needed (e.g. Gibson, 1987).

ADVOCACY, SUPPORT AND INTERVENTION

Part of state strategy in repressing opposition has been to inflict maximum trauma on activists and inspire fear in their organizations and communities, relying on the isolation and secrecy provisions of the security laws to keep human-rights abuses out of the gaze of the rest of the public and the international community. Inevitably, however, small numbers of three professional groups – law, medicine and clinical psychology – have interfaced with these abuses and their effects. In each case a similar pattern has emerged: professionals employed by the state have overwhelmingly tended to turn a blind eye; the established professional bodies and councils have tended to support the political status quo rather than human rights to a point that violates their own codes; and a tiny group of academics or concerned practitioners have provided services to survivors and raised protests, connecting with human rights groups in the international community.

Criticism of the legal profession has been mentioned earlier. None the less, human rights lawyers have worked actively in South Africa, have challenged abuses repeatedly in the courts and in writings, and have operated a range of service organizations for people under repression. The medical profession's primary initial interface with state abuses was through state-employed district surgeons who had medical responsibility for detainees. In the 1970s it became clear that certain practitioners were collaborating with the security police – acting as a 'cover' for torture and brutality by writing false medical reports or autopsies, clearing injured patients for further torture, and neglecting medical care and follow-up. In 1977, at the inquest after activist Steve Biko's death in custody subsequent to sustained assault and torture, it became clear that Drs Lang and Tucker, the district surgeons responsible for Biko's healthy care, had behaved in a grossly neglectful and unethical manner that had contributed to his death.

Faced with the evidence, the South African Medical and Dental Council ruled that there was no *prima facie* evidence of disgraceful or improper conduct – a decision that was echoed by the Medical Association of South Africa (MASA), provoking a public outcry and resignations by some of MASA's members. Unwilling to accept what they saw as dereliction of duty by these bodies, a group of doctors instituted a Supreme Court action and succeeded in having the Council's resolution set aside and corrected. Finally, in 1985, both Lang and Tucker were found guilty of disgraceful and improper conduct and given minimal penalties (Baxter, 1985).

The revelations and publicity associated with this case brought to light the torture and abuse perpetrated under Section 29. It forced the medical profession to acknowledge that doctors' responsibilities to their patients applied fully even when their patients were held by the security police, and that the Medical Council was obliged to uphold the ethical code impartially. It also served notice that official impunity and unaccountability could not be taken for granted indefinitely.

Prior to the Biko case there was a degree of discontent amongst progressive doctors with MASA's easy acquiescence in racial discrimination, but the Association's conduct in this matter directly precipitated the formation of an alternative medical association – the National Medical and Dental Association (NAMDA). It is this small group in the medical profession which has played the major role in providing medical assistance to ex-detainees and denouncing in all available forums the abuses and tortures with which they were faced.

However, the next major public challenge to torture and abuse to come from the medical profession came from Dr Wendy Orr (discussed earlier) who was working with State of Emergency detainees. Her successful application to restrain the security police from assaulting detainees was another blow against the impunity and official indifference of the authorities. Orr's actions were not seen by her as a political act, but as a moral and professional imperative. It was inspiring to people used to professional turpitude; and showed that a stand on conscience could make a difference.

Members of the psychological profession – primarily clinical psychologists – were involved in tiny numbers mainly as individuals in the seventies, offering psychotherapeutic services to individual released detainees. The formation of the Detainees' Parents Support Committee in 1981/82 and its politicization around the torture and death of Dr Neil Aggett in detention focused attention on the need for therapeutic services, as did the DPSC and Institute for Criminology reports. It was at this stage that connections were made with Dr Genefke of the Rehabilitation Centre for Torture Victims (RCT) in Copenhagen, who organized meetings to transfer the skills developed at RCT in the treatment of torture survivors. This contributed to the development of a number of volunteer groups in Johannesburg, Cape Town and Durban, who worked in small detainee treatment teams, usually made up of psychologists or other social service workers together with NAMDA doctors.

Things changed dramatically with the civil conflict that swept across South Africa after the setting up of the 'tricameral' parliament, which definitively excluded blacks from participation in the political process. After the declaration of a State of Emergency in 1985 it became clear that people, including minors, were being detained in huge numbers and tortured and abused as a matter of routine by policemen and soldiers who felt that they were indemnified against the most brutal excesses. In Johannesburg a small group of progressive psychologists concerned with issues of apartheid and mental health calling itself the Organisation for Appropriate Social Services in South Africa (OASSSA) began to expand to offer services. In Cape Town, a small group of staff, clinical psychology trainees and past graduates of the University of Cape Town Child Guidance Clinic set up an organisation of concerned psychologists, using the Clinic as a base to provide therapeutic assistance and workshops in black townships under siege (Swartz, Dowdall & Swartz, 1986). Within a year this group had expanded and decided to link with OASSSA in Johannesburg and form a national body under the name of OASSSA, which eventually incorporated many of the psychological/social service groups actively opposed to apartheid in major cities.

Unsurprisingly, there are no formal care and treatment facilities for torture survivors in South Africa. Therapeutic assistance has been provided almost entirely by volunteer groups. In 1985/6, in an attempt to cope more effectively with the needs of traumatized people, a national 'umbrella' organization called Emergency Services Group was set up to bring together the disparate groups assisting ex-detainees. Funding was obtained to provide a full-time coordinator for each region and premises were rented where members of the organization would render medical and counselling services. Records were coded and care taken to avoid recording 'incriminating' information (which could be no more than the fact that a person was present at a gathering where there was a confrontation with the police), single police raids on these clinics occurred from time to time. In practice, of course, work with ex-detaines sometimes departed from ordinary office interviews. Where a security risk existed, or a person was 'on the run' from the security police, sessions were held at any venue that seemed relatively safe (e.g. Dowdall, 1990a).

TREATMENT METHODS

Psychotherapists naturally bring their own preferred theoretical and practical approaches to their work with tortured ex-detainees. Initial unfamiliarity with the experiences of the ex-detainee and this kind of work led therapists to draw on international experience and literature, and the most usual entry point has been Somnier and Genefke's (1986) work on psychotherapy for victims of torture. This has had to be adapted to local conditions, but the thread of this approach (a cognitively oriented introduction with discussion of what really happened; an 'emotive' phase, where feelings can be expressed in relation to the trauma; and a creative, practical, problem-tackling phase) still underlies a great deal of therapeutic work done in South Africa. As an example, Friedman (1987), discussing work at the detainee counselling service, notes that the first stage involves the establishment of trust, credibility and rapport – a particularly important aspect given the real dangers that many ex-detainees may face. The counsellor's political credibility – established at least in part by organizational links – are frequently a necessary precondition for any work to take place. Clinicians are dealing with casualties of ongoing combat in their own country, in a conflict in which they are implicated and from which they cannot stand aloof; and their personal credibility in this struggle is as real and important an issue as any professional credibility. This differs from centres working with alien refugees, where the staff commonly maintain a politically neutral stance. The second stage involves an explication in accessible language of what counselling is about and how it works – also necessary where it is an alien concept on class or cultural grounds. Stage three explores and 'normalizes' the presenting problems, and stage four and five involve exploration of detention experiences, and a limited and monitored expression of emotion. This moves through to a problem-solving stage, with exploration of future strategies, followed by closure. Straker (1987) presents a detailed, more psychodynamically oriented approach with many similarities. Perkel (1990) has proposed perceived locus of control as a focal point for therapy with detainees which has an eclectic/cognitive–behavioural leaning.

Most counsellors working with abuse and torture survivors in the South African context prefer to contain emotional expression and, in fact, to avoid intense cathartic experiences. Unlike treatment circumstances in a rehabilitation centre in a host country, when the South African ex-detainee walks out the door, he or she frequently walks into a situation fraught with threat. It is simply dysfunctional for him to abandon defences, or become too vulnerable to emotion. Another point that has been experienced across the country is that the most common treatment duration is the single session. Detainees are, for various reasons, often unable to return, and hence a lot of attention has been given to the development of a useful format for a single, usually two-hour session which focuses intensively on stress reduction and coping strategies (e.g. Straker, 1987).

Another approach has been to train activists as lay counsellors (e.g. Green, 1989) and to provide self-help materials such as training or self-help booklets in accessible language. These have normally drawn on limited Rogerian listening skills and some cognitive–behavioural techniques. A general approach of explicit political solidarity and concern with empowerment and the sharing of skills characterises most of these booklets.

Finally, counselling work in a civil conflict situation may place professionals in complex ethical situations (Steere & Dowdall, 1990). Therapy, particularly with children, is often dependent on team work. Do you avoid reporting key information in records in case you cannot guarantee confidentiality and the child is detained? What about the concept of 'dangerousness'? What is your correct course of action if a client tells you of a planned petrol-bomb attack on a police station? Many problematic issues derive from issues of trust, including the issue of political neutrality and the problem of being a white therapist in a country where whites oppress blacks. Others have to do with competence – few whites speak the first language of black ex-detainees, and few have any real idea of the stresses and issues of black township life. And, as yet, the numbers of black psychologists is pitifully small. Attempts have been made from time to time to train people from local communities to act as lay counsellors, but no consolidated programme with a follow-up has been established.

CONCLUSIONS

Two broad issues arise from the discussion of the South African experience. Firstly, torture and abuse flourishes in situations of impunity, unaccountability and secrecy, and it is incumbent on all who encounter abuse to challenge it, preferably in an organized way early on. Exposure and publicity have been crucial in South Africa. Tyrannical regimes seem to be strangely thin skinned when faced with rejection and international attack on their internal policies. The stands made by principled individuals do have a cumulative effect, and in the end they do bring changes (e.g. Dowdall, 1990b). In a court case in 1990, for example, an official complaint was laid by colleagues against a South African psychiatrist who recommended that security police be allowed to continue to interrogate detainee Yusuf Mahomed despite the fact that he was suffering from depression and had tried to kill himself. In a landmark decision in this case the judge has also ruled that doctors – and not the security police – must have the final say on matters concerning the health of the detainee[1]. Detention without trial is not yet gone; but this is yet another nail in the coffin of police unaccountability and impunity.

Secondly, therapeutic practice with torture survivors within a repressive country differs substantially from rehabilitation in a host country. As we have seen in considering legal, medical and psychological issues in South Africa, the political conflicts within the country permeate the operation of the professions and the judgment and modus operandi of the individual professional. The relationship between any given 'helping' professional and detainees will first and foremost be defined in political terms as ally or adversary. The implicit common linkage to a shared set of political beliefs is an important basis for the therapeutic connection. Simultaneously, of course, the professional is defined into an adversarial role in relation to a host of state-linked structures. Political neutrality may, in a sense, be possible in host countries; but in countries under repression there are no neutral players.

REFERENCES

Amnesty International (1978). *Political Imprisonment in South Africa*. Londson, Amnesty International.

Baxter, L. (1985). Doctors on trial: Steve Biko, medical ethics and the courts. *South African Journal on Human Rights*, 1(2) 137–51.

Biko, S. (1978). *I Write what I Like*. London: Heinemann.

Browde, S. (1988). The treatment of detainees. Proceedings of the 1987 National Medical and Dental Association (NAMDA) Annual Conference. Cape Town, NAMDA.

Chaskalson, A. (1985). In A. N. Bell and R. D. Mackie eds, *Detention and Security Legislation in South Africa*. Durban: University of Natal.

De Beer, C. (1984). *The South African Disease*. Johannesburg: South African Research Services.

Detainees' Parents Support Committee (1982). Memorandum on Security Police abuse of political detainees. Johannesburg, DPSC.

Dowdall, T. (1990a). Working with children and their families in civil conflict situations. In *The Influence of Violence on Children*, Cape Town: Centre for Intergroup Studies.

Dowdall, T. (1990b). Repression, health care and ethics under apartheid. Paper delivered at XIX Tromso Seminar in Medicine: Torture and the Medical Profession, Tromso.

Dugard, J. (1985). The judiciary and national security. In A. N. Bell and R. D.

---

[1] *Sunday Star* (Johannesburg) November 4 1990.

Mackie eds. *Detention and Security Legislation in South Africa*. Durban: University of Natal.

Foster, D. & Sandler, D. (1985). A study of detention and torture in South Africa: preliminary report. Institute of Criminology, University of Cape Town.

Foster, D. & Luyt, C. (1986). The blue man's burden: policing the police in South Africa. *South African Journal on Human Rights*, **2**.

Foster, D., Davis, D. & Sandler, D. (1987). *Detention and Torture in South Africa*. Cape Town: David Philip.

Foster, D. H. (1989). Political detention in South Africa: a sociopsychological perspective. *International Journal of Mental Health*, **18**, 21–37.

Friedlander, R. (1986). Stress disorders in former detainees in South Africa. Paper read at the World Psychiatric Association Regional Symposium, Copenhagen.

Friedman, G. (1987). Counselling ex-detainees: themes, problems and strategies in OASSSA: Mental Health in Transition. Proceedings of the OASSSA Second National Conference, Cape Town. OASSSA.

Gibson, K. (1987). Civil conflict, stress and children. *Psychology in Society*. **8**, 4–26.

Green, J. (1989). Evaluation of a Lay Counselling Programme That Trains Lay Counsellors From the Townships. Unpublished M.A. (Clin. Psych.) dissertation, Johannesburg, University of the Witwatersrand.

Human Rights Commission. (1989a). *Anatomy of Repression Information Manual M–I*, Braamfontein: HRC.

Human Rights Commission. (1989b). Detention without Trial. Fact Paper FP1, Braamfontein, HRC.

Human Rights Commission. (1990a). *Children and Repression*: Special Report. Johannesburg: Human Rights Commission.

Human Rights Commission. (1990b). Deaths in Detention. Fact Paper FP7, Braamfontein, HRC.

Mathews, A. (1990). National security, morality and the courts. Paper presented at the 13th South African Law Conference, Durban.

Mathews, A. & Albino, R. (1966). The permanence of the temporary – an examination of the 90 day and 180 day detention laws. *South African Law Journal*, **83**, 16.

Orr, W. (1990). Detention, health and the media. Address given at University of Cape Town Medical School, July 1990.

Perkel, A. (1990). Psychotherapy with detainees: a theoretical basis. *Psychology in Society*, **13**, 4–16.

Rayner, M. (1987). *Turning a Blind Eye? Medical Accountability and the Prevention of Torture in South Africa*. New York committee on Scientific Freedom and Responsibility.

Seedat, A. (1984). *Crippling a Nation: Health in Apartheid South Africa*. London: International Defence and Aid Fund.

Solomons, K. (1989). The dynamics of posttraumatic stress disorder in South African political ex-detaines. *American Journal of Psychotherapy* XLIII, 2.

Somnier, E. & Genefke, I. (1986). Psychotherapy for victims of torture. *British Journal of Psychiatry*, **149**, 323–9.

Steere, J. & Dowdall, T. (1990). On being ethical in unethical places: the dilemmas of South African Clinical Psychologists. *Hastings Center Report*, **20**, 2.

Steere, J. (1984). *Ethics in Clinical Psychgology*. Cape Town: Oxford University Press.

Straker, G. (1987). The continuous traumatic stress syndrome – the single therapeutic interview. *Psychology in Society*, **8**, 48–78.

Swartz, S., Dowdall, T. & Swartz, L. (1986). Clinical psychology and the 1985 crisis in Cape Town, *Psychology in Society*, **5**, 131–8,.

Tucker, R. (1985). Protection of detainees: fact and fiction. In A. N. Bell and R. D. Mackie eds, *Detention and Security Legislation in South Africa*. Durban: University of Natal.

Webster, D. (1987). Repression and the State of Emergency. In G. Moss and I. Obvery, eds, *South African Review 4*. Johannesburg: Raven Press.

Wilson, F. and Ramphele, M. (1987). Children in South Africa. In UNICEF, *Children in the Front Line*. New York: UNICEF.

21
TORTURE IN PAKISTAN
Mahboob Mehdi

PAKISTAN: BACKGROUND INFORMATION

To understand the history of torture in Pakistan better, we need to go briefly through the series of events since the creation of the country. When Pakistan was created in 1947 by the division of British India, as a result of the demand for a separate country for Indian Muslims, the migration of millions of people across the newly created borders of India and Pakistan caused the uprooting of innumerable communities and massive inter-communal massacres. The newly created country with a highly traumatized population was easily taken over by a regime which had no sympathy with the people. The ruling junta governed the country by using religion for political purposes. From the early period of the country's history, human rights have had a low priority in Pakistan. The Police department, established during the colonial period by the Police Act of 1861, continued unchanged and the legacy of torture from the past was inherited by the new state. A number of further statutes were passed which justified torture and preventive detention. Torture remained a normal procedure of inter-rogation and punishment for any activity deemed undesirable by the ruling junta.

The first constitution of Pakistan was framed in 1956. It did nothing to improve the situation, and the government continued to possess wide powers of arbitrary arrest and detention without trial.

In October 1958, the constitution was superseded by the imposition of Martial Law and government was by Martial Law Regulations and Orders. The Military Courts and Tribunals were established with unlimited power to arrest and try political activists.

In 1962, Ayub Khan, the Chief Martial Law Administrator, imposed a new constitution with the help of which he became president. Resentment against this constitution, which, too, was repressive in character, developed into political agitation in 1968. In order to control the situation, a second Martial Law was imposed in March 1969.

The Commander-in-Chief of the army, General Yahya Khan assumed power both as Chief Martial Law Administrator and President. The Martial Law Administration began military action in the eastern part of the country in order to suppress the right of self determination of the people there. The result was the separation of the eastern part of the country as Bangladesh. This situation also resulted in the replacement of General Yahya Khan by Zulfiqar Ali Bhutto, who was the majority party leader from West Pakistan. Zulfiqar Ali Bhutto acted as a Civilian Martial Law Administrator until the imposition of a new constitution which, in its turn, failed to improve the human rights situation in Pakistan. Police atrocities, torture and repression of political opponents continued.

In July 1977, another Martial Law, the longest lasting and most ruthless of all, was imposed on the country by the Army Chief-of Staff Zia-ul-Haq. During this period there was rapid growth and further institutionalization of torture. A fundamentalist interpretation of religion was used to justify torture, cruel and inhuman treatment and punishments (Mahmood, 1989). Under the third Martial Law, political workers were for the first time punished by whipping for political actions such as making a speech, holding a meeting or a demonstration or taking part in a march against the continuance of Martial Law. Political workers, trade unionists, women activists, lawyers and students were arrested from time to time and kept in detention without trial for months and, in some cases, for years. Political trials of hundreds of political activists were held before special or summary military courts, where they were invariably convicted, even though evidence against them was scant and of a most doubtful nature, and given long prison sentences or heavy fines and were sometimes sentenced to whipping. In cases where the arrest of a wanted political worker was not possible, other family members were detained to put pressure on him or her. Detained persons were not always taken to prison but were, on many occasions, taken to special torture dens functioning under both the civil police and the army authorities. Reports of extensive torture inflicted on political workers, including women, have not been uncommon. Many of those who were kept in prison were placed in shackles and bar fetters and remained in isolation for months. Death sentences were passed and carried out in trials held by military courts even though no legal evidence was available to prove the defendant guilty and serious questions about jurisdiction were raised (Amnesty International 1985*a*; Minto, 1986; Petren *et al.*, 1987).

Political detainees and convicts were not treated in accordance with ordinary prison rules. Despite the fact that many political workers were not proved guilty of the charges made against them or had served out their term after conviction, they were not released and were kept in custody for months. Cases occurred where children were detained, imprisoned and whipped (Farani, 1986). Whippings were sometimes carried out publicly.

Torture is interwoven in the socio-economic matrix of Pakistan, and is used as an essential instrument for the survival of the system. Change in government may bring a palliative change in torture but the institutions of torture remain intact. The laws which allow torture remain. Torture cells remain and torturers retain their posts. This is why the death of General Zia in a plane crash in August 1988 did not mark the end of torture in Pakistan. The civilian governments which came to power after the general election could not stop the vast scale of torture conducted in the police stations, prisons and interrogation centres of Pakistan. Torture is endemic in Pakistan but it reaches epidemic proportions from time to time.

METHODS OF TORTURE

Different methods of torture used in Pakistan can be broadly classified into physical and psychological types. Commonly used physical methods include beating which may be unsystematic, such as punching, kicking and indiscriminate beating with different objects, or systematic, such as phalanga, 'telephono' and whipping. In phalanga the soles of the feet are beaten with a rod; in 'telephono' the torturer gives a blow with the flat of his hand against the victim's ear. Whipping is done with a piece of leather or cane on the individual's back. Daang Pherna is a method of torture in which the victim is stripped naked and forced to lie face upwards on his back. A bamboo is firmly pressed on the thighs of the victim by two persons and slowly rolled over the whole length of the lower limbs. Other forms of physical torture include suspending the individual in different ways, such as straight or upside down or 'parrot's perch' style, forcing the individual to stand for prolonged periods or remain in awkward positions, burning with cigarettes and heated metallic rods, strangulation, dental torture, rape and sexual assaults, insertion of foreign bodies into the vagina or rectum and electrical torture. Submarino, the submersion of the victim's head in water contaminated with excreta, etc, until the victim nearly suffocates, is also used, as is dry submarino, when the victim's head is covered with a bag containing foul smelling material, again almost to the point of suffocation. Exposure to cold, such as submersion in ice cold water or forcing the individual to lie naked on a block of ice, is also used as a physical torture.

Commonly used psychological methods of torture include verbal abuse and humiliation, false accusation, witnessing others being tortured, threats of torture to self or relatives and sham executions. Deprivation of food, water or sleep, continuous exposure to powerful light or constant noise are also common, as are the use of solitary confinement or overcrowded cells, and pharmacological tortures. In most cases, the detainee is subjected to both physical and psychological methods of torture (Amnesty International, 1985b; Khan, 1987; Khosa, 1990; Nomani, 1987; Tahir, 1987).

WHIPPING IN PAKISTAN

Whipping as a method of torture and cruel punishment has been internationally identified with Pakistan. It was introduced into the modern judicial punishments of the subcontinent by the British colonialists when they framed the notorious Whipping Act of 1909. This act was incorporated in the system of punishments in Pakistan after the division of the subcontinent. The whipping act has since been amended at various times according to the needs of new rulers. Thus during the rule of General Ayub Khan, the act was amended by the 'West Pakistan Ordinance VI of 1962' and 'West Pakistan Ordinance XLII of 1963' and under General Yahya Khan, by 'Whipping (West Pakistan Amendment) Ordinance of 1969'. General Zia-ul-Haq updated it by enacting 'The Execution of the Punishment of Whipping Ordinance 1979'. The ordinance promulgated by General Zia completely transformed the law of whipping in Pakistan. Under the provisions of the new law, which does not specify the crimes for which whipping should be carried out, the conditions for, and the method of, the punishment of whipping are set out. One important aspect of these provisions is the highly increased role which the doctor is asked to perform during the process of whipping. Before the punishment commences, the authorized medical officer is asked to examine medically the person convicted, to ensure that the execution of the punishment will not cause the individual's death. If the person is ill, execution of the punishment should be postponed until he or she is certified by the authorized medical officer to be physically fit to undergo the punishment. The punishment is executed in the presence of the authorized medical officer at any public place the provincial government may appoint for the purpose. If, after punishment has commenced, the authorized medical officer is of the opinion that there are grounds for concern over the possible death of the person being whipped, the execution of the punishment should be postponed until the authorized medical officer certifies him or her physically fit to undergo the remainder of the punishment (Amnesty International, 1990*a*, *b*; Mahmood, 1989).

At first glance it may seem that the doctor's role in this whole process of whipping is protective and is in the interest of the person convicted. But a careful analysis of the situation would show that quite the reverse is true. The doctor's role in the process of whipping in Pakistan is in contravention of the accepted international standards of medical ethics set out by the World Medical Association in its Tokyo Declaration of 1975 (WMA, 1975). This declaration clearly states that:

1 The doctor should not countenance, condone, or participate in the practice of torture or other forms of cruel, inhuman or degrading procedure, whatever the offence of which the victim of such procedure is suspected, accused or guilty, and whatever the victim's beliefs or motives, and in whatever situation, including armed conflicts and civil strife.
2 The doctor shall not provide any premises, instruments, substances or knowledge to facilitate the practice of torture or other forms of cruel, inhuman or degrading treatment or to diminish the ability of the victim to resist such treatment.
3 The doctor shall not be present during any procedure involving torture or other forms of cruel, inhuman or degrading treatment.
4 A doctor must have complete clinical independence in deciding upon the care of a person for whom he or she is medically responsible. The doctor's fundamental role is to alleviate the distress of his or her fellow men, and no motive whether personal, collective or political shall prevail against this higher purpose.

During this period of the third Martial Law, whipping was extensively used in Pakistan to demoralize and terrorize the people who were opposing the military dictatorship. The Karachi branch of the Pakistan Medical Association, in its resolution of 8 September 1983 stated that whipping 'is not only inhuman and against the dignity of man, but can cause serious physical damage and irreversible psychological trauma especially in young people. It is known that this punishment may activate latent diseases like tuberculosis and precipitate cardiovascular accident besides permanently damaging the personality of the victim' (Pakistan Medical Association, 1983). The participation of doctors in the procedure of whipping was discussed at a seminar organized by 'Voice Against Torture' in Islamabad on 26 September 1988, where it was declared that no one is medically fit for whipping and doctors should refuse to participate in the procedure of whipping whenever they are asked to do so (Iqbal, 1988).

HEALTH PROFESSION AND TORTURE

There are two aspects of this issue in Pakistan: the involvement of health professionals in the process of torture and their role in health care for torture survivors.

The involvement of health professionals in torture is a very serious problem in Pakistan. Some doctors are known to advise torturers about detainee's health and revive the detainee sufficiently to undergo further torture (Corillon, 1989). The code of medical ethics of Pakistan Medical and Dental Council does not deal with doctors' participation in torture, and doctors who are involved in torture do not face any disciplinary action from this body. In fact, their role in torture and degrading and inhuman punishment is usually legal and has been made part of their duties. In many interrogation centres, the doctors examine detainees to declare them fit for interrogation. Doctors are required by law to monitor the execution of the judicial punishment of whipping, and if a court orders the amputaof a hand or foot, this must be carried out in person by an authorized medical officer. Cover-up activities, such as providing false death certificates and false clinical records of the tortured detainees, are very common. Doctors are required to confirm certain offences such as drinking, 'illicit' sexual relations and pregnancy out of wedlock, for which severe and cruel punishments may be imposed. Clearly, doctors should refuse to carry out such examinations.

In Pakistan, the conduct of the prison medical officers is often unethical and falls far short of the United Nations declarations and codes of conduct. Instead of providing the best possible treatment for the prisoners, the prison medical officer behaves as part of the prison administration and takes part in torture. I have interviewed men and women, tortured in different centres and prisons of Pakistan, who gave evidence of the participation of doctors in torture and cruel punishments.

The second aspect of torture relating to health professionals is care of torture survivors. Before the intervention by Voice Against Torture (VAT), the majority of the health professionals in Pakistan were not aware of the health implications of torture. VAT participated in the

'Seventh International Psychiatric Conference' held in Karachi in 1988 by organizing a seminar on torture. Similarly, in 1990, in the 'Eighth International Psychiatric Conference' held in Islamabad a presentation on the medical aspects of torture was given. VAT has also discussed this issue in several clinical meetings of the 'Pakistan Medical Association'. In December 1990, VAT organized an advanced training programme in Lahore for health professionals on 'Health Implications of Torture'. However, enough work has not yet been done. There are thousands of torture survivors and their families who need health care in Pakistan, but the number of health professionals who are engaged in this work is almost negligible. The training of health professionals in the various institutions of Pakistan does not consider the problem of torture and how health professionals should deal with it.

VOICE AGAINST TORTURE (VAT)

Voice Against Torture represents the first organized and systematic effort to combat the serious problem of torture in Pakistan. Founded at the beginning of 1988, it is an interdisciplinary forum for the struggle against all forms of torture and for the treatment and rehabilitation of torture survivors which links together doctors, nurses, psychologists, physiotherapists, scientists, sociologists, lawyers, journalists, intellectuals and social workers.

VAT seeks to raise the public awareness of the aims, methods and consequences of torture and to mobilize opinion against its practice. It aims to impress on doctors the serious challenge that torture poses to the medical profession and to encourage the provision for doctors, physiotherapists, nurses, psychologists and social workers of an adequate education in diagnosing and treating the consequences of torture. By mobilizing medical opinion in favour of the 1975 World Medical Association's Tokyo Declaration and urging the Pakistan Medical and Dental Council to include a clause against torture in its code of medical ethics, VAT hopes to contribute to the prevention of doctors' participation in torture. Doctors should not participate in covering up torture by, for example, providing false death certificates for or false clinical records of tortured detainees. Nor should they monitor torture or in any way assist in its execution. Professional medical skills should not be used to extract information, control the prisoner or merely for punishment. Doctors should, instead, provide the best possible medical treatment for prisoners, without bias. In pursuit of the aim, VAT supports all doctors who refuse to participate in torture and tries to ensure that they and their families are not victimized. VAT's policy *vis-à-vis* those doctors who have chosen to be participants in torture is to collect evidence of their activities, present cases to the Pakistan Medical and Dental Council and to take these cases to court so that the doctors concerned may be tried for their criminal acts and exposed widely in the media. Finally, VAT aims to conduct and participate in fact-finding missions regarding torture and other human rights violations and to maintain good relations with anti-torture organizations abroad, exchanging experiences and participating with them in joint activities. VAT also runs the Rehabilitation and Health Aid Centre for Torture Victims.

The experience of VAT has shown that, though countries with a 'high torture rate' can be individually marked on a map, torture itself is essentially a global phenomenon. Certain governments may claim to be against torture, but they share the responsibility when they support another government which practises torture. One such example is the brutal military dictatorship of General Zia-ul-Haq which was supported by western governments. Torturers, irrespective of faith and ideology, are internationally united, cooperating with each other, teaching each other and learning from each other, exchanging experience and technology, and even handing over people on the so called 'wanted list' to the respective governments (Nomani, 1987). In such a situation, those struggling against torture are in danger of becoming torture victims themselves. It is therefore very important that they too should unite internationally, irrespective of faith and ideology. They should increase their co-operation, teach each other and learn from each other, exchange experience and technology of the struggle against torture, and plan measures for the protection of persons involved in anti-torture work in 'high risk areas'. Such protection is important for the smooth, efficient and safe functioning of anti-torture organisations in 'high risk areas' of the world.

THE REHABILITATION AND HEALTH AID CENTRE FOR TORTURE VICTIMS (RAHAT)

Lack of specialized care for torture survivors in ordinary hospitals has led VAT to establish the Rehabilitation and Health Aid Centre for Torture Victims (RAHAT) in Islamabad. Doctors psychiatrists, psychologists, nurses and social workers experienced in the care of torture survivors provide services at RAHAT, whose staff work as a team assessing and treating the multidimensional problems of torture survivors.

RAHAT, the only centre of its kind so far in South Asia helping people who suffer from the effects of torture, offers a treatment programme which aims at medical, psychological and social rehabilitation of torture survivors and their families. Doctors, other health professionals, hospitals and other organizations can refer survivors to RAHAT for treatment. There is no discrimination on the basis of age, sex, religion, ideology, political affiliation, nationality or ethnic origin and the treatment is free. RAHAT conducts research and educational work and provides health professionals, lawyers, human rights activists and other concerned persons with information on different aspects of torture.

The experience of RAHAT highlights the advantages and disadvantages of having a centre for the treatment of torture survivors in the country where torture was inflicted. In centres located in other countries only those survivors who decide to leave and succeed in reaching foreign countries can be treated. These survivors comprise a very small percentage of the total of those in need of health care. Treating torture survivors in their own country ensures that the maximum number of torture survivors are able to come to the centre and can feel comfortable in the atmosphere of their local culture. Usually, there is no need for interpreters and there is no stress of being in exile. The main disadvantage of indigenous centres is the security risk faced both by the therapist and the survivor.

The risk may be reduced by support from the public, human rights organizations and political parties in the country, although the centre itself should not be affiliated to any political party. Wide media coverage and recognition and support from bodies abroad, such as the UN, affiliated organizations and other anti-torture and human rights groups may also be helpful.

The establishment of RAHAT is a firm step towards the humanizing of medicine in Pakistan. Being, until now, the only centre of its kind in South Asia, RAHAT is responsible for catering for a large variety of torture survivors. Pakistan has a large population of refugees from various countries, forced to leave their homelands because of circumstances threatening their physical and psychological well-being. Thus arrangement has been made for RAHAT to cater for the needs of torture survivors speaking different languages and belonging to different cultures. To date, RAHAT has provided treatment for people from six different countries. Survivors from Pakistan who are at the moment cared for at RAHAT mostly belong to a large group of ex-political prisoners who underwent severe torture during the previous regime of military dictatorship. Many of these released prisoners are in a very bad condition both physically and mentally. Rehabilitation of these persons along with their families is a very serious problem. Despite extreme lack of resources, these persons are given maximum care at RAHAT in order to restore their physical and psychological health.

The situation of torture in Pakistan remains very serious even now that the military dictatorship has gone. Torture of people in police custody and use of different methods of torture during interrogation continue as before. None of the laws which allow torture has been changed, none of the torturers has been brought to the court and none of the institutions where torture takes places has been destroyed. Voice Against Torture and the Rehabilitation and Health Aid Centre for Torture Victims continue to function with very little resources and under unfavourable circumstances.

REFERENCES

Amnesty International (1985a). *Pakistan*. (Index: 33/51/90). Amnesty International: London.

Amnesty International (1985b). *Violations of Human Rights in Pakistan*. (Index: ASA 33/16/85). Amnesty International: London.

Amnesty International (1990a). *Whipping in Pakistan*. (Index: ASA 33/01/90). Amnesty International: London.

Amnesty International (1990b). *Pakistan: Human Rights Safeguards*. (Index: ASA 33/03/90). Amnesty International: London.

Corillon, C. (1989). The role of science and scientists in human rights. In M. E. Wolfgang, ed., *The Annals of the American Academy of Political and Social Science*. Newbury Park: Sage Publishers.

Farani, M. (1986). *Judicial Review of Martial Law Actions*. Lahore: Lahore Law Times Publications.

Iqbal, A. (1988). Nobody medically fit for flogging. *The Muslim*, Sept. 27, Islamabad.

Khan, P. (1987). *Martial Law Kay Qaidee* (Prisoners of Martial Law). Lahore: Daf Publishers.

Khosa, A. S. K. (1990). *Constitution and the Police in Pakistan*. Lahore: Kauser Brothers.

Mahmood, M. (1989). *Enforcement of Hudood: Practice and Procedure*. Lahore: Pakistan Law Times Publications.

Mehdi, M. (1990). Doctors in Pakistan realize that torture is a 'problem'. In *International Newsletter on Treatment and Rehabilitation of Torture Victims*, **1**, 6.

Minto, A. H. (1986). Human rights in Pakistan and the struggle of the lawyers. In C. John (ed.), *Pakistan: Struggle for Human Rights*. Kowloon: Christian Conference of Asia.

Nomani, M. J. (1987). *Jo Mujh Par Guzri [It happened to me]*. Karachi, Shaber Publications.

Petren, G., Cull, H. *et al.* (1987). *Pakistan: Human Rights After Martial Law.* Geneva, International Commission of Jurists.

Pakistan Medical Association (1983). Resolution of Pakistan Medical Association Karachi Branch, September 8.

Tahir, S. (1987) Martial Law: White Paper. Lahore Classics.

World Medical Association (1987). The Declaration of Tokyo: 1975. *Danish Medical Bulletin*, **34(4)**, 203–4.

22
REHABILITATION OF SURVIVORS OF TORTURE AND POLITICAL VIOLENCE UNDER A CONTINUING STRESS SITUATION: THE PHILIPPINE EXPERIENCE

Aurora A. Parong, Elizabeth Protacio-Marcelino, Sylvia Estrada-Claudio, June Pagaduan-Lopez and Victoria Cabildo

This chapter is an exposition on the problem of political torture and the rehabilitation of torture survivors in the Philippines. It presents the essential variables outside the purely personal and clinical framework under which torture and repression occur. It also discusses the various approaches in rehabilitation which are now practised in the country including their limitations and problems.

The various methodologies in rehabilitation herein discussed are seen as in progressive evolution rather than as absolutes. Deeper and better understanding of the variables, both on the individual and societal levels, added experiences in the work and learning more lessons from other countries similarly situated will hopefully result in the development of other varied and more effective approaches.

Since torture rehabilitation is relatively new in the Philippines and given the economic and technical constraints of the existing rehabilitation centers amidst an environment of continuing political conflict, various researches and other materials necessary for a comprehensive discussion of torture and rehabilitation work are not as yet available. Nevertheless, the limited information on rehabilitation work among torture survivors in developing countries and under conditions of continuing stress makes this exposition valuable.

HISTORICAL CONTEXT

Torture occurs in many countries all over the world. Amnesty International in its 1990 Report stated that it happens in one hundred countries including the Philippines.

Generally, throughout the world, torture as it is practised now is 'characterized by the systematic and widespread use of sophisticated scientific techniques against a regime's political opponents. Torture has thus become a tool of regimes seeking to govern by the "reign of terror"' (Lippman, 1979).

'And government by terror is the response of Third World States, which are clients of one or the other superpower, to the stresses of economic development, economic crisis, or the East–West confrontation.'[1] The ideology of terror adopted by governments is justified as necessary to protect the existing governments and for 'national interests' especially when there is economic crisis and there are groups highly critical of the ruling class and government declaring the need to change the existing economic or political system. Thus for national security and to maintain the economic status quo which benefits those in power and the foreign government which supports and props up the ruling regime, individual rights are subverted and torture is practised. 'Equating the political opponent or ideological opponent with an enemy not entitled to respect for the "inherent dignity of the human person", but whose only entitlement is to a combat without quarter, is perhaps the most destructive legacy of the doctrine of national security' (International Commission of Jurists, 1983).

The occurrence of torture in the Philippines, its causes and the political and economic context under which it occurs are best understood from a brief historical review.

The Philippines has been subjected to almost four centuries of colonial rule, first by the Spaniards and then the Americans in the early 1900s and, for a brief period, by the Japanese during the Second World War. The first two have left an indelible colonial legacy on the economy, politics and social psychology of the people. Thus, while granted formal independence in 1946, the country today remains very much a neo-colony of the United States.

In a study of economic development of ten colonies including the Philippines, Professors Thomas Birnberg of Yale and Stephen Resnick of the University of Massachusetts (1975) stated that:

> ... U.S. trade policies facilitated an increase in Philippine exports ... exports were developed to be sold to a developed country in exchange for imports of manufactures, and government expenditures were directed to facilitate and foster this international exchange ... Colonies served the political and economic needs of the developed countries not only by providing assured sources of food and raw materials and markets for their manufactures, but also by providing profitable areas for foreign investment, greater control in response to economic and

[1] Jose W. Diokno, Ending Torture by Governments, 1983.

political rivalry among the countries of the developed world itself.

This economic system, irrelevant to the needs of the Filipinos, persists today. Thus, the majority of the Filipino people live below poverty line while giant multinational companies and a local elite class benefit from the rich resources of the country. The country's technology remains backward and wages are kept incredibly low to attract foreign capital. Meanwhile, in the countryside, the age-old feudal relations remain almost intact.

The people's response to the problems are varied. Many seem to be resigned to fatalism and have left the course of their lives to destiny. A significant number of the population, however, has taken active intervention to change their lives through various, and sometimes conflicting, approaches. The greater part of the population still depend on traditional ways of effecting reforms like elections but a radicalized segment has resorted either to open militant actions or to direct armed confrontation with the state.

Torture in the Philippines occurs within the context of state repression against internal dissent. Thus, while torture is also applied to individuals convicted or suspected of common crime, violations in regular prisons and jails, political torture, or the systematic use of force or violence to obtain information from opposition and dissident suspects, to destroy the individual's personality and/or to create terror in the hearts of opponents and dissidents or potential opponents and dissidents, came to the fore during the time of the late Philippine strongman Ferdinand Marcos.

It was during this period, particularly during the first few months after the declaration of martial law on September 21, 1972, that thousands were rounded up and thrown into jails. In the process, many were tortured while undergoing tactical interrogation by the military.

Repression inevitably intensified as the despot Marcos desperately tried to cling on to power. Amnesty International in its report in 1984 stated that:

> Amnesty International has continued to receive credible reports of systematic torture in the Philippines ... following the pattern established since the proclamation of martial law in 1972 ... evidence of abuses of people taken into custody by military personnel including beatings, forcing individuals to undertake humiliating acts, and other forms of ill treatment ... Despite lifting martial law in 1981, members of the armed forces have

retained extensive powers of arrest and detention in cases involving alleged 'subversives' and other 'public order violators' ... alleged suspects are commonly abducted without warrant and detained incommunicado ... the agencies responsible for arrest were armed forces intelligence branches ... Detainees arrested or abducted by these units were commonly taken to undisclosed and unauthorized interrogation centres, known as 'safehouses', where interrogation was commonly accompanied by torture involving electric shocks, sexual abuse, and beatings ... Amnesty International also knows of instances where detainees in such 'safehouses' have not been seen again and are presumed or known to have died as a result of their ill-treatment.

The health professionals were not exempt from repression. Two Filipino physicians were also arrested and subsequently detained in 1982 and 1985 – one on suspicion of treating dissidents and one for rendering services to political detainees (Claude, 1989).

Fighting hard against the perceived enemies of the state was the dictator's way of bargaining for more support from his foreign bene-factors, particularly the United States government, which generously provided the financial, material and technical know-how for the dictator's bloody counter-insurgency program. Especially during the early days of martial rule, the military establishment employed unmiti-gated violence against opponents, suspected dissidents and their sympathizers.

Long years of dictatorship have geared the state armed forces to the logic of the national security doctrine which essentially disregards human persons. Under the national security doctrine, individuals are 'utilized as tools and tally heads in international competition where aggregate figures count for more than personhood' (Mische, 1977).

The February 1986 'People Power Revolution' did very little to alter the situation. In November 1988, the Philippine Alliance of Human Rights Advocates reported that, for the first 1000 days of the Aquino government, there were 705 persons executed, 480 died in massacres, 11 911 arrested and 1676 tortured, 204 reported missing while 37 132 families became refugees in our own land.[1]

Highly militarized areas in the countryside have become virtual torture zones where victims are abused in their own homes and communities. An atmosphere of fear continues to haunt the populace

---

[1] Philippine Alliance of Human Rights Advocates, *Human Rights Record of the Aquino Government for the First 1,000 Days*, November 1988.

including torture survivors who continue to see those who violated their dignities not only roaming around freely but occupying higher positions of power.

Amnesty International in its 1990 Report declared:

> The authorities frequently labelled non-governmental organizations, including human rights groups, as 'fronts for the CPP (Communist Party of the Philippines) or the NPA (New People's Army, the armed wing of the outlawed CPP)' ... The government's counter-insurgency campaign used regular armed forces, official para-military forces known as the Citizens' Armed Forces Geographical Units (CAFGUs), and armed groups known as 'vigilantes' which have no legal status ... CAFGU forces were reportedly responsible for extrajudicial executions, torture and 'disappearances'.
>
> The bombing and strafing of villages suspected of harbouring NPA and MNLF (Moro National Liberation Front) guerillas resulted in the evacuation of tens of thousands of people.
>
> ... More than 200 critics, opponents or suspected opponents of the government appeared to be victims of extrajudicial executions committed by government or government-backed forces. The dead included church workers, trade unionists, human rights activists and members of various lawful non-governmental organizations accused of being fronts for the CPP or NPA. Dozens of villagers living in areas where the NPA was active were deliberately killed by military and para-military forces. The authorities often claimed that the victims were NPA members who died in 'legitimate encounters', although the victims included elderly people and very young children killed in their homes.
>
> ... Torture and ill-treatment of political detainees during interrogation by police and military personnel were frequently reported.

Furthermore, the Medical Action Group in 1989 reported the harassment, arrest and detention and extrajudicial killing of 102 health workers as well as disruption of 205 community health programs by military, para-military and vigilante forces for the period covering 1987–1989.[1]

---

[1] Medical Action Group, Summary of Cases of Violations of Health and Human Rights, January 1987–October 1989.

REHABILITATION PROGRAMS

It was in 1985, barely a year before Marcos was dislodged from power, that programs for the medical and psychological rehabilitation of torture victims got off the ground. Prior to these, efforts to assist torture survivors in their health needs were unsystematic and erratic.

The Children's Rehabilitation Center (CRC) was established to render psychological and other related assistance to child-victims of political violence.

The Medical Action Group, an organization of health professionals and students working for health and human rights established in 1982, set up the Philippine Action Concerning Torture (PACT) for the rehabilitation of adult torture survivors, either in detention or outside detention.

BALAY was established specifically to assist ex-detainees.

All these were initially based in Metro Manila which is located in Luzon, one of the three big islands of the country but later, each conducted outreach programs outside Metro Manila.

There are various factors which highly affect rehabilitation work in the country. Foremost of these are political repression, economic factors, family and community, culture and subculture. These either serve as obstacles or positive factors for rehabilitation work or important considerations for effective and appropriate intervention.

POLITICAL REPRESSION

Governmental support for the aforementioned rehabilitation programs was zero during the time of Marcos and is still totally absent under the present government. In fact, the current government's 'total war' policy, which is no different from Marcos' counter-insurgency war and also supported by the United States (Lawyers Committee for Human Rights, 1989), constitutes the single biggest obstacle to rehabilitation.

Threats to the security of both the survivors and the health professionals severely limit rehabilitation work.

Survivors fear a repetition of the torture experience while under the custody of the perpetrators of torture while ex-detainees, although freed from detention, continue to suffer from stress, such as fear of recapture or reprisals from the agents of the State who were responsible for their torture experience.

In 1988, two torture survivors informed a physician of the Medical Action Group that after their complaint of torture by their captors in a

Supreme Court hearing for a writ of *habeas corpus* and after being seen with torture marks by health professionals, they again suffered maltreatment by their military custodians.[1] In a survey of 100 ex-detainees in four areas in the Philippines in 1986, 49 respondents gave security reasons as a cause of their difficulties in adjusting to life after imprisonment.[2]

Health professionals rendering services to torture survivors, who are supposed to be protected by universal medical codes and covenants to render service to everyone regardless of their political beliefs, have themselves on many occasions been the victims of military abuses. While visiting detention centers, a number of health professionals were subjected to various kinds of harassments including threats to life, interrogations and actual detention.[3]

A raid on a rehabilitation center, witch-hunting and labelling two rehabilitation centers as communist fronts by the military, have resulted in unnecessary anxieties among those involved in rehabilitation work, deflected possible involvement of more rehabilitation workers as well as disrupted rehabilitation activities (*Manila Chronicle*, 1989; Malaya, 1987).

In the Philippine provinces especially, medical access to torture victims has been very limited. Military restrictions and arbitrary rules regarding detention center visits by non-military physicians make it almost impossible to render medical and rehabilitation services immediately.[4]

The Philippines also does not have the adequate necessary personnel and facilities for treating the victims of conflict like torture survivors. There is an acute inadequacy or virtual absence of health personnel capable of dealing with the physical and mental health problems that arise because of the absence of training centers for rehabilitation work among torture survivors and the government's

---

[1] MAG-PACT Files, 1988. The two survivors (whose names are not divulged for security reasons) are now out of detention and the court charges against them were dismissed for insufficiency of evidence. The government, including the courts, did not take action against the perpetrators of torture.

[2] Samahan ng mga Ex-Detainees Laban sa Detensyon at Para sa Amnestiya (SELDA), Socio-Economic Survey of Ex-Political Detainees in Four Areas of the Philippines, Manila, 1986.

[3] Letter of the Medical Action Group to the Commission on Human Rights, November 19, 1990 regarding harassment of a MAG health team by police authorities at the Navotas Municipal Jail on November 14, 1990 and Affidavits of members of the health team, November 1990.

[4] Notes on the Meeting of the Presidential Human Rights Committee (PHRC) chaired by the Secretary of Justice Franklin Drilon on July 31, 1990. Col. Marciano Bacalla, representative of the Department of National Defense verbally acknowledged arbitrary rules in detention centers in the Philippines.

lack of support for the development of such programs. And when torture occurs in remote and highly militarized areas as in many Philippine villages, there is a total breakdown of the formal medical system.

ECONOMIC CONSTRAINTS

Of the Filipino populace 70% lives below the poverty level and most torture survivors come from the marginalized sectors of Philippine society, specifically workers, peasants and lower petty bourgeoisie.

Those still under detention suffer economic dislocation especially if the detainee is the main breadwinner in the family. Family members, who are outside prison and who can seek assistance from the centers for the health needs of the detainees, are usually fully occupied with survival and financial concerns causing delay or absence of assistance to the survivors of torture. Meanwhile, many of those outside detention either do not have the resources even to visit health professionals for consultation and therapy or are busy looking for jobs.

In 1986, 42 out of 100 ex-detainees surveyed by SELDA gave economic reasons as a cause of their difficulties after release from detention.[1] In a study based on a three year (June 1985–June 1988) experience of the Children's Rehabilitation Center, 44% of the clientele presented financial and economic problems and this topped the list of problems identified.[2]

In this situation, experience showed that providing direct material and economic aid to victims and their families contributed immensely to the victims' overall adjustment. A plus factor in rehabilitation work in the Philippines is the existence of a network of non-governmental organizations (NGOs) which provide some mechanisms for economic support to some torture survivors and their families.

Such organizations and institutions, which have a network in various parts of the country, include Task Force Detainees (TFD), SELDA (means cell; *Samahan ng mga Ex-Detainees laban sa Detensyon at para sa Amnestiya*; an organization of ex-detainees), KAPATID (means brother/sister; an organization of families of political prisoners) and various church institutions. Aid can be in the form of initial capital for income generating projects, assistance in the marketing of detainees,

---

[1] SELDA, *op. cit.*, note 2 p. 489.
[2] Elizabeth Marcelino, Psychological Help to Children Victims of Political Violence, Paper read at the 5th Asian Workshop on Child and Adolescent Development, 24 February 1989, Asian Institute of Tourism, U.P. Systems, Diliman, Quezon City, p. 8.

products, educational scholarships, assistance in job placements as well as support for legal fees. The Free Legal Assistance Group (FLAG), Protestant Lawyers League (PLL), other lawyers' groups and some individual lawyers provide legal services for free or for very minimal fees.

However, given the worsening human rights situation where there is an increasing number of victims of human rights violations, the limited personnel and resources of the aforementioned institutions and groups can only reach and assist a small number of torture survivors.

FAMILY AND COMMUNITY

In the Philippines, family and community resources become primary sources of rehabilitation and healing when skilled medical personnel are unavailable. But, even if trained personnel were available for the victims of human rights violations, the massive restructuring of the social and economic situation of the survivors, including that of their families and relatives, which often occurs, leads to prolonged, repeated, and severe manifold stress. For this reason also, even the most basic rehabilitation framework demands comprehensive understanding and skilled orchestration of interpersonal, family and community variables.

Philippine experience revealed that the typically Asian extended family system is often the main support network that survives in the face of social and economic dislocation of the nuclear family of the victims. In this situation, families who reaffirm, or at the very least, understand the political choices of the victims are much more therapeutic. Economic support to the families from outside groups also becomes crucial because unaffected members of the extended families are themselves pushed into poverty when they take on the support of their displaced relatives. Furthermore, psychological support and rehabilitation of the individual must be worked out with the extended families.

Issues such as strained interpersonal relationships, changes in primary caregiver for the children, differences in political perspectives, communal sharing of resources and changes in primary breadwinners, and the need for the entire extended family network to face up to and live with the traumatic effects of the human rights violations are important variables in the therapy. In cases of children handled by the CRC, the majority of the problems of the children were due to the breakdown of the family after exposure to human rights violations, thereby necessitating the inclusion in its rehabilitation programs the revitalization and strengthening of the family as the basic and primary support system.[1]

Communities, too, play a significant role in the rehabilitation of the victims. This is specially true in the provinces where the barrios are of the Gemeinschaft society type. A member of the community is treated in many ways like a member of the family. Thus, in areas marked by intense conflict, failure of the community to respond to the needs of a torture survivor for fear of military reprisal, is very painful indeed for the survivor. There are even situations where survivors have no more communities to go back to since the communities themselves have broken down under military bombings and prolonged military operations.

CULTURE AND SUBCULTURE

Cultural understanding is most important in rehabilitation work. This has been recognized by rehabilitation workers in various countries after much work with refugees from other nations and cultures coming into exile in another host country. Cultural differences have been noted in various refugee groupings which necessarily have implications regarding assessment of mental health, interpretation of a respondent's behaviour or response and in the treatment or rehabilitation technique (Hauff, 1987).

Recognition of the importance of cultural differences for objective and effective work has resulted in the use of interpreters. But interpretation is not just a simple matter of translating since 'the task is not only to be faithful to the original version, but also to achieve connotative equivalence with the source language' (Hauff, 1987).

The relevance of the above mentioned considerations comes to focus because 'many contrasts or conflicts between Filippino values or ideals and actual behavior have been noted by various authors who suggest that this dichotomy may be due to interrelated urban–rural, traditional–modern distinctions and influences of social class' (Marcelino, 1990).

Bartolome (1990) declares that it is not correct to apply observed values, traits and virtues uncritically across all strata in a highly stratified society like the Philippines. He further says that generalizations are usually made by those who, living comfortably within it, are most interested in preserving the status quo where there is tremendous inequality in the distribution of wealth.

---

[1] Ibid.

Long years of colonization have produced the prevailing subservient culture and consciousness among Filipinos. This is usually described as a culture of silence and colonial mentality.[1] Filipinos are also observed to be family and small group oriented, paternalistic, with a strong need for acceptance and emotional security but reticent about undergoing psychotherapy (Marcelino, 1990).

This, however, is divergent even among Filipinos – divergences mostly arising from differences in class, social standing, urbanization, and experience. Also, this has not been static as there is an evolution of a counter-culture and counter-consciousness with the growing movement for social change in the Philippines.

Thus, there is a mixture of sometimes even conflicting subcultures in Philippine society. There are those who want to maintain the status quo but there are a growing number who are actively involved in creating a counter-culture, a liberating culture that is of the greatest importance for the movement for change in the country. And most survivors of political torture come from this counter-culture.

There have been efforts to characterize torture survivors. Some observations among ex-detainees include the following: they are committed individuals with a lot of strength; therapy is not the ex-detainee's priority; the ex-detainee is concerned about security; it is possible that they are primarily verbal in cognitive style; they are used to testing theory in practice (Decentecco, 1989). It has to be noted, however, that further studies are necessary to validate, amend or change these conclusions.

Torture survivors ask questions, not just the whats but the whys and the wherefores. Even the peasants and the urban poor, who may be unschooled and usually described as meek and subservient, do not just accept things as they are without any analysis of situations. Many psychiatrists who trained in the Philippine health schools and sometimes even in foreign countries, find themselves in a dilemma as their clients are not the usual run of the mill patients encountered in their clinics.[2]

In rehabilitation work among torture survivors, therefore, it is most important to consider the presence of a prevailing culture, subcultures and even counterculture and counterconsciousness. This is a problem in the Philippines as not everyone involved in rehabilitation work may be aware of all these. Moreover, except for a few, rehabilitation workers have undergone studies and training in schools that adopt

[1] What is foreign is best and what is indigenous is inferior.
[2] Testimonies of psychiatrists to whom the Medical Action Group referred torture survivors in 1988.

Western or foreign orientation. There is a dearth of materials and books from the Filipino perspective in libraries and bookstores compared to a flood of foreign materials written from an alien perspective. It is primarily through venues initiated by individuals and non-government organizations that most rehabilitation workers learn of all these most important considerations for culture-relevant therapies.

Because of the Western orientation of many Filipinos, pitfalls in interpretation of values are widespread. Enriquez (1990) says that 'the analysis and interpretation of Filipino values is substantially keyed to a foreign language and perspective ... More often than not ... the studies fail to see the values in terms of the Filipino world view, experience and milieu. The organization and logic of the value as it is viewed from the indigenous perspective is ignored.'

Samson (1990) says that the 'interpretative scheme' should be 'critically evaluated' – 'from whose national interest should Philippine culture be evaluated? The culture of a dependent society like the Philippines is oftentimes interpreted in terms of the interests and the standards of its "director" country'.

It has been noted that attempts to formulate appropriate techniques in therapy suited to the Filipino personality are minimal. Bulatao in 1990 made an attempt and described 'transpersonal counselling'. His main assumptions were: 1) Filipinos are freer to be themselves when in a sympathetic group of friends than in a one-on-one situation; 2) when supported by the group, Filipino clients prefer paternalistic counselors to non-directive ones who are perceived as detached, and non-caring; 3) the Filipino character is contemplative, patient, and accepting of things as they are; and 4) Filipino subjects readily enter into altered states of consciousness.

Among others, the *Akademya ng Sikolohiyang Pilipino* (Philippine Psychology Research and Training House, a group of concerned social scientists and professionals) and other non-governmental institutions including MAG, CRC and BALAY are now actively involved in developing culture-relevant therapies.

PHILIPPINE ACTION CONCERNING TORTURE: PROGRAM OF THE MEDICAL ACTION GROUP

There were large numbers of torture survivors during Marcos' rule. The very few health professionals willing to assist survivors, whether in their clinics or in detention centers, were only able to help a very small percentage of those needing assistance because of the lack of organizations or institutions coordinating and systematizing health services for victims of repression.

To systematize the delivery of services to more survivors, the Medical Action Group, with the assistance of the United Nations Voluntary Fund for Torture Survivors, established the Philippine Action Concerning Torture (PACT) shortly before the fall of the Marcos dictatorship. Thus, the Medical Action Group, guided by the Declaration of Tokyo approved by the World Medical Assembly in 1975 and the Principles of Medical Ethics approved by the United Nations General Assembly in 1982, set to work in assisting the torture survivors regain independence and go back to the mainstream of life.

Initially, the PACT staff and volunteers simply had their basic knowledge of medicine, counselling, psychotherapy and rehabilitation gained from formal schooling, attendance at a seminar in the Philippines with the assistance of the Rehabilitation Center for Torture Survivors-Denmark and participation in a few international conferences on torture rehabilitation. There was therefore a recognized need to develop and evolve culture-relevant and specific-client population – relevant therapies.

MAG-PACT's program include out-patient services at the clinic and health services in detention centers. It also conducts education activities relevant to torture (i.e. the nature and objectives of torture and the various coping mechanisms) among health professionals and among high risk groups. The high risk groups are those who are not assured safety and freedom because of their active involvement in the movement for social change (Medical Action Group, 1986).

Initially, in the delivery of services at the out-patient clinic, a standard survivor(patient)-flow was instituted regardless of the survivor's presenting complaint. The survivor saw all the members of the team (composed of a nurse, a physician, a psychologist or psychiatrist and a social worker) in succession as much as possible during the first visit. This was to ensure complete data on the survivor which were not only important for therapy but for research.

However, after several months and especially in the second year of operation, it was noted that there was poor patient follow-up. When human rights violations continued despite the change in government, survivors and their relatives expressed reservations over seeking consultation at the clinic for fear of rearrest or reprisals from the military. This heightened when MAG was labeled as a communist front.

MAG, therefore, assessed its approach and noted the following:[1]

[1] Assessment of the Medical Action Group's program on rehabilitation of torture survivors in 1986 and 1987.

1. Under conditions of continuing repression where even the physical security of the survivors and the health workers were not assured, the center-based approach was not very effective since the center could serve as a fixed point for military surveillance or re-arrest. It was also deficient in terms of gathering a comprehensive data on the survivors and their families since most of them were fully occupied with economic concerns and clinic visits would deprive them of precious time.

2. The inflexibility of the patient-flow meant a delay in the relief of the complaint or a delay in satisfying the survivor's needs. The succession of interviews by people, not all of whom directly tackle or help resolve the presenting problem, was physically and mentally exhausting. Perhaps, it may have served as a reminder of the survivor's helplessness during the torture experience.

Thus the approach was modified with the following guiding principles:[1]

1. It must be problem-oriented and action-oriented. Immediate attention should be given to the presenting problem or felt need so that relief of the complaint or the resolution of the problem is not delayed. Patient satisfaction encourages follow-up or return.

2. It must be comprehensive and systematic but flexible. The team approach is still applicable but the gathering of comprehensive information about the survivor may not be done on the first visit. Survivors, however are informed of the need to see the whole team for comprehensive assessment, appropriate therapies and research.

3. It must be individual, family and community oriented. The primary focus of therapy is the torture survivor presenting with a problem. Assistance to survivors must necessarily include investigations not only of the nature of violence inflicted upon them – the extent it has left physical, emotional and social scars on the individual – but also of their organizational backgrounds. This is even more evident in the case of torture survivors who carry with them a very strong political and ideological subculture. A grasp of the values and prescribed ways of coping within this subculture is essential in whatever therapeutic method is chosen.

However, given the fact that some of the individual's problems may arise because of poor interpersonal relationships in the family, involvement of the family members in therapy is important in order to work out resolutions to the problems. Also, the family is usually the

---

[1] Ibid.

main support system for the survivor in Philippine society. Moreover, the community often serves as an extension of the family.

A purely individual oriented approach limits the information gathered about the survivor and restricts involvement of other support systems which are vital in rehabilitation. Follow-up visits to the clinic are maintained but in combination with home and community visits, where the family and community members are more easily available.

If there is a security risk for a patient over follow-up at the clinic, alternative methods such as follow-up at the health professional's private clinic or home visit may be established.

4. It must assist the survivor to regain independence and to go back to the mainstream of life. There are many harsh realities in life which confront the survivor especially in a society undergoing economic and political crisis. Although at the early stage, reminders of the torture experience should be avoided as much as possible, therapy should not encourage dependence and should not be over-protective towards the survivor. In fact, participation of the survivor in working out resolutions to the presenting problems is in itself therapeutic for a person used to joint or collective efforts. For a person who has invested his life in the movement for social change prior to the torture experience, going back to the mainstream of society would most probably mean participating again in the movement for societal change.

5. It must consider the social, political and cultural situation of the country. This is based on the recognition that a person's behavior is largely influenced, if not a product of, the society in which he or she lives. Thus, to understand a survivor better, the societal conditions – including the worsening economic conditions and continuing repression – should be considered. Moreover, it should not be forgotten that it is the existing socio-economic-political system which gave rise to the survivor's problems.

The patient flow was thus revised. The survivor sees the nurse who, in turn, refers him or her to the member of the rehabilitation team who can immediately give attention to the presenting complaint or felt need, unless a life-threatening problem not recognized by the survivor is identified. Other team members will be seen but with some flexibility in schedule considering both concerns of the survivor and the team member. Nevertheless, discipline, which is most important in daily life, should not be compromised for flexibility.

The program uses various methods, usually in combination, to assist the survivors and promote their physiological and psychological well-being. The methods used for each survivor vary according to the

T

complaints and problems presented by the survivor and those identified by the therapist apart from the other important variables such as
political situation, economic factors, family and community, and
culture and subculture. The program also continues with its education
activities regarding torture among the high risk groups which include
members and staff of organizations and institutions as well as communities involved in the movement for change.

Activities of the program include:

1. Individual counselling or psychotherapy – This is primarily done
by a psychologist or a psychiatrist but supplemented by the other team
members. Good rapport and trust between the survivor and therapist
are most important especially since information given may have
security implications.

At the Medical Action Group Out-Patient Clinic only 15 out of 158
torture survivors and their relatives (9%) and 37 out of 300 patients
(12%) sought psychological assistance from January to June 1990 and
July to December 1990, respectively, despite harrowing tales of torture.[1] This may be explained by the fact that individuals belonging to
this specific client population have been steeped in a spartan way of
life, have strong coping mechanisms and thus were not emotionally
broken by torture.

SELDA's survey showed that 59% of 100 respondents coped on their
own. Some simply coped with the assistance of family and friends.
With the sense of collectivity developed in the movement for social
change, the 'mga kasama' (comrades) also served as support system. In
fact, feelings of isolation, depression and helplessness, even while
inside detention, are easily overcome when others, who are important,
such as family, friends and 'mga kasama' show understanding,
concern and acceptance for the survivor. For the ex-detainees interviewed by SELDA, about half of those who did not have adjustment
problems after release declared that it was because of acceptance by
family, friends and community.[2]

However, further studies are necessary to investigate the relationships between the social stigma Filipinos attach to being under
psychological treatment and these findings. Psychological help is
widely perceived as only for the weak or people supposed to be crazy
or lunatic. Moreover, for the Filipino male in a chauvinist society, it is
not 'acceptable' to reveal and discuss emotions in public, particularly
with strangers.

[1] Medical Action Group, Report of Activities on Rehabilitation of Torture Survivors,
January–June 1990 and July–December 1990.
[2] SELDA, *op. cit.*, Table 8.

The building of rapport or trust between therapist and survivor had not been much of a problem. MAG has earned credibility from among those involved in the movement for social change because of its track record on the defense and promotion of human rights. Thus the first step in building trust between therapist and survivor has been achieved. Therapists, who are either staff, members or part of the network of MAG are easily accepted by survivors who are assured that information about them will be treated in the strictest confidence and that their political decisions will, at the very least be understood, if not accepted and validated.

A continuing problem, however, is that there are very few health professionals who can be relied on and some of those who are capable and reliable only spend part of their time in the rehabilitation work for torture survivors because of financial considerations.

2. Group therapy – This is handled by the psychologist and involves several survivors who are willing to share their problems and views with other people. This is most effective for those who have a high regard for collective discussions, cooperative efforts and concerted actions. This provides a venue for each participant to relate to one another, help solve another person's problems and realize that problems are not limited to him or herself. This greatly assists the survivor to recover self confidence and to get back to the mainstream of life.

This is used in combination with individual therapy to ensure that feelings not expressed in the group and reactions to the group therapy are known and acted upon accordingly by the therapist.

MAG's experience showed that group therapy facilitated improvement in most of those who participated. However, for security reasons, some torture survivors expressed their anxieties and reservations in revealing highly confidential information to a group and a few even rejected group therapy. For these survivors, individual therapy may be used or the torture survivors may be encouraged to join the group therapy with caution – that is, by just revealing information they are comfortable to give to a group – and this can be complemented by individual counselling or therapy. As much as possible, group therapy is encouraged as it provides the survivor with a venue to improve relations with others and develop trust, away from the therapist, in preparation to going back to the mainstream of society.

3. Stress Tension Reduction Therapy (STRT) – This consists of breathing and physical exercises and manual treatment after detection of tense muscle groups in survivors. The techniques reduce stress reactions as patients undergo relaxation and help facilitate group cohesiveness since some of the exercises are done by groups.

An exploratory study by Larsen and Lopez on three Filipino women subjected to sexual abuse showed that the manual method of stress reduction produced significant relief of both physical and psychological problems. Moreover, they also surmised the potential of manual stress reduction therapy for survivors 'not suited to psychotherapy' and its inherent non-verbal and self-reliant approach to the management of stress and tension.[1]

It has been noted that a few torture survivors who presented with muscle tension at the MAG clinic benefited from the manual and physical exercises conducted by the MAG staff who learned the technique from Larsen.

4. Medical and surgical services – These are most often needed by torture survivors not only for the immediate physical or physiological effects of torture but due to health problems caused by inadequate nutrition and very poor detention conditions. In fact, many survivors visit the clinic for these problems.

Special care should be taken in assessing patients who present with physical symptoms. It has been noted that Filipinos have a strong tendency to somatize psychological stress – a reactive depression may present as bodily pains, headache or malaise instead of verbal expressions of sadness, guilt or worthlessness.[2]

5. Dental services – These are also provided for, whether in the detention centers or in the clinic. Most of the detainees visited and ex-detainees seen at the clinic had dental problems. This is part of the wholistic approach to rehabilitation of torture survivors.

6. Occupational therapy – This facilitates recovery of self-esteem and confidence by the survivors. Through activities like writing, painting, handicraft-making or carpentry, the survivors express their interests, capabilities and even feelings. The activities help many realize that they can still be productive individuals even if the torturers tried to destroy them. The activities also help some overcome feelings of helplessness and regain their self-esteem as they are able to augment the family's finances apart from having an income of their own. Financial assistance to start the project is given by other concerned groups.

7. Home visits and community outreach – They are undertaken to get a more comprehensive background of the survivors and to solicit

[1] Helle Larsen and June Pagaduan-Lopez, Stress Tension Reduction in the Treatment of Sexually Tortured Women – An Exploratory Study, Manila, 1986.
[2] June Pagaduan-Lopez, The Psychological Aspects of Torture as Seen Among Filipino Torture Victims, paper presented to the World Psychiatric Association Regional Meeting, Athens, 1985.

family and community assistance in rehabilitation. Signs, symptoms and sequelae of torture as well as various ways of coping are discussed with the family and community.

8. Discussions on the nature, objectives of and coping mechanisms for the problem of torture – These are conducted among high risk individuals and groups, which include those involved in the struggle for change in Philippine society so that they are psychologically prepared if and when torture happens. This is a stop-gap measure while the conditions that breed the occurrence of torture remain. For the staff of health and human rights organizations and institutions, this is an attempt to disseminate information on how one can assist a torture survivor to cope with the torture experience (Cabildo *et al.*, 1988).

One big obstacle in the rehabilitation of torture survivors is the fact that torture continues under the present government. The incommunicado status of many political detainees especially during the first days of detention when torture occurs, the maintenance of secret 'safehouses' which serve as torture houses by the military and the arbitrary detention rules restricting medical visits to torture survivors are problems that continue. Also, the remoteness of communities where mass arrests and beatings occur coupled by the still relatively few people involved in rehabilitation of torture survivors are problems that remain to be confronted. Those who are willing to assist torture survivors experience various ways of harassment by military authorities and personnel, discouraging some from continuing to serve victims of repression.

Another big constraint is the limitations of financial resources. Because of the increasing number of survivors, the limited number of personnel afforded by the program focuses basically on action-oriented activities so that research is relegated to the periphery.

CHILDREN'S REHABILITATION CENTER

Intensified repression launched by the Marcos regime led to widespread abuses not only of adults but also of children. It was for this reason that the Children's Rehabilitation Center (CRC) was set up to meet systematically the psychological and other needs of child-victims of political violence in the hope that they could grow up to be productive members of the society.

Child-victims of political violence include those who are directly tortured or whose parents or families are forcibly arrested and detained, executed extrajudicially, strafed or dislocated. Children of human rights workers who are harassed and threatened by the rising political tension are classified as 'potential victims.'[1]

Cases seen at CRC in a period of three years showed that most were suffering from emotional disorders and social maladjustment. Symptoms such as withdrawal behavior, depression, irritability, sleep disturbances, extreme anxieties and fears triggered off by specific stimuli such as armed men, loud noise and sudden motions were very common. Socialization difficulties gave rise to school problems while poverty complicated the emotional problems.[2]

The treatment procedure follows a general methodological flow with specific objectives for the three stages – data gathering and diagnosis, treatment, monitoring and evaluation. The specific objectives aim to support the long term objective of assisting the family in joining the mainstream of society.

Assessment and diagnosis of the problems of the child is a continuing process throughout the entire relationship but it is specially important in the beginning when the child care worker establishes rapport not only with the child but with the family as well. The holistic view of the child demands that assessment be done of the non-verbal and verbal actions of the child on the emotive, cognitive and behavioral levels. The cooperation of the family is a necessary ingredient in the identification of the child's problems as well as for possible solutions to the problem.

Various therapeutic methods have been developed and refined by the CRC over the past years. In its treatment method, CRC has applied 'Sikolohiyang Pilipino' (Filipino psychology) in terms of looking at the problem of the child at two levels. The first level focuses on the individual needs and problems of the child to ensure proper physical, emotional, intellectual and social development while the second level is societal. The second focuses on the socio-economic and political roots of the child's problems and their consequences on the child's rights and welfare.[3]

In group therapy, the approaches include:
1. Intrafamily counselling – This is accomplished during home visits. Possible repercussions of certain behaviors of the child or the parent are analyzed and explained to assist the family as a unit in responding to the problem. Family disintegration which is a common consequence of war is dealt with by the program so that smooth family

[1] Elizabeth Marcelino, *op. cit.*, note 2 p. 490.   [2] Ibid.
[3] Elizabeth Marcelino, Psychological Help to Children Victims of Political Armed Conflict, paper presented at the National Conference of the Philippine Psychiatric Association, Manila, 1986.

relations can pave the way for faster recovery of the family from the crisis situation.

2. Interfamily counselling – Adults from different families get the chance to exchange their views on handling problems which they may share in common.

3. Children's play activities – This method provides venues for the children to relate, express and share with one another their experiences. The activities provide the staff with venues for natural observation of each child to monitor his or her progress and development.

Initially, in its one and a half years of operation, CRC adopted a topic-centered curriculum for group therapy where the children were passive recipients in the whole learning process. There was very little feedback elicited from the children. Thus, it was modified to become a skills-centered program where the children engage in arts and sports activities. The skills-oriented approach enables the children to develop new skills which boosts their self-confidence and makes them have a more positive image of themselves. Moreover, the activities allow for deeper and sustained interaction among the children which help them overcome withdrawal behavior. It also allows the CRC staff to interact with the children continuously and observe them under various conditions. The meaningful relationships established over time between and among the children and the staff members enhance the emotional support system for each child and facilitate the opening up of fears and apprehensions and lead to alternative sources of comfort and hopefulness.

Because of the stress and psychological trauma of the children, the program also conducts individual treatment of patients. This is done through home visits and constant observation and documentation of the progress of each child. A special program is likewise designed for children with particular behavior or socio-emotional problems, implemented either in their homes or at the center.

The program also gives other support services to the families of the victims in order to unburden them of economic problems and thus help them slowly develop self-reliance through their income-generating projects. Although support services serve as an integral part of the individual therapy procedures, it can be taken as a separate program activity because of its significant contribution to rehabilitation.

Several models regarding psychological events that follow a period of trauma like the death of a loved one, natural disasters and accidents, generally postulate a clearcut period of stability for a discrete and short period after the traumatic event occurs. A study on 25 Filipino children shows that there is no discrete, peaceful pre- and post-traumatic period – there had been stresses suffered by the children long before the actual death or disappearance of parents and the stress situation continues after that for weeks, months or years.[1] The continuing repression giving rise to continuing stressful situations prevents us from using such models to label behavioral problems of the Filipino child-victims of political violence.

One specific concern encountered in the rehabilitation of children is the withholding of information or truth regarding what happened to the lost parent. There were cases where the remaining parent or surrogate parent withheld the truth for fear of not being able to explain the traumatic life situation in a way understandable to the child. This resulted in the denial of one important ingredient for a healthy and normal emotional growth of the child – the truth.

When half-truths about the parents are fed to the child, fragmented and distorted images of parents are built up while the continued absence of the parents remain a mystery. Sooner or later, the child may exhibit strange behavior to attract attention. Unfortunately, the strange actuations are what the family members will notice so that the child's real message does not get across.

Experience of the CRC has shown that more often than not, information and knowledge of the truth helps the children cope with stressful life events. With cognitive mastery, the children are able to understand life situations at their own pace and level and thus are able to process whatever stressful life events occur on the basis of this knowledge and then cope accordingly. When children start confronting problems, then they can begin to grow enhanced by the strength of support systems. Therapy and rehabilitation must therefore strike a balance between strengthening the child and revitalizing the existing support systems.[2]

JUSTICE, HUMAN RIGHTS AND REHABILITATION WORK

It is evident from our experiences in the Philippines that the socio-cultural, economic and political context under which torture and political violence occurs, must be identified, defined and understood if one is to be scientific and holistic when dealing with the problem. Failure to do this would mean a failure to clearly define the problem

[1] Sylvia Estrada-Claudio, Jose Bartolome, Grace Aquiling-Dalisay, A Pilot Study on Children in Crisis, 1989, pp. 8 & 15.
[2] Elizabeth Marcelino, Psychological Help to Children Victims of Political Violence, pp. 9–10 *op. cit.*, note 2, p. 490.

and the realities surrounding it which would definitely serve as obstacles in effective rehabilitation.

Development of effective rehabilitation approaches and programs for victims of political violence must necessarily continue in order to minimize, if not totally eliminate horrifying and lasting effects. This should be of utmost concern for health professionals and social workers, most especially for those who have the skills and resources to effectively conduct studies and developmental work. In the Philippines, research remains very limited because most of the activities of the rehabilitation programs remain action-oriented, given the increasing number of survivors seeking assistance vis-a-vis the dearth of professionals involved in rehabilitation work. Thus the evaluation of existing approaches and techniques as well as the development of culture-relevant and specific client population-relevant therapies remain inadequate.

Another important concern, which some may immediately consider as outside the purview of rehabilitation work, is obtaining justice for the survivor. Justice denied is a persistent irritant to the psychological wounds of a torture survivor. Given this logic, the importance of working for justice must not and cannot be underrated especially since justice has been very elusive in the country. Amnesty International (1990) stated that for perpetrators of torture, the 'stiffest punishment in practice was discharge from military service and that only three officers had received this under President Aquino's administration'.

The usefulness and significance of intervention after the fact, such as services to survivors of torture, is very easily understood and not much subject to controversy. But there is one controversial but vital aspect of rehabilitation work: prevention.

The prevention of the occurrence of torture and political violence is part and parcel of human rights work which is also within the framework of the progressive movement for social change. Human rights advocacy is vital because psychological and physical scars of torture and political violence heal, but the scars remain in the hearts and minds of torture survivors or reflected in the hearts and minds of the people. If the society in which they live continue to breed, sustain or perpetrate human rights violations, rehabilitation can never be achieved fully. If human rights violations escalate, our society may just end up organizing more rehabilitation programs instead of maximizing efforts and resources for development and improving the life of humanity.

Work for the promotion of human rights, within the framework of the progressive movement for meaningful societal change, is controversial among many health professionals who want to veer away from 'political' concerns and just concentrate on purely 'health' concerns. To veer away from 'politics' is in effect to escape from the reality that the problem of torture is not purely a psychological or medical concern but that in Philippine society, it is only a symptom of a decaying socio-economic-political order where the government makes up in repression what it lacks in legitimate authority.

The challenge is there for health professionals, social workers and scientists, and students to be involved in human rights advocacy and the struggle for justice, democracy and sovereignty in the Philippines. For the sake of humanity, the challenge should not be left unheeded.

REFERENCES

Amnesty International (1984). *Torture in the Eighties.* London: Pitman Press.
Amnesty International (1990). *1990 Report.* London: AI Publications.
Bartolome, J. M. (1990). The Pitfalls of Filipino Personality. In V. Enriquez, ed., *Indigenous Psychology.* Quezon City: Akademya ng Sikolohiyang Pilipino.
Birnberg, T. & Resnick, S. (1975). *Colonial Development – An Economic Study.* Yale: Yale University Press.
Bulatao, J. (1990). Filipino Transpersonal World View. In V. Enriquez, ed., *Philippine World Views.* Manila: Philippine Psychology Research House.
Cabildo, V., Claudio, S. E., Jimenez, A. L. & de la Paz, S. C. (1988). *Pagtulong sa mga Biktima ng Tortyur (Isang Gabay).* Manila: Medical Action Group.
Claude, R. (1989). The Right to Health: Transnational Support for the Philippines. In *Human Rights and Development.* Macmillan Press.
Decentecco, E. (1989). Therapy with ex-detainees: some preliminary considerations. In *Ex-Political Detainees, Psychological Aspects of Rehabilitation, The BALAY Experience.* Manila: Crossroads Publications, Inc.
Enriquez, V. (1990). Indigenous personality theory. In V. Enriquez, ed., *Indigenous Psychology.* Quezon City: Akademya ng Sikolohiyang Pilipino.
Hauff, E. (1987). Assessment of mental health in refugee populations. In *Health Hazards of Organized Violence.* Rijswijk: Ministry of Welfare, Health and Cultural Affairs.
International Commission of Jurists (1983). *States of Emergency. Their Impact on Human Rights.* Geneva: International Commission of Jurists.
Lawyers Committee for Human Rights (1989). *Human Rights and U.S. Foreign Policy, Linking Security Assistance and Human Rights,* 1988 Project Series No. 3.
Lippman, M. (1979). The Protection of Universal Human Rights: the Problem of Torture. *Universal Human Rights,* 1(4), October–December.
Malaya (1987). *Military Names 25 Red Front Groups.* Manila: People's Independent Media.
Manila Chronicle (1989). Cops fail to find Rowe killers in safehouse. *Manila Chronicle.* Manila.

Marcelino, E. P. (1990). Towards understanding the Filipino psychology. In L. Brown and M. Root, eds, *Diversity and Complexity in Feminist Therapy*. New York: Harrington Park Press.

Medical Action Group (1986). Philippine Action Concerning Torture (PACT), A Project of the Medical Action Group, Inc. *Medical Action Group Magazine*, **III(1)** January–March, 9–10.

Mische, G. and P. (1977). *Toward a Human World Order*. New York: Paulist Press.

Samson, L. (1990). The politics of understanding Philippine culture. In V. Enriquez, ed., *Indigenous Psychology*. Quezon city: Akademya ng Sikolohiyang Pilipino.

Part VII

MODERN ETHICS AND
INTERNATIONAL LAW

23
MODERN ETHICS AND INTERNATIONAL LAW
Bent Sørensen

DEFINITIONS

In the following, the word 'modern' should be understood as the time after World War II; the term 'ethics' primarily ethics for health personnel; 'international law' indicating declarations, conventions, convenants or other regulations which have been introduced by the United Nations or other very large groups of states, e.g. the Council of Europe.

INTERNATIONAL LAW

United Nations

When World War II was about to end the United Nations was created and as early as 1948 the General Assembly adopted the *Universal Declaration of Human Rights*. Article 5 of this Declaration reads:
'No one shall be subjected to torture or to cruel, inhuman or degrading treatment or punishment'.

- A phrasing of words which can be refound unchanged or almost unchanged up till now and which will probably remain unchanged.

This universal declaration was followed by regional ones:

1950, The European Convention on Human Rights, Article 3, which however omits the word 'cruel'.

1969, The American Convention on Human Rights, Article 5, par. 2 with practically unaltered phrasing.

1969, The African Charter on Human and People's Rights, Article 5, which – naturally enough – in addition to the above phrasing adds some words concerning degradation of man, in particular slavery etc.

Torture in the world continued. It was recognized that torture was practised to a great and frequent extent and the United Nations elaborated on the problem. On 9th of December 1975 the General Assembly adopted without voting:

Declaration on the Protection of all Persons from being subjected to Torture and any other Cruel, Inhuman or Degrading Treatment or Punishment.

The Declaration consists of 12 Articles, most of which can be refound in the Convention Against Torture and which will be dealt within this context.

The General Assembly recommended that the Declaration serve as a guideline for all states and other entities exercising effective power.

However, this did not have the desired effect. The problem was further elaborated upon and after a great preparation with lengthy and difficult negotiations and with many compromises the General Assembly adopted on 10th of December 1984:
The Convention Against Torture and Other Cruel, Inhuman or Degrading Treatment or Punishment.

It came into force when 20 states had ratified it, which was the case on 26th June 1987. Presently – June 1990 – 52 states of the 163 member states of the United Nations have ratified the Convention.

The Conventions is the singular law being valid at present.

In Article 1 torture is defined thus:
'For the purposes of this Convention, the term "torture" means any act by which severe pain or suffering, whether physical or mental, is intentionally inflicted on a person for such purposes as obtaining from him or a third person information or a confession, punishing him for an act he or a third person has committed or is suspected of having committed, or intimidating or coercing him or a third person, or for any reason based on discrimination of any kind, when such pain or suffering is inflicted by or at the instigation of or with the consent or acquiescence of a public official or other person acting in an official capacity. It does not include pain or suffering arising only from, inherent in or incidental to lawful sanctions.'

Thus, the definition has been laid down on an historical basis and is rather limiting. The key-words are: pain, purpose and official, whereas a number of other aspects are excluded.

Articles 2 – 16 then describe the various obligations of the participating states.

Article 2 maintains that the states shall take 'effective legislative, administrative, judicial or other measures to prevent acts of torture' . . ., and paragraph 2 adds that there are no excuses whatsoever to practise torture, and par. 3 states that 'an order from a superior officer or a public authority may not be invoked as a justification of torture'.

Article 3 lays down that no person may be expelled, 'refouler' to another state where there are substantial grounds for believing that he would be in danger of being subjected to torture.

Articles 4 – 9 are of less interest for Medical Ethics, but are probably of considerable preventive value.

The Articles at first lay down that the States through their legislation must ensure that torture is to be punished. Furthermore, legal authority must be established to prosecute foreign citizens, even if the crime has been committed outside the territory of the country in question and against persons other than the country's own citizens.

Viewed from an international legal angle these demands are quite far-reaching and the result is that torturers have become outlawed.

Article 10, par. 1 reads:
'Each state party shall ensure that education and information regarding the prohibition against torture are fully included in the training of law enforcement personnel, civil or military, medical personnel, public officials and other persons who may be involved in the custody, interrogation or treatment of any individual subjected to any form of arrest, detention or imprisonment.'

In other words, the state party has an *obligation* to incorporate the torture-concept into the medical curriculum for doctors, dentists, nurses, physiotherapists, etc.

Articles 11, 12 and 13 are to ensure the individual: There must be fixed rules for arresting persons, imprisonment and the like; there must be a possibility of impartial investigation of complaints and any person must have the right to put forth such complaints.

In Article 14 the tortured is given: ... 'an enforceable right to fair and adequate compensation, including the means for as full rehabilitation as possible ...'.

Article 15 maintains, that '... any statement which is established to have been made as a result of torture shall not be invoked as evidence in any proceedings ...'.

Article 16 deals with aspects other than torture viz.: cruel, inhuman or degrading treatment or punishment. This too, must be prohibited in the State Party and there is special reference to Articles 10, 11, 12 and 13 which also cover these acts.

As mentioned, many of the above-mentioned decisions can also be found in The Declaration Against Torture from 1975, which evidently did not have sufficient effect. And in order to ensure that the Articles mentioned are now fulfilled, the Convention has created a Committee – Articles 17 and 18.

The Committee consists of '... 10 experts of high moral standing and recognized competence in the field of human rights, who shall serve in their personal capacity ...'.

The members of the Committee are elected for a period of 4 years by secret ballot between the states that have ratified the Convention, but they do not necessarily represent the states. Thus they are *'personae designatae'*.

The task of the Committee is to survey that the Convention is being implemented. According to Article 19 the state parties must forward reports (an initial report upon entering, thereafter supplementary reports every 4th year). The reports must contain a general description of the conditions in the country as well as a detailed description – according to Articles 2 – 15 of the Convention – of the initiatives made by the states to implement the Convention.

The written report is supplemented with an oral presentation by senior civil servants and the Committee raises further questions and receives answers. This entire procedure takes place in open meetings. The Committee then concludes whether they can accept the report, whether supplementary written information is needed or whether they desire a totally new report, not after 4 years but after 1 year.

The state parties' written reports are publicly accessible. The Committee's debate of the reports, questions and answers, is public and is made into a report on each single state party. This report is incorporated into the Committee's Annual Report which is submitted to the General Assembly of the United Nations.

Article 20 yields the Committee a right to act, if 'it receives reliable information which appears to it to contain well-founded indications that torture is being systematically practised in the territory of a state party ...'. The Committee shall then start negotiations with the country and possibly start investigations in the country on their own.

This is a rather far-reaching decision and the State Parties have the possibility of opting out.

About 20 states have accepted Article 20 and about 30 have opted it out.

At the Committee's fourth session in May 1990, the first information referring to Article 20 was received.

Article 21 gives a state the possibility of accusing another state before the Committee and Article 22 gives single persons (tortured as well as their relatives or lawyers) the possibility of presenting cases of torture before the Committee.

The state parties may choose not to recognize the two latter Articles as well – just under half of the member states have recognized the Articles and just over half have not.

The Committee has until now not had any cases with reference to Article 21, but a few with reference to Article 22.

All meetings and negotiations on cases with reference to Articles 20,

21 and 22 are closed and confidential until they are completed, whereafter a Communiqué is made on the case.

In summary, it may be concluded:

In contrast to the *recommendation* in the Declaration of 1975, the Convention of 1984 has established an *obligation* for the state parties and has created a 'machinery' the task of which is to survey that the implementation of the Convention actually *takes place*. Lenin's words come to the mind: 'To trust is all very well, to control is better'.

Europe

The European Convention for the Prevention of Torture and Inhuman or Degrading Treatment or Punishment came into force on 1st of February 1989, three months after seven members had ratified it.

In May 1990, 23 States had signed and 18 States had ratified, of the total of 23 States in the Council of Europe.

The machinery to implement the aims of the Convention is a *Committee* consisting of one member from each of the member states. 'The member shall be chosen among persons of high moral character, known for the competence in the field of human rights or having professional experience in the areas covered by this Convention ... They shall serve in their individual capacity, shall be independent and impartial and shall be available to serve the Committee effectively.'

The method of implementation are visits.

The Committee has a right to visit all places where persons are detained against their own will: police stations, prisons, refugee camps, military barracks, certain psychiatric institutions and the like.

Periodical visits are obligatory, and *ad hoc* visits are possible. These are made as urgent visits, induced by specific petitions.

Three to five persons from the Committee take part in the visits, accompanied by secretarial staff, interpreters and experts if necessary.

The Committee deals with torture and inhuman or degrading treatment or punishment.

Intentionally, the Convention does not give a definition of torture: the Committee members themselves set the limits for ill treatment.

The Committee cannot receive and consider singular complaints. The work of the Committee is solely of a preventive nature for which reason *co-operation* between the states and *confidentiality* is necessary. All meetings take place in camera and all negotiations are confidential. However, the Committee can present communiqués against the wish of a single member state if two-thirds of the members of the Committee approve.

Thus, there is a great difference between the fields of work and aims of the United Nations Committee and that of the European Council. They supplement each other but do not in any area overlap.

Internationally, efforts are made to create systems like the European one in other continents – either in the form of independent regional conventions or by means of a further extension of the United Nations Convention against Torture.

MEDICAL ETHICS

Although the topic of this chapter is 'Modern Ethics' it is natural to emphasize that medical ethics are based on principles from the ancient Greek culture and the first ethical rules are in fact the Hippocratic Oath. This has been presented in many versions and has been interpreted in many ways. In some countries, e.g. Denmark, taking the oath is a condition to practise as a doctor. The oath used there was drawn up in 1815. It contains a paragraph on confidentiality and quality but also a quite modern social–medical paragraph, which reads: ' ... I will always in my practice as a doctor zealously use my knowledge to the best of my judgment to the benefit of society and my fellow beings ...', and further: '... I shall attend the poor as conscientiously as the rich ...'.

Modern medical ethics are expressed by official organizations, like the United Nations as well as by professional organizations, first of all the World Medical Association (WMA).

On the 18th of December 1982 the United Nations' General Assembly adopted:
'Principles of medical ethics relevant to the rôle of health personnel, particularly physicians, in the protection of prisoners and detainees against torture and other cruel, inhuman or degrading treatment or punishment'. The following six principles are listed:

1 It is the doctors' duty to treat prisoners and detainees at the same quality and standard as is afforded to those who are not imprisoned or detained.
2 It is a gross contravention of medical ethics to participate in torture or other cruel, inhuman or degrading treatment or punishment.
3 The only professional relationship between prisoners or detainees and medical personnel is solely to evaluate, protect or improve their physical or mental health.
4 It is prohibited to 'assist in the interrogation of prisoners or

detainees in a manner that may adversely affect their physical or mental health ...', just as it is forbidden to 'certify ... the sickness of prisoners and detainees for any form of treatment or punishment that may adversely affect their physical or mental health ...'.

5 It is prohibited to '... participate in any procedures for restraining a prisoner or detainee ...'.

6 There may be no derogation from the foregoing principles on any ground whatsoever ...'.

Over the years the United Nations have worked on:
Standard minimum rules for the treatment of prisoners and related recommendations – the latest revision of these rules took place in 1977.

It is a rather comprehensive work which in detail gives the minimum demands for a long row of circumstances – a total of 95 articles. It is actually more a listing of demands rather than dealing with ethics as such. Some of the articles are hardly in accordance with the present ethics of the medical profession. This is especially the case with article 32, the first paragraph of which reads:
'Punishment by close confinement or reduction of a diet shall never be inflicted unless the medical officer has examined the prisoner and certified in writing that he is fit to sustain it'. Paragraph 3 of the article orders daily attending this category or prisoners.

In the 1990s the medical profession is probably going to dissuade doctors from participating in such procedures entirely.

WORLD MEDICAL ASSOCIATION

The World Medical Association (WMA) has adopted a long series of ethical rules ranging from rules for recommendations concerning medical care in rural districts to the *Sydney Declaration* on the statement of death.

Of paramount importance for all medical work on torture is the *Tokyo Declaration* adopted by the 29th World Medical Association's Assembly in 1975. After a preamble the declaration itself follows which is found essential enough to be quoted *in toto*:

1 The doctor shall not countenance, condone or participate in the practice of torture or other forms of cruel, inhuman or degrading procedures, whatever the offence of which the victim of such procedures is suspected, accused or guilty, and whatever the victim's beliefs or motives, and in all situations, including armed conflict and civil strife.

2 The doctor shall not provide any premises, instruments, substances or knowledge to facilitate the practice of torture or other forms of cruel, inhuman or degrading treatment or to diminish the ability of the victim to resist such treatment.

3 The doctor shall not be present during any procedure during which torture or other forms of cruel, inhuman or degrading treatment is used or threatened.

4 A doctor must have complete clinical independence in deciding upon the care of a person for whom he or she is medically responsible. The doctor's fundamental role is to alleviate the distress of his or her fellow men, and no motive whether personal, collective or political shall prevail against this higher purpose.

5 Where a prisoner refuses nourishment and is considered by the doctor as capable of forming an unimpaired and rational judgment concerning the consequences of such a voluntary refusal of nourishment, he or she shall not be fed artificially. The decision as to the capacity of the prisoner to form such a judgment should be confirmed by at least one other independent doctor. The consequences of the refusal of nourishment shall be explained by the doctor to the prisoner.

6 The World Medical Association will support, and should encourage the international community, the national medical associations and fellow doctors to support the doctor and his or her family in the face of threats or reprisals resulting from a refusal to condone the use of torture and other forms of cruel, inhuman or degrading treatment.

COMITÉ PERMANENTE

Medical initiatives are also being taken regionally. The Comité Permanente (The Union of Medical Associations within the EEC) adopted *The Statement of Madrid – Recommendations concerning Doctors, Ethics and Torture* at their meeting in Madrid on November 24 and 25, 1989.

The Statement first of all maintains that the Tokyo Declaration is the basis for doctors' ethical conduct – even in this context. It recommends that training on the Tokyo Declaration receives a place in the medical curricula of all countries and that its principles be integrated in the statutes of all scientific and professional medical bodies. Furthermore, it recommends the establishment of a reimbursement system concerning the violation of ethical rules and finally that international support is given to doctors 'who take action to resist the involvement of doctors in such procedures ...'.

SUMMARY

On the whole, there is accordance between international law and modern ethics.

One of the few areas where disagreements can be expected is that of hunger strikes:

The law profession is mostly of the opinion that life should be kept at any cost and that a doctor therefore has a duty to feed persons by force who are unconscious because of refusal of nourishment and who would die if not treated.

Modern medical ethics places the individual's right to self-determination higher than this demand, cf. please the last paragraph of the Tokyo Declaration (pt. 5). The Madrid Statement must be interpreted as a strong support of the views expressed in the Tokyo Declaration.

The Court decision of the various countries on this problem may be expected with some suspense.

However, the divergence on hunger strike constitutes only a small part of the large picture. Possibilities of eliminating torture must be considered to exist. International law has created the Conventions and the implementation seems possible. The medical profession (WMA) has laid down ethical rules which in complete global agreement support all of the initiatives.

INDEX

Printed in the United States
by Bookmasters

Printed in the United States
By Bookmasters